An aid to the MRCP PACES
VOLUME 1
STATIONS 1, 3 AND 5

'*MRCP; Member of the Royal College of Physicians . . .*
They only give that to crowned heads of Europe'.
From *The Citadel* by A.J. Cronin

An Aid to the MRCP PACES

THIRD EDITION
VOLUME 1
STATIONS 1, 3 AND 5

**R.E.J. Ryder, M.A. Mir
and E.A. Freeman**

*Departments of Medicine, City Hospital, Birmingham,
University Hospital of Wales and
University of Wales College of Medicine, Cardiff
and Department of Integrated Medicine,
Royal Gwent and St Woolos Hospitals, Newport*

Blackwell
Publishing

One-third of the royalties from this book will be donated to the Missionaries of Charity of Mother Teresa of Calcutta

First published as An Aid to the MRCP Cases 1986
Reprinted 1988, 1989, 1990, 1991, 1992, 1993, 1994, 1996, 1997
Second edition 1999
Reprinted 2000, 2002, 2003
Third edition 2003

ISBN 1-4051-0768-5

Catalogue records for this title are available from the British Library and Library of Congress

Set in 9.5/12.5 pt Minion by SNP Best-set Typesetters Ltd., Hong Kong
Printed and bound in Denmark by Narayana Press, Odder

Commissioning Editor: Alison Brown
Editorial Assistant: Elizabeth Callaghan
Production Editor: Julie Elliott
Production Controller: Kate Charman

For further information on Blackwell Publishing, visit our website: http://www.blackwellpublishing.com

Contents

Preface

The second edition of *An Aid to the MRCP Short Cases* comprehensively dealt with the old MRCP short cases exam. Stations 1, 3 and 5 of the MRCP PACES exam (Practical Assessment of Clinical Examination) have replaced this exam. Though the new exam is more structured and potentially more fair in several important ways, it is, in its essence, fundamentally the same exam, testing the same things. The skills and experience required to pass it remain the same, as do the many ways of failing it. Thus the third edition of *An Aid to the MRCP Short Cases* has become *An Aid to the MRCP PACES*, vol. 1 and we have been able to focus all that was helpful in the first two editions on the new format of the exam. This book deals with stations 1, 3 and 5 of the MRCP PACES exam.

At the time of writing the exam remains relatively new, but we have already been able to undertake an initial survey. As with our previous editions this forms the basis of the book. Though smaller than previous surveys, candidates were again aware of our book and poured out information to us. On reflection it is not surprising that we have found that the same old short cases continue to occur with frequencies that are not dissimilar. This is inevitable because the same patient pools are being tapped and the same patients lend themselves to testing the clinical skills that the College wishes to assess. In terms of frequency of occurrence there are some notable exceptions. For example the wider and earlier use of cardiac surgery has led to 'prosthetic valves' becoming the commonest cardiac case with 'mitral stenosis', which was the commonest at the time of our first survey in the 1980s, now relegated to sixth commonest as patients with this condition get fewer and are operated on earlier. The new format of the exam has also had its effect. For example the fact that there 'must be' a 'skin' case in station 5 has meant that the majority of the small number of new short cases we have had to create for the new edition are 'skin' cases. Nevertheless we have yet again found from the feedback from candidates in our survey that overall the cases seen, mistakes made or avoided, accounts of triumphs, tragedies and downward spirals, remain remarkably constant as each sitting comes and goes. We have during the first year of PACES been able to amass enough questionnaires from candidates to update the 'frequency of occurrence' figures and apply them to each of the subsections of station 1, 3 and 5. Because the new survey is as yet not great enough to cover all the less common short cases, we have adapted the figures from earlier surveys where there was inadequate data from the new surveys. In acknowledgement of the creation of station 5, locomotor, in PACES, we have created for this new edition two new examination *routines*, 'Examine this patient's knee' and 'Examine this patient's hip'.

In the guide notes for host examination centres, the College states: 'The patients attending the clinical stations should exhibit mainstream medical conditions. Patients with esoteric conditions are not suitable.' There is a problem, however, as to what constitutes an 'esoteric' condition. One physician's esoteric condition is another's extremely interesting and important one. Our survey suggests that the spectrum of patients being selected remains unchanged. Presumably the more there is a tendency to a consensus that a condition tends towards the esoteric end of things, the less likely such a patient is to be selected. On the other hand less likely does not necessarily mean never, and this is reflected in the frequency of occurrence rates, which are sometimes very low indeed. Our own view remains that it would be a shame if clinical awareness of uncommon conditions was extinguished from the physicians of the future just because these conditions are rare or considered by some to be esoteric. What about the patient with an 'esoteric' condition? — would he/she not be horrified to learn that there was a policy that his/her condition no longer had to be studied and recognized in the way it had been by physicians in the past? We maintain our belief that failure to recognize a rare condition would never be an important pass/fail factor. On all types of cases, both 'easy' and 'hard', observation shows that some candidates perform well and others badly and all types of case can act as discriminators in one way or another. There is potential, with rarities, to show a breadth of clinical diagnostic skills which may distinguish a candidate from his/her peers. Before coming to terms with rarities, however, you should ensure you can perform well with the more commonly occurring short cases. As our overriding principle remains to translate the standards set by the Colleges we have covered them all in this book — the common and rare with rates of frequency of appearance in the clinical exam given so that you can ensure that you establish your priorities appropriately.

Stations 2 and 4 are dealt with in a new book *An Aid to the MRCP PACES*, vol. 2. The PACES survey has enabled us to further expand our collection of experiences and anecdotes that are now presented in vol. 2. We have been able to present a number of hardly edited complete PACES accounts written in the first person. At the same time the similarity of stations 1, 3 and 5 to the old short cases exam has meant that most of our older collection of experiences and anecdotes from our previous editions are as valuable now as ever and they have been retained.

Medical Short Cases for Medical Students

In previous editions we encouraged medical students to use this book and many did. We have therefore written a medical student version. *Medical Short Cases for Medical Students*. We invite all of you who find this book useful to draw the attention of your medical students to the medical student version, to help with their clinical exams, whether OSCE or the traditional short case format.

Acknowledgements

We are extremely grateful to the following for reviewing some or all of the second edition short cases and/or examination routines related to their speciality. Many of these devoted a considerable amount of their valuable time to this task for no reward other than the accolade of 'Speciality advisor to *An Aid to the MRCP PACES*, Volume 1'. We should stress that we did not necessarily always take the advice given but we hope the errors of fact are minimal. They are acknowledged in order according to the number of short cases they dealt with: S. Sturman (neurology), C. Tan (dermatology), T. Millane (cardiology), D. Banerjee (respiratory), S. Jones (endocrinology), D. Carruthers (rheumatology), P. Wilson (gastroenterology), P. Dodson (medical ophthalmology), J. Wright (haematology) and T. Pankhurst (renal). We are grateful to D. Banerjee who wrote the first drafts of two of the new short cases—stridor and lung transplant; and to D. Carruthers who wrote the first drafts of the new examination *routines*, 'Examine this patient's knee' and 'Examine this patient's hip'.

We are grateful to so many candidates for their encouragement and enthusiasm and especially the many who have filled in questionnaires and to colleagues for their tolerance and support. Finally, we once again reinforce the gratitude, expressed at the end of previous prefaces, to our long suffering families without whose forbearance and help the whole venture would never have happened.

Bob Ryder
Afzal Mir
Anne Freeman

Preface to the second edition

Following publication of the first edition, my co-authors continued making surveys of candidates and accumulated an overwhelming number of questionnaires finding that many candidates, now aware of our book, poured out information to us. These greatly reinforced the information found in our original surveys and presented in the first edition. We found another 50 short cases which we present in this new edition, yet overall the cases seen, mistakes made or avoided, accounts of triumphs, tragedies and downward spirals, remain remarkably constant as each sitting comes and goes. Our much more limited time, now that I have also become a consultant, meant that we were not able to analyse the new surveys to anything like the same extent as in the original edition. Therefore we have not altered the 'frequency of occurrence' figures used in the first edition for the 150 short cases of that edition as we do not believe that a more superficial analysis of the new surveys would be as accurate. It is possible that, for instance, 'old tuberculosis' is occurring in the exam less often than it did as fewer patients who had a thoracoplasty all those years ago are still available (patients with similar signs due to partial or complete pneumonectomy may appear instead, however, and indeed this is one of the new short cases); similarly Fallot's tetralogy with a Blalock shunt. Nevertheless the vast majority of cases seem to maintain a remarkably constant rate of occurrence.

We were able to assign an approximate occurrence rate for each of the additional 50 short cases so that they could be merged in with the original 150. One of the new short cases has come into existence since the first edition because of new College guidelines ('Resuscitation Annie') and one because of the spread of a new condition ('AIDS related'). Some of the new cases are relative rarities which appear in the exam just occasionally. We do not believe that such cases should be excluded from the exam. It would be a shame if clinical awareness of uncommon conditions was extinguished from the physicians of the future just because these conditions are rare. At the same time we do not believe that failure to recognize a rare condition would ever be an important pass/fail factor in the MRCP short cases. A candidate seeing such a case is also likely to see a number of other more usual cases on which the main pass/fail decisions would be made.

Nevertheless there is potential, with rarities, to show a breadth of clinical diagnostic skills which may distinguish a candidate from his/her peers. Before coming to terms with rarities, however, you should ensure you can perform well with the more commonly occurring short cases. In this book we cover them all—the common and rare with rates of frequency of appearance in the clinical exam so that you can ensure that you establish your priorities appropriately. The new surveys have enabled us to considerably expand the experiences and anecdotes in Section 4 and because candidates often 'knew what they were writing for', we have been able to present a number of hardly edited accounts written in the first person.

Acknowledgements

We are grateful to the following for reviewing some or all of the first edition short cases and/or examination routines related to their speciality. We should stress that we did not necessarily always take the advice given but we hope the errors of fact are minimal. G.S. Venables (neurology), S. Sturman (also neurology), K.S. Channer (cardiology), E.E. Kritzinger (medical ophthalmology), P. Stewart (endocrinology), C. Tan (dermatology), D. Honeybourne (respiratory medicine), T. Iqbal (gastroenterology), M. El Nahas (renal medicine), D. Situnayke (rheumatology), D. Bareford (haematology), P. Harper (medical genetics), K.G. Taylor (lipids) and E. McLoskey (Paget's disease). There was also a contribution from A. Jackowski (neurosurgeon). We thank C. Tan for Figs 3.114b and c, and C. Ellis for Fig. 3.156b.

I am particularly grateful to my co-authors for their tolerance with regard to my contribution to the tardiness of the new edition; to colleagues, in particular Ken Taylor and Sharon Jones for their support; to Anne's family, Pete, Lizzie and Jonathan Williams for what they have had to put up with; similarly to Lynda, Farooq, Deborah and Joanne Mir (especially for their wonderful hospitality during some crucial sessions over several days at Afzal's house); similarly and more so to my children Bobby and Anna for what they have had to put up with, but most of all sincere thanks to my wife Anne, without whose support and tolerance, well beyond the call of duty, none of it could ever have happened.

Bob Ryder

Preface to the first edition

The short cases part of the examination for the Membership of the Royal College of Physicians (MRCP) is, by tradition, considered to be the most critical test of bedside behaviour and diagnostic competence. It forms an important milestone in the development of practicing physicians. There is, however, no formal syllabus or tutoring and, despite the high failure rate, there is a notable lack of books specifically written to help candidates with this test.

The spectrum of clinical conditions used in the short cases examination is determined by a variety of interchanging factors such as the availability of patients with demonstrable physical signs, the prejudice of the doctors choosing the cases, that of the examiners taking part in the examination and, occasionally, the speciality bias of the examination centre. The cases chosen by the examiners from those assembled on the day in turn determine the problems presented to the candidates and the clinical skills required of them. For this reason we decided to build this book around an extensive survey conducted amongst successful candidates. Our questionnaires yielded information about the cases presented, the questions asked, answers given and the reactions of the examiners. We have thus been able to identify the chief difficulties of candidates in dealing with this practical examination and have attempted to help with these. The advice in Section 1 on how to prepare for the short cases is based on, and illustrated by, the comments received from the candidates. Section 2 is written around the clinical instructions given by the examiners to the candidates, the likely diagnoses under each instruction as revealed in the survey, and details of the examination steps suitable for each command. Section 3 forms the bulk of the book and presents the clinical features of 150 short cases in order of the frequency of their occurrence in the examination as derived from our survey. Thus, priorities are sorted out for the candidates preparing for the examination. In the final section we pass on the experiences and advice of some of the candidates in our survey which we felt would be of interest.

In fulfilling our main task of helping candidates to improve their performance in clinical examinations we have used three learning techniques which are rather novel to this field. Firstly, the iterative approach which exploits the retentive potential of reinforcement by repeating the main clinical features of a number of conditions whenever any reference to these is made. It is hoped that this method will not only reinforce, but will also alert the candidates to other diagnostic possibilities when looking at a related condition. Secondly, in the examination methods suggested by us we have individualized the inspection to the examination of each subsystem, and have provided a *visual survey* to note the features most likely to be present. This enriches the usual advice to look for everything which often accomplishes nothing unless a specific sign is being looked for. Thirdly, we have reduced our suggested clinical methods to simple steps (*checklists*) which, if practised, may become spontaneous clinical habits, easy to recall and execute.

In the age of superspecialization, the task of summarizing and streamlining a subject as vast and diverse as general medicine to the needs of the short cases examinee has been formidable. We are in no doubt that our attempt will have its inadequacies and would be pleased if you would write to us (c/o Blackwell Scientific Publications) about any errors of fact, or with any suggestions which might be helpful for a future edition, or indeed with any other comments. We would also be interested to hear of any short cases which have occurred in the examination and which are not included on our lists (please give us an idea of your confidence that the case was indeed the condition concerned and why—clinical details, invigilator's confirmation, etc.) or of any Membership experiences which might be of interest.

Medical student note

Although this book has concentrated exclusively on the needs of MRCP candidates, it is noteworthy that the cases included in undergraduate medical short cases examinations are drawn from the same pool as those used in the MRCP examination. Furthermore, physicians are all MRCP trained and tend to use the MRCP style in these examinations. Though clearly the required standard of performance is lower, we feel that medical students preparing for their short cases examinations would also benefit from using this book. It would be a supplement to information gained from more comprehensive textbooks (we assume much basic knowledge) and an aid to practice on the wards.

Acknowledgements

We are indebted to the late Dr Ralph Marshall and his team (especially Paul Crompton, Keith Bellamy, Steve Young and Adrian Shaw) in the Department of Medical Illustration at the University Hospital of Wales, and Nigel Pearce and Steve Cashmore at the Department of Medical Illustration at the Royal Gwent Hospital. A large proportion of the photographs in the book are from the archives of these departments.

We are grateful to all the patients who gave their consent to the publication of the photographs depicting their medical conditions. Our thanks are due to many colleagues who have allowed us to use photographs from their own collections and photographs of their patients including: T.M. Hayes, the late C.E.C. Wells, M.S.J. Pathy, R. Marks, the late R. Hall, J.G. Graham, B.H. Davies, P.J.A. Holt, J. Jessop, M.H. Pritchard, N.W.D. Walshaw, I.S. Petheram, J.M. Swithenbank, M.D. Mishra, B.D. Williams, I.N.F. McQueen, P.E. Hutchinson, J. Rhodes, C.A.R. Pippen, A.J. Birtwell, P.M. Smith, A.G. Knight, S. Richards, A.G. Karseras, J.P. Thomas, C.N.A. Matthews, P.J. Sykes, M.L. Insley, P.I. Williams, B.S.D. Sastry, J.H. Jones, M.Y. Khan, the late J.D. Spillane, K. Tayton, G.M. Tinker, A. Compston, B.A. Thomas, H.J. Lloyd, G.B. Leitch, the late B. Calcraft, O.M. Gibby, G.O. Thomas, E. Graham Jones, Byron Evans, D.J. Fisher, G.S. Kilpatrick, L.E. Hughes, P. Harper, G. Griffiths, A.D. Holt-Wilson, D.B. Foster, D.L.T. Webster, J.H. Lazarus, D. Beckingham, J.E. Cawdery, R. Prosser, M.F. Scanlon, M. Wiles, I.A. Hughes, the late O.P. Gray, E. Waddington and L. Beck. Figure 3.42b has already been published in *An Atlas of Clinical Neurology* by Spillane and Spillane (Oxford University Press) and Figs 3.97b and 3.114 from the UHW Medical Illustration archives are also published in *A Picture Quiz in Medicine* by Ebden, Peiras and Dew (Lloyd-Luke Medical Books Ltd). Figures 3.115a (i) and (ii) are published with the permission of the Department of Medical Photography, Leicester Royal Infirmary and Fig. 3.110 with the permission of the University of Newcastle upon Tyne, holders of the copyright.

Our thanks go to colleagues who advised us on points of uncertainty in their fields of interest; especially A.C., B.H.D., M.J.D., L.G.D., R.H., T.M.H., M.H., T.P.K., I.N.F.M., M.D.M., M.F.S., H.S., P.M.S., S.S. and B.D.W.

We are obliged to: Andrea Hill for typing and retyping the manuscript; Janet Roberts for secretarial help with the survey; Jill Manfield for telephoning, chasing and writing again in pursuit of patient consents and for numerous minor secretarial chores; Alan Peiras for some nifty detective work in Edinburgh during the survey; Steve Young for the cover photograph for the book; and to certain pharmaceutical companies for financial assistance (including Astra Pharmaceuticals Ltd, CIBA Laboratories, May and Baker Ltd, Roche Products Ltd, Merck Sharp and Dohme Ltd and Thomas Morson Pharmaceuticals). Our particular thanks to Bayer UK Ltd for sponsoring the colour photographs.

Most of all we thank our long-suffering families without whose forebearance and help the book would never have been finished.

Bob Ryder
Afzal Mir
Anne Freeman

Introduction

'The result comes as a particular shock when you have been sitting exams for many years without failing them.'*

From June 2001, the Royal College of Physicians replaced the traditional MRCP 'clinical' examination, consisting of 30 minutes of short cases, a long case lasting 1 hour and 20 minutes and a viva lasting 20 minutes, with the MRCP PACES exam (Practical Assessment of Clinical Examination). The candidate who reaches the MRCP PACES examination has already demonstrated considerable knowledge of medicine by passing the MRCP Part I and MRCP Part II written examinations. The PACES exam is divided into five stations each of which is timed for precise periods of 20 minutes. Stations 1 and 3 are divided into two substations of 10 minutes each. The stations are:

Station 1 respiratory system
           abdominal system
Station 2 history taking skills
Station 3 cardiovascular system
           central nervous system
Station 4 communication skills and ethics
Station 5 skin, locomotor, eye and endocrine

Stations 2 and 4 are commonly referred as the 'new' stations because they represent developments that are very different from the old exam. These stations are dealt with in volume 2 of *An Aid to the MRCP PACES*. Stations 1, 3 and 5 represent a more structured version of the old MRCP short cases exam that we dealt with in the first two editions of *An Aid to the MRCP Short Cases*. Examples of the mark sheets used in stations 1, 3 and 5 of PACES are shown in Appendix 4. On each short case, each examiner gives an independent mark between 1 and 4 where 1 = clear fail, 2 = fail, 3 = pass and 4 = clear pass. In order to pass PACES your average mark for all examiners on all five stations needs to be ≥3. Thus a 2 scored by an examinee anywhere in PACES needs to be compensated for by the scoring of a 4 somewhere else in the exam. The scoring of only 1 anywhere in PACES needs to be compensated for by the scoring of a 4 twice at some other part of the exam. Over the years all have been agreed that the short cases examination is the major hurdle in MRCP Part II and with the advent of PACES the cases appearing in stations 1, 3 and 5 remain as challenging as ever, and for many who do fail it is the first examination they have ever failed and it may also be the only examination they have taken that does not have some form of syllabus.

The exam in stations 1, 3 and 5 is a practical test which assesses various facets of clinical competence in many subtle ways. Although it is generally accepted that clinical competence cannot be acquired from textbooks, a book such as this can provide indirect help towards that objective. We hope that the examination *routines* (Section B) together with the *checklists* (Appendix 1) may assist candidates in developing a keen sense of clinical search and detection. The short case *records* (Section C) should provide the framework, i.e. the main clinical features, the discipline of how to look for them, how to differentiate the diagnostic from the incidental or associated findings, and how and when to be alert to other possibilities. By basing our book on the results of a survey of successful MRCP candidates (see below) we have *created a form of syllabus* which we hope will be of value to future candidates. Not only do the results of the survey advise as to what you are required to know and do, but they also grade these requirements in order of importance.

The examination in Stations 1, 3 and 5

'I am sure they assess you very quickly . . . and decide whether they would like you to be in charge of their patients.'†

Two examiners will each take you for half of each 20-minute station. They each record a separate mark. At each case you will be given a written instruction, e.g.: 'This 48-year-old man has had a heart valve operation. He complains of recent shortness of breath on exertion but not at rest. Examine the cardiovascular system to see if you can establish the cause.' Nevertheless it is clear from our PACES survey that candidates translate the instruction into the traditional one: 'Examine this patient's heart'. We would counsel you to be careful on this point.

* Vol. 2, p. 369

† Vol. 2.

Sometimes there is an important clue in the instruction. For example one candidate in our survey (p. 289) was asked to look at the patient and then listen to the heart. The diagnosis was Marfan's syndrome with a prosthetic heart valve and the clue in the instruction was that the candidate was specifically asked to look before examining. In the case of the acromegalic with homonymous hemianopia described on page 9, the candidates were given the written instruction to inspect the patient and then undertake a visual field assessment. Many undertook their visual field examination without spotting the acromegaly and then got into difficulty accordingly.

During the examination the examiners are constantly testing your ability to *elicit and interpret physical signs*. Many examiners say that, in the final analysis, whether a candidate will pass or fail depends very much on the general air of competence or incompetence which prevails during his/her clinical performance. Many candidates who fail feel that the exam is unfair in one way or another (e.g. first person experience 31, p. vol. 2, p. 356). However, candidates are not in a good position to judge their performance. A candidate who diagnosed a patient with aortic stenosis (which the last three candidates before him all diagnosed correctly) as having mitral stenosis may never know of his error. Furthermore, it is more than just a question of getting the right diagnosis. One candidate who failed complained that he knew, because he had a contact at the examination centre, that he had got the right diagnosis in all except two of the cases he saw. He was reporting this during the feedback session of a subsequent mock exam which he had also failed. During that mock exam, after examining the wasted legs of a patient with myotonic dystrophy, his first suggestion as to the cause of the signs in the legs was 'canda equina lesion'. He eventually got to the correct diagnosis but his initial responses left a poor impression on the mock examiners, especially since other candidates in the same mock exam noticed, at once and without prompting, that the patient had gross generalized wasting, indicating that the problem was not one confined to the legs. In similar ways he had performed poorly on many of the other cases in the mock exam and as a mock examiner one could easily see how he failed in the real exam whilst believing that he usually got the right diagnosis. Most agree that the move to PACES has increased the fairness of the exam, in particular because of the break between stations followed by 'starting again' with two new examiners who are not influenced by what occurred on the previous occasion. It is clear from our survey that this may have interrupted in

some cases what may otherwise have gone on to become a 'downward spiral' disaster (see comments on PACES experience 1, vol. 2, p. 283; comments on PACES experience 3, vol. 2, p. 287; comments on PACES experience 11, vol. 2, p. 301.). Nevertheless some continue to feel unfairly treated (see comments on PACES experience 7, vol. 2, p. 295; comments on PACES, experience 14, vol. 2, p. 304). However, experience suggests, as one senior membership examiner put it, that the MRCP will usually pick out those who should fail; it will also usually pick out those who should pass — but not necessarily on the current attempt! Given the importance of clinical competence and the fact that this can only be assessed through a clinical exam (and clinical exams by their very nature will always have some in-built inadequacies), it seems unlikely that one could ever improve on this situation. In the old short cases exam the mark for each case was out of 12. As testimony to the precision of the marking system, it was an impressive fact that examiners, though marking independently, rarely differed by more than one mark in the scores out of 12 that they gave. The degree to which, generally, the examiners' marks concur suggests that the exam is probably as good as it can be. Our aim in this book, if you are one of those who should pass, is to try to help you to let the examiners know this on the current attempt or the next, rather than on the next attempt or the one after!

The surveys of MRCP short cases

'Certain "favourite" topics seem to recur. Make sure you know these.'

First edition

This survey has been introduced in the preface to the first edition (p. xii). In the first part of this survey, questionnaires were obtained from a number of doctors who had gained the MRCP during the previous 10 years. In the second part all the successful candidates at a single sitting were circulated. The questionnaires obtained in the two parts of the survey included both the pass and the previous fail attempts of those candidates. Altogether we collected accounts of 248 attempts at the MRCP short cases, covering over 1300 'main focus' short cases as well as over 500 'additional' short cases (see p. 68 for an explanation of these terms). The diagnoses given by these candidates were graded according to the confidence each candidate had in his retrospective assessment. Pass attempt diagnoses were given more weight than fail attempt ones. As a result we hope that the rather complex analysis per-

* Vol. 2, p. 369.

formed produced a picture which is as near to the truth as possible. Analysis of the first part of the survey covering candidates' attempts over several years was essentially the same as analysis of the second part. This suggests that the cases used and the skills tested tend to remain constant. This comparison also gives some support to the accuracy of our method of analysis. The figures are used wherever they may be helpful throughout this volume. Apart from figures, the organization of our suggested examination *routines* (Section B) and the contents of our short case *records* (Section C) have been closely guided by this original, as well as subsequent, surveys. For light entertainment, but with ingrained lessons, a number of experiences, anecdotes and quotations from the survey are given in volume 2 of *An Aid to the MRCP PACES*.

Second edition

As discussed in the preface to the second edition (p. xi), the original surveys were embellished for the second edition with several surveys conducted between the two editions. We collected accounts of a further 379 attempts covering nearly 2300 additional 'main focus' short cases.

Though the second edition surveys were more extensive than those for the first edition, the analysis of them was more superficial and, therefore, the analysis from the first edition surveys remained the bedrock of the book.

Current (PACES) edition

As discussed in the preface to the current edition (p. ix), we have been able to undertake a small initial PACES survey which has provided, despite its size, considerable valuable information for us to modify our book accordingly. We used for the survey the first 50 PACES questionnaires that we received during the 12 months. This has given us accounts of 400 short cases—200 from stations 1 and 3 and 200 from station 5. The questionnaires gave accounts from the first three PACES sittings with one questionnaire from the fourth sitting. Wherever the data from this survey was sufficient to supersede that from previous surveys it was thus used. We have also been able to give a number of complete PACES experiences written in the first person at the end of volume 2 of *An Aid to the MRCP PACES*. By studying these the first timer in particular can be given considerable insight into what the exam is actually like.

Section A
Preparation

'Expressionless and without comment they led me away.'*

The clinical skills required for the MRCP examination, particularly in relation to the short cases, can only be acquired by thoughtful preparation, experience and purposeful practice. Tutors and examiners alike agree that it is more important to spend time examining patients than reading textbooks. The examiners are not looking for encyclopaedic knowledge, they are just anxious to ascertain that you can be trusted to carry out an adequate clinical examination and make a competent clinical assessment. This book aims to help you organize your overall preparation to meet that objective. We have provided preparatory aids including examination *routines* and short case *records* (see below). We also aim to give you some insight into what most candidates experience in the examination and we hope to help you prepare psychologically. We would like to stress that though the written examination may appear a formidable hurdle, it often turns out to be less of an obstacle than PACES. You would be wise to err on the side of safety and prepare for the PACES before, during and after your preparations for the written exam. Thus, we begin with some basic principles of practice and preparations at work.

Clinical experience in everyday work

'Imagine you are seeing the cases in a clinic and carrying out a routine examination.'*

The intention of the College in the examination is to gain a reflection of your usual working day clinical competence for the examiners to judge. In arriving at their final verdict the examiners may take particular note of factors such as your approach to the patient, your examination technique, spontaneity of shifting from system to system in pursuit of relevant clinical signs, fluidity in giving a coherent account of all the findings and conclusions, and your composure throughout. Though you can acquire all this for the day only, as some successful candidates do who are experts at passing examinations, it would be preferable if you could adopt many of these good habits into your everyday clinical approach. In either event, a long, diligent and disciplined practice is required if your aim is to be able to perform a smooth and polished clinical examination, to display the subtle confidence of a skilled performer, and to suppress signs of anxiety.

One simple approach to the task is that, whatever your job, you should consider all the patients you see as PACES patients from one station or another. Such a practice should not only improve your readiness for the examination but also improve your standard of patient care — the primary objective of every clinician. Look out for all the 'good signs' passing through your hospital and use as many of these as possible as practise short cases. Ask your colleagues to let you know of every heart murmur, every abnormal fundus, every case with abnormal neurology, etc. If you are in, or can get to, a teaching hospital, make regular trips not only to clinical meetings and demonstrations but also, more importantly, to *visit the specialist wards* — neurology, cardiology, chest, rheumatology, dermatology, etc. It is useful to study the signs and conditions even when you know the diagnosis in order to further familiarize yourself with them. It is also a good practice to see cases 'blind' to the diagnosis and to try to simulate the examination situation. Imagine that two examiners are standing over you and there is a need to complete an efficient, once-only examination followed by an immediate response to the anticipated question: 'What are your findings?' or 'What is the diagnosis?'

Simulated examination practice

'I had a lot of practice presenting short cases to a "hawk" of a senior registrar. This experience was invaluable.'†

If a constant effort is made to improve your clinical skills by seeing as many cases as possible, there is no reason why the spontaneity and competence so acquired should not show up on the day. As with all examinations, however, much can be learned about the deficiencies requiring special attention when you put your composite clinical ability to the test in 'mock' examinations. In most district, general, and all teaching, hospitals the local postgraduate clinical tutors organize Membership teaching and 'mock' examination sessions, and you should find out about, and join in, as many of these as you can manage. Unfortunately, a lot of these, though useful, tend to teach in groups and discuss management or look at X-rays, rather than provide the intensive 'on the spot' practise on patients that is the ideal preparation for PACES. It is, therefore, advisable to supplement these sessions with simulated examination practise arranged by yourself. This requires the cooperation of a 'mock' examiner (consultant, experienced registrar and, on occasion, a fellow examinee) on a *one-to-one basis*. If you can practise with a variety of 'mock' examiners, you will not only broaden the assessment of your imperfections but also learn to respond to the varied approaches of different examiners.

---

* Vol. 2, quotation 91, p. 373.

† Vol. 2, quotation 19, p. 370.

Examination *routines*

'The most important point is to look professional — as if you have done it a hundred times before.'*

The short cases part of the test is very important for the Membership examination because it is designed to test critically two major areas of clinical competence. The first and more important of these is your ability to detect abnormal physical signs, interpret them correctly and put them together into a reasonable diagnosis or differential diagnosis. The second is your competence to conduct a professional and efficient clinical examination (see experience 34, vol. 2). As said above, these are generally considered to arise from day-to-day work and your conduct in the examination will reflect your experience in performing clinical tasks, presenting your assessments of patients to your seniors and getting their constant constructive criticism. If you are lucky enough to have worked with a good teacher you may have acquired a firm foundation upon which you could build a structured clinical examination for all systems. As most candidates are engaged in busy clinical jobs and their seniors are often overburdened by administrative chores, etc., useful clinical dialogue between them may be limited. As a result there may be little improvement in the weaknesses acquired during the undergraduate years. The enormous task of preparing for the Membership examination provides an ideal opportunity to remedy any deficiencies in one's clinical methods. We would suggest that you work out the exact number and sequence of clinical steps for the examination of each subsystem, particularly those you would need to take in response to a particular command from the examiner; then practise going through these steps. Practise them over and over again† on your spouse, or any other willing person, until all the steps become as automatic as driving a car. Practise them on patients until you are confident of being able to pick up or demonstrate any abnormal physical signs. You should be able to maintain the same sequence and run through it rapidly and comprehensively in a way that is second nature to you. The sequence of clinical steps required for the examination of each system or subsystem is collectively referred to as the examination *routine* in this book. In Section B we suggest various examination *routines* (which you may wish to adopt or adapt) for you to practise in response to particular commands. In Appendix 1 we provide *checklists* which summarize the major points in each examination *routine*. The *checklists* are designed to help in practising the *routines*.

Short case *records*

'The more practice at presenting short cases the better.'‡

A knowledge of the possible short cases that may be used in the examination is important so that you can become familiar with the physical signs associated with each, and know what you are looking for as you work through the examination *routine*. Having a good grasp of the clinical features of the case may enable you to score extra marks by looking for additional signs that may be present. Such extra marks identify the above-average candidate from the average ones. Furthermore, by becoming acquainted with descriptions of typical cases you will find it easier to present the case to the examiner using acceptable descriptive terms. In this book, under each short case, we have presented the typical clinical features for you to remember, and to 'regurgitate' what you see (hence the descriptive term *record*), omit what you do not find, and add what you find new. Thus, when confronted with the face of a man with Parkinson's disease which you diagnose at once on seeing his tremor, instead of stuttering and stumbling as you try to think of the right words to describe his face, the terms depressed, expressionless, unblinking, drooling and titubation will immediately surface for you to use. In Section C, under the headings of each PACES substation, we have covered the overwhelming majority of cases which could occur and we have put them in order of priority according to the likelihood of occurrence as assessed from our surveys.

Getting 'psyched up'

'Do not be distracted by mistakes made (or imagined) in preceding cases or the examiners' mannerisms or approach (I was and suffered for it). Being very nervous does not necessarily fail you and one bad case should not put you off.'§

It is common to hear candidates agonizing over their feeling that they failed to give a performance commensurate with their actual capabilities, simply because they were discouraged by the 'examination ordeal'. Though it is true that knowledge and competence tend to generate confidence and capability, it is also true that extreme anxiety can seriously impair the performance of even the most knowledgeable and competent candidate.

The downward spiral syndrome

'After the first case there was a long pause as if they were waiting for me to say more — I went to pieces after this.'¶

* Vol. 2, p. 369.

† MRCP = Methods Require Constant Practice.

‡ Vol. 2, p. 370.

§ Quotations 47–54 and 81, Vol. 2, pp. 371, 372.

¶ Vol. 2, p. 371, see also experience 2, Vol. 2, p. 283.

The candidate, an otherwise able and experienced doctor, enters the PACES examination room extremely anxious and lacking in confidence. He is just hovering on the edge of despair and the slightest upset is going to push him over. On one or more of the cases he convinces himself that he is doing badly (whether or not he actually is) and over the edge he goes. The first stage of a rapid 'downward spiral' sets in; the dispirited candidate gets worse and worse and actually gives up before the end in the certainty that he has failed. Months of intensive bookwork and bedside practice, not to mention the examination fee, go to waste because of *inadequate psychological preparation*. To avoid this there are four basic rules that are well worth noting.

1 You never know you have failed until the list is published

'Don't be put off if you get a few things wrong. I made a lot of mistakes that I know of and still passed.'*

In the same way as it is said of the greatest saints that they considered themselves to be the greatest sinners, many successful candidates leave the examination centre feeling certain that they have failed. Good candidates may have a heightened awareness of the imperfections of their performance and thereby may exaggerate the impact of their mistakes on the examiner. Furthermore, the 'hawk' examiner may make you feel that you are doing badly, or you may deduce it from his mannerism, regardless of your performance. By the same token the newcomer may slide through the stations unaware of any errors and with the examiners acting benignly, and then express great surprise as the inevitable 'thin' envelope arrives. It is not really important whether or not you think you have failed during the days between the examination and the arrival of the result. However, if you become convinced that you are failing while you are still sitting the examination, the thought can be disastrous and impair your performance to the extent that your conviction becomes a reality (e.g. see experiences 1 and 2, anecdote 24 and quotation 52, vol. 2).

2 Do not be put off by the examiners or their reactions

'The most off-putting aspect of each case is the lack of feedback from the examiners as to whether you are right or wrong. This is much more disconcerting than outright criticism.'†

Many first-timers, despite excellent clinical experience, are stunned by the sombre and restrained atmosphere of the examination, which is unlike anything in their past experience (except perhaps the driving test!). It is as well, therefore, to be aware that the examiners tend to wear a 'poker-face' and usually give no feedback or encouragement. The 'hostile hawk' may appear dissatisfied with everything you do and say, but this is not necessarily a guide as to whether you are doing badly or not. A positive atmosphere is no guide either: the smiling ('smiling death'!) and pleasant ('deadly dove'!) examiner (and the apparently uninterested one), can be as deadly as a black widow spider if you get yourself into a diagnostic maze! Bear in mind that 'hawks' and 'doves' tend to have similar rates of passing and failing candidates. Disregard the atmosphere and concentrate on what the examiner asks you to do rather than on what he looks like, and recall your *routines* and *records*.

3 The cases are easy and you have seen it all before

'My cases were more straightforward than I had been led to believe. Nothing was particularly rare.'‡

The psychological scenario of the examination is such that many candidates enter it with the distorted view that behind every case and every question there will be some catch, some clever trap, something never seen before, or a diagnosis never heard of. In fact these suspicions are rarely justified. The *vast majority* of cases and questions are straightforward and a realization of this is likely to produce a confident, straightforward answer from the start instead of the hesitancy born of a mind filled with suspicion and struggling to solve the hidden catch. A study of membership short cases§ reveals that there are two broad groups. The first group includes common conditions which you are well used to seeing in everyday clinical practice such as rheumatic heart disease, cirrhosis of the liver, rheumatoid hands and so on. These should surely present little difficulty (especially if you have tailor-made *routines* and *records*). In the second broad group are the rarities with good physical signs such as Osler–Weber–Rendu syndrome, pseudoxanthoma elasticum, Peutz–Jeghers syndrome, etc. You should be well used to these from the study of colour atlases, etc. that you will have done in preparation for the MRCP written examination. These too, therefore, should be easy (once you recognize the condition all you have to do is 'play the *record*'!).

4 You have already passed and you have just got to keep it that way

'It's like skating on thin ice—if you keep going and don't fall through, you make it.'*

Confidence in one's ability is a very important ingredient in any form of competition. As you go into the examination imagine that you have a clean sheet with a 100% mark and that you just have to keep it that way as the examiners show you a few simple short cases as you pass through stations 1, 3 and 5† such as fibrosing alveolitis, splenomegaly, mitral stenosis, cerebellar signs, psoriasis, systemic sclerosis, acromegaly and diabetic retinopathy (a typical combination). Such an attitude should replace the more usual: 'Everybody fails this examination; it's too difficult; how can I possibly pass'. The examination on clinical short cases for MRCP has been well described (Royal Northern course) as 'like walking up a path full of puddles without stepping in the puddles; and you make the puddles yourself'. Remember the way to success is '*Readiness, Routines, Records* and *Right frame of mind*'.

---

* Vol. 2, p. 371.

† With an interesting interlude in stations 2 and 4 in between!

Section B
Examination *Routines*

'Work out the best method for examination and practise it until it is second nature to you.'*

* Vol. 2, p. 369.

In this chapter *routines* are suggested for the clinical assessment of various subsystems. These are readily adaptable to your individual methods. The subsystems are arranged according to the examiners' standard instructions (e.g. examine the heart, abdomen, hands, etc.). We have retained the original choice of subsystems which was governed by our first edition surveys. In addition to this, in acknowledgement of the creation of station 5, locomotor, in PACES, we have created for this new edition two new examination *routines*, 'Examine this patient's knee' and 'Examine this patient's hip'. The extent to which candidates are, or are not, challenged with these new instructions remains to be determined. Examples of variations of the instruction are given both from our original survey and from our PACES survey. Under each subsystem a list of the possible short cases is presented in order of their occurrence in either the PACES survey (where there were sufficient data) or the original survey according to what was most appropriate. The percentages given represent our estimate of your chances of each diagnosis being present when you hear the particular instruction.* These lists of diagnoses have guided our suggested *routines*. The latter are broken down into numbered constituents to aid memory and *checklists* are given in Appendix 1 which match up to the numbered points in the examination *routine*. The *checklists* are to help your practice with each subsystem. The idea is to develop a controlled, spontaneous and flawless technique of examination for each subsystem, so that you do not have to keep pausing and thinking what to do next and so that you do not miss out important steps (see experience 35, vol. 2, p. 330). Often you will not need the complete sequence in the examination (for example, with regard to the 'Examine this patient's chest' *routine*, often the examiner will ask you to only examine 'the back of this patient's chest') but it will certainly increase your confidence if you enter the examination armed with the complete *routines* so that you can adapt them as necessary. The examination methods are supplemented with appropriate hints to avoid common pitfalls and to simplify the diagnostic maze.

The *routines* are presented in a single section without necessarily being associated with a particular station because our PACES survey has confirmed that many of the routines may be called upon in more than one station. For example, assessment of visual fields may be required in station 3 for a patient with a hemiplegia who might have homonymous hemianopia, or station 5 for a patient with acromegaly who might have a bitemporal hemianopia. It is essential that you bear in mind the station you are in when you are given the particular instruction and adapt it accordingly, but you also need to be wary of jumping to conclusions. For example we are aware of the anecdote from a PACES pilot of a patient with acromegaly who had had a cerebrovascular accident secondary to acromegalic hypertension, her visual fields were required to be examined in station 5 and showed homonymous hemianopia! Similarly the only radial nerve palsy patient to occur in any of our surveys since the 1980s turned up in station 5, locomotor, of a PACES sitting. In experience 10, vol. 2, p. 298, an account is given of a patient with Marfan's appearing in station 1, respiratory, so it is important to remain open to many possibilities whilst taking into account the station you are in.

---

* As with all our survey analyses, we graded the confidence of each candidate in his retrospective diagnosis of each short case seen. The percentages are not meant to add up to 100% because: (i) there are always missing percentages representing those short cases we could not be certain about; (ii) sometimes more than one diagnosis was considered worth counting for one instruction (for example, in order to give you the percentage of 'heart' cases with clubbing, when clubbing was present it was counted as well as the underlying cardiac condition). The figures are best used to give an index of the *relative importance* of the different conditions in terms of frequency of occurrence when you hear a given instruction.

Before dealing with the individual subsystems we would make some general points. You should avoid repeating the instruction or echoing the last part of it. Refrain from asking questions like: 'Would you like me to give you a running commentary or give the findings at the end?' Such a response wastes invaluable seconds which could be used running through the *checklist* and completing your *visual survey*. It is like a batsman asking a bowler in a cricket match whether he would like his ball hit for a six or played defensively! You must do what you are best at and hope that the examiner does not ask you to do otherwise. As suggested below, a well-rehearsed procedure suited to each sub-system should make it possible for you to start purposefully without delay. Your approach to the patient is of great importance, you should introduce yourself to him and ask his permission to examine him. Permission should also be sought for various manoeuvres, such as adjusting the backrest when examining the heart, or before removing any clothing. These polite exchanges will not only please most examiners and patients, but will also provide you with an opportunity to calm your nerves, collect your thoughts and recall the appropriate *checklist*. Although we have continually emphasized the value of looking for signs peripheral to the examiner's instruction (e.g. examine this patient's heart, abdomen, chest), we would like to emphasize too that *dithering* may be counterproductive. In the *visual survey* you should be scanning the patient rapidly and purposefully with a trained eye, not gazing helplessly at him for a long period while you try to decide what to do next. While you are feeling the pulse (heart) or settling the patient lying flat (abdomen), a quick look at the hands should establish whether there are any abnormalities or not. Pondering over normal hands from all angles at great length looks as unprofessional as, indeed, it is. It is of paramount importance to be gentle with the patient. Rough handling (e.g. roughly and abruptly digging deep into the patient's abdomen so that he winces with pain) can bring you instantly to the pass/fail borderline or below it (see experience 82, vol. 2, p. 334). Make sure that you cover the patient up when you have finished examining him, and thank him.

1 | 'Examine this patient's pulse'

Stations 3 and 5
Variations of instruction from original, pre PACES, survey
Feel this pulse
Examine this patient's pulse — look for the cause
Examine this patient's pulses.

Diagnoses from our original, pre PACES, survey in order of frequency
1 Irregular pulse 44%
2 Slow pulse 12%
3 Graves' disease 12%
4 Aortic stenosis 9%
5 Complete heart block 9%

6 Brachial artery aneurysm 9%
7 Impalpable radial pulses due to low output cardiac failure 9%
8 Tachycardia 6%
9 Takayasu's disease 3%
10 Hypothyroidism 3%
11 Fallot's tetralogy with a Blalock shunt 3%.

Examination *routine*

As you approach the patient from the right and ask for his permission to examine him you should

1 look at his **face** for a *malar flush* (mitral stenosis, myxoedema) or for any signs of *hyper-* or *hypothyroidism*. As you take the arm to examine the right radial pulse, continue the *survey* of the patient by looking at

2 the **neck** (Corrigan's pulse, raised JVP, thyroidectomy scar, goitre) and then the *chest* (thoracotomy scar). Quickly run your eyes down the body to complete the *survey* (ascites, clubbing, pretibial myxoedema, ankle oedema, etc.) and then concentrate on

3 the **pulse** and note

4 its **rate** (count for at least 15 seconds), volume and

5 its **rhythm.** A common diagnostic problem is presented by *slow atrial fibrillation* which may be mistaken for a regular pulse. To avoid this concentrate on the *length of the pause* from one beat to another and see if each pause is equal to the succeeding one (see also p. 153). This method will reveal that the pauses are variable from beat to beat in controlled slow atrial fibrillation.

6 Assess whether the **character** (waveform) of the pulse (information to be gained from radial, brachial and carotid) is normal, *collapsing, slow rising,* or jerky. To determine whether there is a collapsing quality put the palmar aspect of the four fingers of your left hand on the patient's wrist just below where you can easily feel the radial pulse. Press gently with your palm, lift the patient's hand above his head and then place your right palm over the patient's axillary artery. If the pulse has a *water-hammer* character you will experience a flick (a sharp and tall up-stroke and an abrupt down-stroke) which will *run* across all four fingers and at the same time you may also feel a flick of the axillary artery against your right palm. The pulse does not merely become palpable when the hand is lifted but its character changes and it imparts a sharp knock. This is classic of the pulse that is present in haemodynamically significant aortic incompetence and in patent ductus arteriosus. If the pulse has a collapsing character but is not of a frank water-hammer type then the flick runs across only two or three fingers (moderate degree of aortic incompetence or patent ductus arteriosus, thyrotoxicosis, fever, pregnancy, moderately severe mitral incompetence, anaemia, atherosclerosis). A *slow rising* pulse can best be assessed by palpating the brachial pulse with your left thumb and, as you press *gently*, you may feel the anacrotic notch (you will need practice to appreciate this) on the up-stroke against the pulp of your thumb. In mixed aortic valve disease the combination of plateau and collapsing effects can produce a bisferiens pulse. Whilst feeling the brachial pulse look for any catheterization *scars* (indicating valvular or ischaemic heart disease).

7 Proceed to feel the **carotid** where either a slow rising or a collapsing pulse can be confirmed.

8 Feel the **opposite radial pulse** and determine if both radials are the same (e.g. Fallot's with a Blalock shunt—p. 163), and then feel

9 the **right femoral pulse** checking for any *radiofemoral delay* (coarctation of the aorta). If you are asked to examine the pulses (as opposed to the pulse) you should continue to examine

10 all the other **peripheral pulses**. It is unlikely that the examiner will allow you to continue beyond what he thinks is a reasonable time to spot the diagnosis that he has in mind. However, should he not interrupt continue to look for

11 **additional diagnostic clues**. 'Thus, in a patient with atrial fibrillation and features suggestive of thyrotoxicosis you should examine the thyroid and/or eyes. In a patient with atrial fibrillation and hemiplegia or atrial fibrillation and a mitral valvotomy scar, proceed to examine the heart.

For *checklist* see p. 527.

2 | 'Examine this patient's heart'

Station 3
Variations of instruction in initial PACES survey (resultant diagnoses in brackets)
Examine this patient's heart (mitral stenosis)

Examine this patient's cardiovascular system (mitral valve disease and aortic regurgitation; mitral valve disease; mixed aortic valve disease; prosthetic valves; aortic stenosis; atrial fibrillation and prosthetic mitral valve; corrected Fallot's)

Examine this gentleman's heart. He has been complaining of palpitations (atrial fibrillation and mitral stenosis)

The GP has referred this 72-year-old lady with a murmur. Please examine her (mitral regurgitation)

This patient has been having palpitations—can you find a cause? (atrial fibrillation and mitral stenosis)

This patient is short of breath. Please examine the heart (mixed aortic valve disease)

You are seeing this elderly lady in the cardiology clinic which she has been attending for some time (prosthetic valve)

This young lady presented with increasing shortness of breath on exertion. Examine the cardiovascular system (aortic incompetence)

This lady has a heart murmur. Please examine her cardiovascular system (mitral stenosis and cerebrovascular accident)

This patient had a myocardial infarct 1 year ago. Please examine the cardiovascular system (aortic stenosis)

This man has been complaining of chest pain and palpitations. Please examine the cardiovascular system (aortic stenosis)

This patient has had an acute episode of breathlessness. Please examine the cardiovascular system (aortic stenosis)

This patient presented with shortness of breath. Please examine the cardiovascular system (mixed mitral valve disease and atrial fibrillation; aortic incompetence)

This gentleman came in on the take 2 days ago and he was breathless. Examine his cardiovascular system (atrial fibrillation and mitral regurgitation)

This man has just returned from ITU. Please examine his cardiovascular system (prosthetic valves)

This woman, who is about 60 years of age, is becoming increasingly breathless. Can you examine her cardiovascular system and see if you can find a reason (atrial fibrillation and mitral senosis)

Look at this patient and describe what you see. Then listen to the heart (Marfan's and prosthetic aortic valve)

The GP has noted a murmur—can you tell me what you think (mixed aortic valve disease)

This man has a heart murmur. Please examine him (mitral regurgitation)

Examine the cardiovascular system (hypertrophic cardiomyopathy).

Diagnoses from survey in order of frequency

1. Prosthetic valves 17%
2. Mitral incompetence (lone) 13%
3. Mixed aortic valve disease 9%
4. Mixed mitral valve disease 9%
5. Other combinations of mitral and aortic valve disease 8%
6. Mitral stenosis (lone) 7%
7. Aortic stenosis (lone) 7%
8. Aortic incompetence (lone) 5%
9. Ventricular septal defect 3%
10. Irregular pulse 2%
11. HOCM 2%
12. Marfan's 2%
13. Eisenmenger's syndrome 2%
14. Mitral valve prolapse 2%
15. Patent ductus arteriosus 2%
16. Tricuspid incompetence 2%
17. Fallot's tetralogy/Blalock shunt 0.9%
18. Raised jugular venous pressure 0.9%
19. Coarctation of the aorta 0.9%
20. Slow pulse 0.9%
21. Dextocardia 0.5%
22. Pulmonary stenosis 0.5%
23. Cannon waves 0.5%
24. Subclavian-steal syndrome 0.3%
25. Pulmonary incompetence 0.3%
26. Infective endocarditis 0.3%
27. Atrial septal defect 0.1%.

Other diagnoses were: chronic liver disease due to tricuspid incompetence (<1%), pulmonary stenosis (<1%), cor pulmonale (<1%), complete heart block (<1%), transposition of the great vessels (<1%), repaired thoracic aortic aneurysm (<1%) and left ventricular aneurysm (<1%).

Examination *routine*

When asked to 'examine this patient's heart' candidates are often uncertain as to whether they should start with the pulse or go straight to look at the heart. On the one hand it would be absurd to feel all the pulses in the body and leave the object of the examiner's interest to the last minute, whilst on the other hand it would be impetuous to palpate the praecordium straight away. Repeating the examiner's question in the hope that he might clarify it, or asking for a clarification, does nothing but communicate your dilemma to the examiner. You should not waste any time. Bear in mind that our survey has confirmed that the diagnosis is usually mitral and/or aortic valve disease. Approach the right-hand side of the patient and adjust the backrest so that he reclines at 45° to the mattress. If the patient is wearing a shirt you should ask him to remove it so that the chest and neck are exposed. *Meanwhile*, you should complete a *quick*

1 *visual survey*. Observe whether the patient is
 (a) breathless,
 (b) *cyanosed*,
 (c) pale, or
 (d) whether he has a *malar flush* (mitral stenosis).
 Look briefly at the earlobes for creases* and then at the *neck* for *pulsations*:
 (e) forceful carotid pulsations (Corrigan's sign in aortic incompetence; vigorous pulsation in coarctation of the aorta), or
 (f) tall, sinuous venous pulsations (congestive cardiac failure, tricuspid incompetence, pulmonary hypertension, etc.).
 Run your eyes down onto the chest looking for
 (g) a *left thoracotomy scar* (mitral stenosis†) or a *midline sternal scar* (valve replacement‡), and then down to the feet looking for
 (h) ankle oedema. As you take the arm to feel the pulse complete your *visual survey* by looking at the hands (a quick look; don't be ponderous) for
 (i) clubbing of the fingers (cyanotic congenital heart disease, subacute bacterial endocarditis) and splinter haemorrhages (infective endocarditis).
If the examiner does not want you to feel the pulse he may intervene at this stage—otherwise you should proceed to

2 note the *rate* and *rhythm* of the **pulse**.

3 Quickly ascertain whether the pulse is **collapsing** (particularly if it is a large volume pulse) or not (make sure you are seen lifting the arm up—see experience 35, vol. 2, p. 330).
Next may be an opportune time to look for

---

* Frank's sign: a diagonal crease in the lobule of the auricle: grade 3 = a deep cleft across the whole earlobe; grade 2A = crease more than halfway across the lobe; grade 2B = crease across the whole lobe, but superficial; grade 1 = lesser degrees of wrinkling. Earlobe creases are associated statistically with coronary artery disease in most population groups.

† NB Experiences 4 and 7, vol. 2, pp. 326–327.
‡ Other scars may also be noted during your *visual survey*—those of previous cardiac catheterizations may be visible over the brachial arteries.

4 radiofemoral delay (coarctation of the aorta), though this can be left until after auscultation if you prefer and if you are sure you will not forget it (see experience 1, vol. 2, p. 325).

5 Feel the brachial pulse followed by the carotid pulses to see if the pulse is a **slow rising** one, especially if the volume (the upstroke) is small.

If the pulsations in the neck present any interesting features you may have already noted these during your initial *visual survey*. You should now proceed to confirm some of these impressions. The Corrigan's sign in the neck (forceful rise and quick fall of the carotid pulsation) may already have been reinforced by the discovery of a collapsing radial pulse. The individual waves of a large venous pulse can now be timed by palpating the opposite carotid. A large *v* wave, which sometimes oscillates the earlobe, suggests tricuspid incompetence and you should later on demonstrate peripheral oedema and the pulsatile liver using the bimanual technique. If the venous wave comes before the carotid pulsation it is an *a* wave suggestive of pulmonary hypertension (mitral valve disease, cor pulmonale) or pulmonary stenosis (rare). After

6 assessing the height of the **venous pressure** in centimetres vertically above the sternal angle you should move to the praecordium* and

7 localize the **apex beat** with respect to the mid-clavicular line and ribspaces, firstly by inspection for visible pulsation, and secondly by *palpation*. If the apex beat is vigorous you should stand the index finger on it, to localize the point of maximum impulse and *assess* the extent of its thrust. The impulse can be graded as just palpable, lifting (diastolic overload, i.e. mitral or aortic incompetence), thrusting (stronger than lifting), or heaving (outflow obstruction).

8 Palpation with your hand placed from the lower left sternal edge to the apex will detect a tapping impulse (left atrial 'knock' in mitral stenosis) or *thrills* over the mitral area (mitral valve disease), if present.

9 Continue palpation by feeling the **right ventricular lift** (left parasternal heave). To do this place the flat of your right palm parasternally over the right ventricular area and apply *sustained* and gentle pressure. If right ventricular hypertrophy is present you will feel the heel of your hand lifted by its force (pulmonary hypertension).

10 Next, you should **palpate** the pulmonary area for a *palpable second sound* (pulmonary hypertension), and the aortic area for a palpable *thrill* (aortic stenosis).†

If you feel a strong right ventricular lift quickly recall, and sometimes recheck, whether there is a giant *a* wave (pulmonary hypertension, pulmonary stenosis) or *v* wave (tricuspid incompetence, congestive cardiac failure) in the neck. A palpable thrill over the mitral area (mitral valve disease), or palpable pulmonary second sound over the pulmonary area (pulmonary hypertension) should make you think of, and check for, the other complementary signs. You should by now have a fair idea of what you will hear on auscultation of the heart but you should keep an open mind for any unexpected discovery.

11 The next step will be **auscultation** and you should only stray away from the heart (examiner's command) if you have a strong expectation of being able to demonstrate an interesting and relevant sign (such as a pulsatile liver to underpin the diagnosis of tricuspid incompetence). *Time* the first heart sound with either the apex beat, if this is

---

* The *visual survey* and the examination steps 2–6 should be completed *quickly* and efficiently, particularly if you have been asked to examine the *heart*.

† The thrill of aortic stenosis is best felt if the patient leans forwards with his breath held after expiration.

palpable, or by feeling the carotid pulse (see experience 78, vol. 2, p. 334). It is important to listen to the expected murmurs in the most favourable positions. For example, mitral diastolic murmurs are best heard by turning the patient *onto the left side*, and the early diastolic murmur of aortic incompetence is made more prominent by asking the patient to *lean forwards* with his breath held after expiration.* For low-pitched sounds (mid-diastolic murmur of mitral stenosis, heart sounds) use the bell of your chest-piece but do not press hard, or else you will be listening through a diaphragm formed by the stretched skin! The high-pitched early diastolic murmur of aortic incompetence is very easily missed (see anecdote 29, vol. 2, p. 364). Make sure you specifically listen for it.

If the venous pressure is raised you should check for

12 **sacral oedema** and, if covered, expose the feet to demonstrate any *ankle oedema*.

Auscultation over

13 the **lung bases** for inspiratory crepitations (left ventricular failure), though an essential part of the routine assessment of the cardiovascular system, is seldom required in the examination. You may make a special effort to do this in certain relevant situations such as a breathless patient, aortic stenosis with a displaced point of maximum impulse or if there are any signs of left heart failure (orthopnoea, pulsus alternans, gallop rhythm, etc.). Similarly, after examination of the heart itself it may (on rare occasions only) be necessary to

14 palpate the **liver**, especially if you have seen a large *v* wave and heard a pansystolic murmur over the tricuspid area. In such cases you may be able to demonstrate a *pulsatile* liver by placing your left palm posteriorly and the right palm anteriorly over the enlarged liver.† Finally, you should offer to

15 measure the **blood pressure**. This is particularly relevant in patients with aortic stenosis (low systolic and narrow pulse pressure), and aortic incompetence (wide pulse pressure).

For *checklist* see p. 527.

3 | 'Examine this patient's chest'

Station 1

Variations of instruction in initial PACES survey (resultant diagnoses in brackets)

Examine this patient's chest (bronchiectasis; pleural effusion with chest drain; pleural effusion; bilateral lower lobectomy and fibrosis)

This gentleman is breathless on climbing stairs. Examine his respiratory system (chronic obstructive pulmonary disease)

---

* With the diaphragm of your chest-piece *ready* in position: 'Take a deep breath in; now out; hold it'. Listen intently for the absence of silence in early diastole. Ask the patient to repeat the exercise if necessary.

† An alternative and useful way of demonstrating a pulsatile liver is to place the knuckles of your closed right fist against the inferior border of the liver in the right hypochondrium (warn the patient beforehand!). Your fist will oscillate with each pulsation of the liver.

Examine this patient's respiratory system (lung transplant and bronchiolitis obliterans; lung cancer)

This gentleman presented with a cough and shortness of breath. Please examine his respiratory system (pleural effusion)

This is a 56-year-old lady who has been dyspnoeic for a long time. Examine her respiratory system (Marfan's and pulmonary fibrosis)

This patient is complaining of shortness of breath. Please examine the chest (pleural effusion)

Examine this man's chest from the back (reduced expansion with reduced breath sounds and increased vocal resonance)

This patient presented with worsening shortness of breath. Please examine his chest (pulmonary fibrosis)

This lady is short of breath, please examine her respiratory system (pulmonary fibrosis)

This man has a long history of breathlessness. Please examine his respiratory system (pulmonary fibrosis)

Examine this lady's respiratory system from the front. About half a minute later I was asked to examine her chest from the back (carcinoma of the lung)

This gentleman has been getting more breathless in recent months. Please examine his chest (thoracotomy)

This lady is breathless. Please examine her chest (emphysema)

This man has noisy breathing. Please examine his chest to find out why (upper airways obstruction)

This man has developed a productive cough. Please examine his chest and suggest a cause (aspergillosis and old tuberculosis)

Examine this patient's respiratory system and comment on positive findings as you go (pulmonary fibrosis)

This young man is breathless. Please examine his chest (chronic obstructive pulmonary disease and α_1-antitrypsin deficiency)

This man has a cough. Please examine his chest (bronchiectasis)

This man has been becoming increasingly breathless over the past 2 years. He is a non-smoker. Please examine his respiratory system to determine a cause (no diagnosis reached)

This man complains of shortness of breath. Examine him and find out why (no diagnosis reached).

Diagnoses from survey in order of frequency
1. Interstitial lung disease (fibrosing alveolitis) 21%
2. Pneumonectomy/lobectomy 16%
3. Bronchiectasis 12%
4. Dullness at the lung bases 10%
5. Chronic bronchitis and emphysema 8%
6. Rheumatoid lung 8%
7. Old tuberculosis 6%
8. Stridor 4%
9. Superior vena cava obstruction 3%
10. Kartagener's 2%
11. Marfan's 2%

12 Lung transplant 2%

13 Cor pulmonale 2%

14 Chest infection/consolidation/pneumonia 1%

15 Obesity/pickwickian syndrome 1%

16 Tuberculosis/apical consolidation 1%

17 Carcinoma of the bronchus <1%

18 Pneumothorax <1%

19 Cystic fibrosis <1%

Examination *routine*

While approaching the patient, asking for his permission to examine him and settling him reclining at 45° to the bed with his chest bare, you should observe from the end of the bed

1 his **general appearance**. Note any evidence of *weight loss*. The features of conditions such as superior vena cava obstruction (p. 90), systemic sclerosis (p. 393) and lupus pernio (p. 316) may be readily apparent as should be severe kyphoscoliosis. However, *ankylosing spondylitis* is easily missed with the patient lying down (see experiences 3 and 30, vol. 2, p. 326 and p. 329). Observe specifically whether the patient

2 is **breathless** at rest or from the effort of removing his clothes,

3 **purses** his lips (chronic small airways obstruction), or

4 has central **cyanosis*** (cor pulmonale, fibrosing alveolitis, bronchiectasis). Central cyanosis may be difficult to recognize; it is always preferable to look at the oral mucous membranes (see below). Observe:

5 if the **accessory muscles** are being used during breathing (chronic small airways obstruction, pleural effusion, pneumothorax, etc.),

6 if there is generalized **indrawing** of the intercostal muscles or supraclavicular fossae (hyperinflation), or if there is indrawing of the lower ribs on inspiration (due to low, flat diaphragms in emphysema). Localized indrawing of the intercostal muscles suggests bronchial obstruction.

Listen to the breathing with unaided ears whilst you observe the chest wall and hands (but do not dither). This will allow a dual input whereby a collaboration of what you hear and what you see may help you form a diagnostic impression. You should listen to whether *expiration* is more *prolonged* than inspiration (normally the reverse), and difficult (chronic airways obstruction), whether it is *noisy* (breathlessness) and if there are any additional noises such as *wheezes* or *clicks*. Difficult and noisy inspiration is usually caused by obstruction in the major bronchi (mediastinal masses, retrosternal thyroid, bronchial carcinoma, etc.) while the more prolonged, noisy and often wheezy expiration is caused by chronic small airways obstruction (asthma, chronic bronchitis). Note the character of any cough, whether it is productive (?bronchiectasis) or dry. While you are listening observe

7 the *movement* of the **chest wall**. It may be mainly *upwards* (emphysema), or *asymmetrical* (fibrosis, collapse, pneumonectomy, pleural effusion, pneumothorax). In the

---

* Occurs with mean capillary concentration of $\geq 4\,g\,dl^{-1}$ of deoxygenated haemoglobin (or $0.5\,g\,dl^{-1}$ methaemoglobin). Alternatively, the presence of cyanosis may be supported by demonstrating a low arterial oxygen saturation (<85%) non-invasively with an ear oximeter applied to the antihelix of the ear.

Central cyanosis is more readily detected in patients with poly-cythaemia than in those with anaemia—because of the low haemoglobin, patients with anaemia require a much lower oxygen saturation to have $4\,g\,dl^{-1}$ of unsaturated haemoglobin in capillary blood.

context of the examination it is particularly important to look for localized *apical flattening* suggestive of underlying fibrosis due to old tuberculosis (p. 83) or pneumonectomy (p. 73). You may also note a thoracotomy or thoracoplasty *scar* (pp. 83 and 73) or the presence of *radiotherapy field markings* (Indian ink marks) or radiation *burns* on the chest (intrathoracic malignancy, p. 341).

Before touching the patient, ensure that you have looked for any peripheral clues, such as sputum pots for haemoptysis or purulent sputum, nebulizer therapy, inhaler therapy, oxygen (what rate per minute?), temperature chart, peak flow chart or transplant pagers.

Check the hands for

8 clubbing (p. 312), *tobacco staining*, coal dust tattoos, or other conditions which affect the hands and may be associated with lung disease such as rheumatoid arthritis (nodules, p. 384) or systemic sclerosis (p. 393).

9 Feel the **pulse** and if it is bounding, or if the patient is cyanosed, check for a *flapping tremor* of the hands (CO_2 retention) or a fine tremor due to β-agonist therapy (salbutamol or terbutaline). If there is doubt about the presence of cyanosis you could at this point check the tongue and the buccal mucous membranes over the premolar teeth before moving to the neck to look for

10 raised venous pressure (cor pulmonale) or fixed distension of the neck veins (superior vena cava obstruction). Next examine

11 the **trachea**. Place the index and ring fingers on the manubrium sternae over the prominent points on either side. Use the middle finger as the exploring finger to gently feel the tracheal rings to detect either *deviation* or a *tracheal tug* (i.e. the middle finger being pushed upwards against the trachea by the upward movement of the chest wall). Check the *notch–cricoid* distance.*

12 Feel for **lymphadenopathy** (carcinoma, tuberculosis, lymphoma, sarcoidosis) in the cervical region and axillae. As the right hand returns from the left axilla look for

13 the **apex beat** (difficult to localize if the chest is hyperinflated) which in conjunction with tracheal deviation may give you evidence of mediastinal displacement (collapse, fibrosis, pneumonectomy, effusion, scoliosis).

14 To look for **asymmetry** rest one hand lightly on either side of the front of the chest to see if there is any diminution of movement (effusion, fibrosis, pneumonectomy, collapse, pneumothorax). Next grip the chest symmetrically with the fingertips in the rib-spaces on either side and approximate the thumbs to meet in the middle in a straight horizontal line in order

15 to assess **expansion** first in the inframammary and then in the supramammary regions. Note the distance between each thumb and the midline (may give further information about asymmetry of movement) and between both thumbs and try to express the expansion in centimetres (it is better to produce a tape measure for a more accurate assessment of the expansion in centimetres). Comparing both sides at each level

16 percuss the chest from above downwards starting with the supraclavicular fossae and over the clavicles† and do not forget to percuss over the axillae. Few clinicians now regularly map out the area of cardiac dullness. In healthy people there is dullness be-

---

* The length of trachea from the suprasternal notch to the cricoid cartilage is normally three or more finger breadths. Shortening of this distance is a sign of hyperinflation.

† Percussion on the bare clavicle may cause discomfort to the patient.

hind the lower left quarter of the sternum which is lost together with normal liver dullness in hyperinflation. Complete palpation by checking for

17 tactile vocal fremitus with the ulnar aspect of the hand applied to the chest.

18 Auscultation of the **breath sounds** should start *high* at the apices and you should remember to listen in the *axillae*. You are advised to cover both lung fields first with the bell* before using the diaphragm (if for no other reason than that this allows you a chance to check the findings without appearing to backtrack!). In the nervousness of the examination harsh breathing heard with the diaphragm near a major bronchus (over the second intercostal space anteriorly or below the scapula near the midline posteriorly) may give an impression of bronchial breathing, particularly in thin people. Compare corresponding points on opposite sides of the chest. Ensure that the patient breathes with the mouth open, regularly and deeply, but not noisily (see experience 53, vol. 2, pp. 331–332). Auscultation is completed by checking

19 vocal resonance in all areas; **if** you have found an area of bronchial breathing (the sounds may resound close to your ears — aegophony) check also for whispering pectoriloquy. The classic timings of crackles/crepitations of various origins are:

(a) *early inspiratory*: chronic bronchitis, asthma,

(b) *early and mid-inspiratory and recurring in expiration*: bronchiectasis (altered by coughing),

(c) *mid/late inspiratory*: restrictive lung disease (e.g. fibrosing alveolitis†) and pulmonary oedema.

20 To examine the back of the chest sit the patient forward (it may help to cross the arms in front of the patient to pull the scapulae further apart) and repeat steps 14–19. You may wish to start the examination of the back by palpating for cervical nodes from behind (particularly the scalene nodes between the two heads of the sternomastoid).

Though with sufficient practice this whole procedure can be performed rapidly without loss of efficiency, often in the examination you will only be asked to perform some of it — usually 'examine the back of the chest'. As always when forced to perform only part of the complete *routine*, be sure that the partial examination is no less thorough and professional. Be prepared to put on your 'wide-angled lenses' so as not to miss other related signs (see experience 1, p. 325 and anecdotes 7 and 8, vol. 2, p. 363).

Though by now you will usually have sufficient information to present your findings, occasionally you will wish to check other features on the basis of the findings so far. Commonly, you will wish to inspect the ankles for oedema and, if relevant and available, the peak flow chart and temperature chart. Further purposeful examination gives an impression of confidence but it should not be overdone. For example, looking for evidence of Horner's syndrome, or wasting of the muscles of one hand‡ in a patient with apical dullness and a deviated trachea, will suggest professional keenness; whereas routinely looking at the eyes and hands after completion of the examination may only suggest to the examiner that you do not have the diagnosis and are hoping for inspira-

---

* Many physicians prefer to use the diaphragm in their routine examination of the chest, though purists believe that as the respiratory auscultatary sounds are usually of low pitch, the bell is preferable.

† In fibrosing alveolitis late inspiratory crackles may become reduced if the patient is made to lean forward; thereby the compressed dependent alveoli (which crackle-open in late inspiration) are relieved of the pressure of the lungs.

‡ A good *visual survey* may reveal such signs at the beginning.

tion! If you suspect airways obstruction the examiner may be impressed if you perform a bedside respiratory function test—the *forced expiratory time* (FET).*

For *checklist* see p. 527.

4 | 'Examine this patient's abdomen'

Station 1
Variations of instruction in initial PACES survey (resultant diagnoses in brackets)

Examine this patient's abdomen (transplanted kidney; hepatomegaly and lymph nodes; ascites and chronic liver disease; ascites and hepatosplenomegaly)

This gentleman was found collapsed. Examine his abdomen and give a differential as to the cause of his collapse (alcoholic liver disease)

This gentleman has lost weight and is experiencing fullness in his abdomen. Please examine the abdomen (hepatosplenomegaly and axillary lymph nodes)

This lady has thrombocytopenia. Examine her abdomen and come up with a likely diagnosis (splenomegaly)

This patient is complaining of tiredness, examine his abdomen (hepatosplenomegaly and rheumatoid hands)

Examine this gentleman's abdomen (alcoholic liver disease, tender hepatomegaly and encephalopathy)

This man has pain on walking. Please examine his abdomen (hepatosplenomegaly and polycythaemia rubra vera)

This patient's abdomen has shown intermittent swelling—what could one cause be? (alcoholic liver disease)

Examine this abdomen (jaundice, parotid swelling and liver; hepatosplenomegaly and ascites; hepatosplenomegaly and Dupuytren's)

This patient has been referred from the cardiology clinic with sweats and a mass in the abdomen. Please examine (infective endocarditis)

Please examine this gentleman's abdominal system and comment on the findings (alcoholic liver disease)

I was given some haematology results which were suggestive that the patient might have a spleen palpable. Examine the abdomen (splenomegaly)

This patient attends the renal clinic with hypertension. Please examine his abdominal system (transplanted kidney)

* Ask the patient to take a deep breath in and then, on your command (timed with the second hand of your watch), to breathe out as hard and as fast as he can until his lungs are completely empty. A normal person will empty his lungs in less than 6 seconds (1 second for every decade of age, e.g. a normal 30-year-old will do it in 3 seconds). An FET of >6 seconds is evidence of airways obstruction. You need to practise this test with patients if it is to be slick. As with peak flow rate (PFR) and forced expiratory volume in 1 second (FEV$_1$), etc., it is important to make sure that certain patients, particularly females, *are* blowing as hard and as fast as they can ('don't worry about what you look like—give it everything you've got—like this' and give a demonstration) and empty their lungs completely ('keep going, keep going . . . keep going, well done!')

This 62-year-old man has a lymphocytosis. Please examine his abdomen (splenomegaly)

This lady has been having abdominal pain. Please examine and suggest a cause (polycystic kidneys and polycystic liver)

Examine this man's abdomen commenting on what you are doing (hepatosplenomegaly)

Please examine the abdomen of this man who is complaining of pruritus (polycystic kidneys)

This man has high blood pressure. Please examine his abdomen (heart transplant and dialysis fistula)

This 43-year-old man failed a routine medical examination for insurance purposes. Please examine the abdomen and suggest if you can find a reason why (hepatomegaly)

Examine this man's abdomen and tell me what you find (chronic liver disease).

Diagnoses from survey in order of frequency

1 Chronic liver disease 21%
2 Hepatosplenomegaly 17%
3 Polycystic kidneys 14%
4 Splenomegaly (without hepatomegaly) 13%
5 Transplanted kidney 9%
6 Hepatomegaly (no splenomegaly) 5%
7 Ascites 4%
8 Polycythaemia rubra vera 4%
9 Abdominal mass 2%
10 Carcinoid 2%
11 Crohn's disease 1%
12 Idiopathic haemochromatosis 1%
13 Nephrotic syndrome <1%
14 Hereditary spherocytosis <1%
15 Felty's syndrome <1%
16 Generalized lymphadenopathy <1%
17 Single palpable kidney <1%
18 Primary biliary cirrhosis <1%.

Other diagnoses were: aortic aneurysm (1%), haemochromatosis (<1%), polycystic kidneys and a transplanted kidney (<1%), splenomegaly and generalized lymphadenopathy (<1%), abdominal lymphadenopathy (<1%), postsplenectomy (<1%) and normal abdomen (<1%).

Examination *routine*

Analysis of the above list reveals that in over 80% of cases the findings in the abdomen relate to a palpable spleen, liver or kidneys. Bearing this in mind you should approach the right-hand side of the patient and position him so that he is lying supine on one pillow (if comfortable), with the whole abdomen and chest in full view. Ideally the genitalia should also be exposed but to avoid embarrassment to patients, who are volunteers and whose genitals are usually normal, we suggest that you ask the patient to lower his garments and ensure that these are pulled down to a level about halfway between the iliac crest and the symphysis pubis. While these preparations are being made you should be performing

1 a *visual survey* of the patient. Amongst the many relevant physical signs that you may observe in these few seconds are pallor, pigmentation, jaundice, spider naevi, xanthelasma, parotid swelling, gynaecomastia, scratch marks, tattoos, abdominal distension, distended abdominal veins, an abdominal swelling, herniae and decreased body hair. If you use the following *routine* most of these will also be noted during your subsequent examination but at this stage you should particularly note any

2 **pigmentation**. As the patient is being correctly positioned,

3 *quickly* **examine the hands*** for:

    (a) Dupuytren's contracture,

    (b) clubbing,

    (c) leuconychia,

    (d) palmar erythema, and

    (e) a flapping tremor (if relevant).

After asking you to examine the abdomen many examiners would like, and *expect*, you to concentrate on the abdomen itself without delay, and yet they will not forgive you for missing an abnormal physical sign elsewhere. This emphasizes the importance of a good *visual survey*; a trained eye will miss nothing important on the face or in the hands while the patient is being properly positioned with the hands by his side. Thus, steps 1–3 need not occupy you for more than a few seconds; you may wish to omit steps 5 and 6 if there is no visible abnormality, and steps 7–11 can be completed as part of the *visual survey*.

4 Pull down the lower eyelid to look for *anaemia*. At the same time check the sclerae for *icterus* and look for *xanthelasma*. The guttering between the eyeball and the lower lid is the best place to look for pallor or for any discoloration (e.g. cyanosis, jaundice, etc.).

5 Look at the lips for cyanosis (cirrhosis of the liver) and shine your pen torch into the mouth† looking for swollen lips (Crohn's), telangiectasis (Osler–Weber–Rendu), patches of pigmentation (Peutz–Jeghers) and mouth ulcers (Crohn's).

6 **Palpate the neck** and supraclavicular fossae for *cervical lymph nodes*.‡ If you do find lymph nodes you should then proceed to examine the axillae and groins for evidence of generalized lymphadenopathy (lymphoma, chronic lymphatic leukaemia). As you move from the neck to the chest, check for:

7 **gynaecomastia** (palpate for glandular breast tissue in obese subjects),

8 **spider naevi** (may have been noted already on hands, arms and face and may also be present on the back), and

9 **scratch marks** (may have been noted on the arms, and may also be found on the back and elsewhere). Next,

10 look at the chest (in the male) and in the axillae for **paucity of hair** (if diminished note facial hair in the male; pubic hair if not visible, may be noted later).

---

* For a full list of the signs that may be visible in the hands in chronic liver disease, see p. 106.

† Though a brief examination of the mouth is usefully included as part of the full 'examine the abdomen' *routine*, it is worth noting that in our survey when there were the findings mentioned, the candidates were given a more specific instruction such as 'Look at this patient's mouth'.

‡ The supraclavicular lymph nodes, particularly on the left side, may be enlarged with carcinoma of the stomach (*Troisier's sign*; NB *Virchow's node* behind the left sternoclavicular joint) or carcinoma of any other abdominal organ or with carcinoma of the bronchus.

11 Observe the abdomen in *three segments* (epigastric, umbilical and suprapubic) for any visible signs such as *pulsations*, generalized *distension* (ascites) or a *swelling* in one particular area. Note any scars or fistulae (previous surgery; Crohn's). Look for distended *abdominal* veins (the flow is away from the umbilicus in portal hypertension but upwards from the groin in inferior vena cava obstruction).

With practise the examination to this point can be completed very rapidly and will provide valuable information which may be overlooked if proceeding carelessly straight to palpation of the abdomen (see experience 2, vol. 2, p. 326). If the examiner insists that you start with abdominal palpation* it suggests that there is little to be found elsewhere, but you should nevertheless be prepared to use your 'wide-angled lenses' in order not to miss any of the above features.

12 Palpation of the abdomen should be performed in an orthodox manner; any temptation to go straight for a visible swelling should be resisted. Put your palm gently over the abdomen and ask the patient if he has any tenderness and to let you know if you hurt him. First systematically examine the whole of the abdomen with *light palpation*. Palpation should be done with the *pulps* of the fingers rather than the tips, the best movement being a gentle flexion at the metacarpophalangeal joints with the hand flat on the abdominal wall. Next, examine specifically for the *internal organs*. For both liver and spleen start in the right iliac fossa (you cannot be frowned upon for following this orthodox procedure†), working upwards to the right hypochondrium in the case of the *liver* and diagonally across the abdomen to the left hypochondrium in the case of the *spleen*. The organs are felt against the radial border of the index finger and the pulps of the index and middle fingers as they descend on inspiration, at which time you can gently press and move your hand upwards to meet them. The *kidneys* are then sought by bimanual palpation of each lateral region. The lower pole of the normal right kidney can sometimes be felt, especially in thin women. Palpation of the internal organs may be difficult if there is ascites. In this case the technique is to press quickly, flexing at the wrist joint, to displace the fluid and palpate the enlarged organ ('dipping' or 'ballotting'). In a patient well chosen for the examination, a mass in the left hypochondrium may present a problem of identification (see experiences 22 and 39, and anecdotes 24 and 28, vol. 2, p. 329); the examiner (testing your confidence) may ask you if you are sure that it is a spleen and not a kidney or vice versa. Do not forget to establish whether you can *get above* the mass and *separate* it from the costal edge, whether you can *bimanually* palpate it and whether the percussion note over it is *resonant* (all features of an enlarged kidney, see also p. 111). Palpate *deeply* with the pulps to look for the *ascending* and *descending colons* in the flanks, and use *gentle* palpation to feel for an *aortic aneurysm* in the midline. Complete palpation by feeling for *inguinal lymph nodes*, noting obvious herniae and, at the same time, adding information about the distribution and thickness of pubic hair to that already gained about the rest of the body hair.

13 Percussion must be used from the nipple downwards on both sides to locate the upper edge of the liver on the right and the spleen on the left (NB the left lower lateral

---

* Some examiners admit to being irritated at seeing candidates examine normal hands for a long time after being asked to examine the abdomen. They argue that the information obtainable from the face, mouth and hands can be gathered without delay during the inspection part of the examination (see anecdote 18, vol. 2, p. 363).

† Even though it is the time-honoured, orthodox procedure, many clinicians, these days, are opposed to this practice. They argue that a grossly enlarged spleen will be picked up on the initial light palpation which makes the approach from the right iliac fossa unnecessary. If they do not feel a mass in the left hypochondrium on initial palpation, they start deep palpation a few centimetres below the left costal edge.

chest wall may become dull to percussion before an enlarged spleen is palpable). The lower palpable edges of the spleen and liver should be defined by percussion in an orthodox manner, proceeding from the resonant to dull areas. If you suspect free fluid in the peritoneum you must establish its presence by demonstrating

14 **shifting dullness**. Initially check for *stony dullness* in the flanks. There is no need to continue with the procedure of demonstrating shifting dullness if this is not present. By asking the patient with ascites to turn on his side you can shift the dullness from the upper to the lower flank. Before you conclude the palpation and percussion of the abdomen, ask yourself whether you have found anything abnormal. If there are no abnormal physical signs make sure that you have not missed a polycystic kidney or a palpable splenic edge (or occasionally a mass in the epigastrium or iliac fossae); during your auscultation listen carefully for a bruit over the aorta and renal vessels. Generally speaking

15 **auscultation** has very little to contribute in the examination setting, but as part of the full *routine* you should listen to the bowel sounds, check for renal artery bruits and for any other sounds such as a rub over the spleen or kidney or a venous hum (both excessively rare).

Examination of the

16 **external genitalia** is not usually required in the examination for the reasons given above, and we have never heard of a case where

17 **a rectal examination** was required. You should, however, comment that you would like to complete your examination of the abdomen by examining the external genitalia (especially in the male with chronic liver disease—small testes; or cervical lymphadenopathy—drainage of testes to para-aortic and cervical lymph nodes) and rectum. You may of course never get this far since the examiner may interrupt you at an appropriate stage to ask for your findings. If you are allowed to conclude the examination and you have found nothing abnormal despite your careful search, on rare occasions the diagnosis of a normal abdomen will be accepted (see p. 135).

For *checklist* see p. 527.

5 | 'Examine this patient's visual fields'

Stations 3 and 5
Variations of instruction from original, pre PACES, survey
Examine this patient's visual fields and fundi*

Diagnoses from original, pre PACES, survey in order of frequency
1 Homonymous hemianopia 25%
2 Optic atrophy 21%
3 Bitemporal hemianopia 21%
4 Unilateral hemianopia 7%

* See also Introduction, page xv.

5 Partial field defect in one eye due to retinal artery branch occlusion 7%
6 Bilateral homonymous quadrantic field defect 4%
7 Acromegaly 4%

Examination *routine*

Ask the patient to sit upright on the side of the bed while you position yourself in visual confrontation about a metre away. This apposition will help you to test the visual fields of his left and right eyes against those of your right and left respectively. As he is doing this perform

1 a **visual survey** (acromegaly, hemiparesis, cerebellar signs in multiple sclerosis) of the patient. Test both temporal fields together so that you do not miss any *visual inattention*. Ask the patient to look at your eyes while you place your index fingers just inside the outer limits of your temporal fields. Then move your fingers in turn and then both at the same time, and ask him:

'Point to the finger which moves'.

If there is visual inattention, the patient will only point to one finger when you move both at the same time. Next test each eye individually and ask him to cover his right eye with his right hand, and close your left eye:

'Keep looking at my eye'.

2 Examine his **peripheral visual fields**. Test his left temporal vision against your right temporal by moving your wagging finger from the periphery towards the centre:

'Tell me when you see my finger move'.*

The temporal field should be tested in the horizontal plane and by moving your finger through the upper and lower temporal quadrants. Change hands and repeat on the nasal side. By comparing his visual field with your own, any areas of field defect are thus mapped out. The visual fields of his right eye are similarly tested.

3 **A central scotoma** is tested for with a red-headed hat pin. If you have already found a field defect which does not require further examination, or if the examiner does not wish you to continue, he will soon stop you. Otherwise comparing your right eye with his left, as before, move the red-headed pin from the temporal periphery through the central field to the nasal periphery, asking the patient:

'Can you see the head of the pin? What colour is it? Tell me if it disappears or changes colour'.

Patients with optic neuropathy may report altered colour vision even if there is no absolute central loss of vision. If there is no scotoma find his blind spot and compare it with your own. The blind spot may be enlarged in chronic papilloedema or consecutive optic atrophy.

Having found the field defect, look for

4 **additional features** (e.g. acromegaly, hemiparesis, nystagmus and cerebellar signs) if appropriate. Recall the possible causes for each type of field defect as this question, at the end of the case, is almost inevitable (see p. 194).

For *checklist* see p. 528.

* This will pick up most gross visual field defects rapidly. Moving objects are more easily detected and therefore your moving finger will be immediately noticed by the patient as it moves out of the blind area into his field of vision. Remember that his area of blindness to a stationary object may be greater than that to a moving object. In the dysphasic patient you should ask him to point at the moving finger when he sees it rather than telling you he sees it.

6 | 'Examine this patient's cranial nerves'

Station 3
Variations of instruction in initial PACES survey (resultant diagnoses in brackets)
Examine this patient's cranial nerves (right homonymous hemianopia)
Examine this patient's cranial nerves and check the reflexes in the lower limbs as this
   patient has had a noticeable weakness of both legs (multiple sclerosis).

Diagnoses from our MRCP, surveys
Right homonymous hemianopia with macula sparing
Bulbar palsy
Internuclear ophthalmoplegia — multiple sclerosis
Cerebellopontine angle syndrome
Myasthenia gravis
Ocular palsy and dysarthria
Unilateral VIth, VIIth nerve palsies and nystagmus and possibly a XIIth nerve palsy*
Unilateral IXth, Xth, XIth and XIIth nerve lesions (suggesting jugular foramen
   syndrome†).

Examination *routine*

Perhaps surprisingly this instruction was comparatively rare in our surveys before
PACES, but seems to have experienced a slight increase in popularity in the PACES era,
appearing in 4% of the PACES survey reports we have received (pp. 289 and 294). It is
one of the most feared instructions but at the same time it can provide an opportunity
to score highly. More than in any other system, the well-rehearsed candidate can appear
competent and professional compared with the unrehearsed. Detailed examination of
the individual nerves is not usually required but rather a quick and efficient screen like
that used by neurologists at the bedside or in out-patients (it is well worth attending
neurology out-patients to watch quick and efficient examination techniques, if for
nothing else). Not only can you look good but also the abnormalities are usually easy to
detect. Although it is to be hoped that your practised *routine* will not miss out any
nerves, it is preferable to perform a smooth, professional examination, which accidentally misses out a nerve, than to test your examiner's patience through a hesitant and
meditative examination which takes a long time to start and may never finish! Since the
examination is most easily carried out face to face with the patient it is best, if possible,
to get him to sit on the edge of the bed facing you. First
   1 take a good general and *quick* **look** at the patient; in particular his face, for any
obvious abnormality. Next ask him about
   2 his sense of **smell** and **taste**:
   'Do you have any difficulty with your sense of smell?' (I). Although you should have
the ability to examine taste (VII, IX) and smell formally if equipment is provided, usually questioning (or possibly the judicious use of a bedside orange) is all that is required.

---

* The candidate diagnosed a XIIth nerve palsy and passed (experience 1 vol. 2, p. 325) but see footnote, p. 28.

† This diagnosis was not made by the candidate.

All the examination referable to the eyes is best performed next. Unless there is a Snellen's chart available ask the patient to look at the clock on the wall or some newspaper print to give you a good idea of his

3 **visual acuity:**

'Do you have any difficulty with your vision?'

'Can you see the clock on the wall?' (if he has glasses for long sight he should put them on).

'Can you tell me what time it says?' (II).

A portable Snellen's chart will enable you to perform a more formal test (see Appendix 3). Now test the

4 **visual fields** (see p. 25), including for *central scotoma*, with a red-headed hat pin. Follow this by examining

5 **eye movements** (move your finger in the shape of a cross, from side to side then up and down):

'Look at my finger; follow it with your eyes' (III, IV, VI),

asking the patient at the extremes of gaze whether he sees one or two fingers. If he has diplopia establish the extent and ask him to describe the 'false' image. As you test eye movements note at the same time any

6 **nystagmus** (VIII, cerebellum or cerebellar connections — see Fig. C3.15, p. 231) or

7 **ptosis** (III, sympathetic).

Remember that either extreme abduction of the eyes or gazing at a finger that is too near can cause nystagmus in normal eyes (optikokinetic). Now examine

8 the **pupils** for the direct and consensual *light reflex* (II → optic tract → lateral geniculate ganglion → Edinger–Westphal nucleus of III → fibres to ciliary muscle) and for the *accommodation–convergence* reflex (cortex → III) with your finger just in front of his nose:

'Look into the distance'.

'Now look at my finger' (see also footnote, p. 46).

Finally examine the optic discs (II) by

9 **fundoscopy** (this can be left until last if you prefer). Having finished examining the eyes examine

10 **facial movements:**

'Raise your eyebrows'
'Screw your eyes up tight'
'Puff your cheeks out'   } VII
'Whistle'
'Show me your teeth'

'Clench your teeth' — feel masseters and temporalis   } motor V
'Open your mouth; stop me closing it'

11 then **palatal movement:**

'Keep your mouth open; say aah' (IX, X)

12 and **gag reflex*** — touch the back of the pharynx on both sides with an orange stick (IX, X). Look at

---

* This can be unpleasant, so ask the examiner's permission, explain
to the patient and ask for his permission as well.

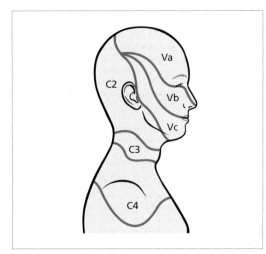

Figure B.1 Dermatomes in the head and neck.

13 the **tongue** as it lies in the floor of the mouth for *wasting* or *fasciculation* (XII):
  'Open your mouth again'
then get the patient to:
  'Put your tongue out' — note any deviation* — 'waggle it from side to side' (XII).
14 Test the **accessory nerve**:†
  'Shrug your shoulders; keep them shrugged' — push down on the shoulders (XI).
  'Turn your head to the left side, now to the right' — feel for the sternomastoid muscle
    on the side opposite to the turned head (XI).
Finally test
15 hearing:
  'Any problem with the hearing in either ear?'
  'Can you hear that?' — rub finger and thumb together in front of each ear in turn
    (VIII — proceed to the Rinné and Weber tests‡ if there is any abnormality, and
    look in the ear if you suspect disease of the external ear, perforated drum, wax,
    etc.), and
16 test **facial sensation** including *corneal reflex* (sensory V — Fig. B.1).

For *checklist* see p. 528.

---

* In unilateral facial paralysis the protruded tongue, though otherwise normal, may deviate so that unilateral hypoglossal paralysis is suspected (see p. 211). In unilateral lower motor neurone XIIth nerve palsy there is wasting (? fasciculation) on the side of the lesion and the tongue curves to that side.
† Painless neck weakness has only four causes: myasthenia gravis (p. 242), myotonic dystrophy (p. 182), polymyositis (p. 254) and motor neurone disease (p. 190).

‡ *Weber test*: sound from a vibrating tuning fork held on the centre of the forehead is conducted towards the ear if it has a conductive defect (e.g. wax or otitis media) and away from the ear if it has a nerve deafness. *Rinné test*: a positive test (normal) is when the sound of the tuning fork is louder by air conduction (prongs by external auditory meatus) than by bone conduction (base of fork on mastoid process). Negative is abnormal.

7 | 'Examine this patient's arms'

Stations 3 and 5

Variations of instruction in initial PACES survey (resultant diagnoses in brackets)

This elderly lady has had some falls and difficulty with mobility. Please examine her upper limbs (drug-induced dystonia)

This patient has a worsening tremor of his upper limbs. Please give some reasons (intention tremor and patchy peripheral sensory neuropathy)

This patient has a 20-year history of weakness in the right arm and shoulder (C5 radiculopathy)

Examine this patient's upper limbs. There has been a weakness for about the last 5 years (motor neurone disease)

This lady has difficulty doing the housework, especially taking things out of cupboards. Look at her face and examine her hands (myotonic dystrophy)

This man had an operation which is unrelated to the case, then woke with a weak left arm. Why? (radial nerve palsy)

This 50-year-old lady has problems driving. Examine her arms to find out why (arthritis secondary to ulcerative colitis).

Diagnoses from original, pre PACES, survey in order of frequency

1 Wasting of the small muscles of the hand 26%
2 Motor neurone disease 19%
3 Hemiplegia 7%
4 Cerebellar syndrome 6%
5 Cervical myelopathy 6%
6 Neurofibromatosis 4%
7 Muscular dystrophy 4%
8 Psoriasis 4%
9 Purpura due to steroids 4%
10 Parkinson's disease 3%
11 Syringomyelia 3%
12 Hemiballismus 3%
13 Lichen planus 3%
14 Pseudoxanthoma elasticum 3%
15 Old polio 3%
16 Rheumatoid arthritis 3%
17 Axillary vein thrombosis 3%
18 Contracture of the elbow in a case of haemophilia 3%
19 Ulnar nerve palsy 1%
20 Pancoast's syndrome 1%
21 Herpes zoster 1%
22 Mycosis fungoides 1%
23 Polymyositis 1%.

Examination *routine*

Consideration of the above list from the survey reveals that the vast majority (over 80%) of conditions behind this instruction are neurological with a handful of spot diagnoses which will usually be obvious. If the diagnosis is not an obvious 'spot' (and you should make sure that you would recognize each on the list—see individual short cases) your *routine* should commence in the usual way by scanning the whole patient but in particular looking at

1 the **face** for obvious abnormalities such as *asymmetry* (hemiplegia), *nystagmus* (cerebellar syndrome), *wasting* (muscular dystrophy), sad, immobile, unblinking facies (*Parkinson's* disease), or *Horner's* syndrome (syringomyelia, Pancoast's syndrome). You may return to seek a less obvious Horner's or nystagmus later, if necessary. In search of obvious abnormalities run your eyes down to

2 the **neck** (pseudoxanthoma elasticum, lymph nodes), and then scan down the arms looking in particular at

3 the **elbows** which should be particularly inspected for *psoriasis, rheumatoid nodules* and *scars* or *deformity* underlying an ulnar nerve palsy. Before picking up the hands look for

4 a **tremor** (Parkinson's disease), then briefly inspect

5 the **hands** in the same way as you have practised under 'Examine this patient's hands' (p. 48), looking at

   (a) the joints (swelling, deformity),

   (b) nail changes (pitting, onycholysis, clubbing, nail-fold infarcts), and

   (c) skin changes (colour, consistency, lesions).

If you have not already been led towards a diagnosis requiring specific action, start a full neurological examination by studying first

6 the **muscle bulk** in the upper arms, lower arms and hands, bearing in mind that in about one-quarter of cases there will be wasting of the small muscles of the hands (see p. 226), and in one-fifth of cases there will be motor neurone disease which means wasting and

7 **fasciculation.**

8 Test the **tone** in the arms by passively bending the arm (with the patient relaxed) to and fro in an irregular and unexpected fashion, and in the hands by flexing and extending all the joints, including the wrist in the classic 'rolling wave' fashion used to detect cog-wheel rigidity (Parkinson's disease).

9 Ask the patient: '**Hold your arms out in front of you**' (look for *winging* of the scapulae, involuntary movements or the *myelopathy hand sign**); 'Now close your eyes' (look for *sensory wandering*—parietal drift or pseudoathetosis (see Fig C3.18c, p. 237)).

Next test

10 **power:**

   (a) 'Put your arms out to the side' (demonstrate this to the patient yourself—arms at 90° to your body with elbows flexed); 'Stop me pushing them down' (deltoid—C5),

---

* With the hands outstretched and supinated, passive abduction of the little finger indicates a pyramidal lesion or ulnar nerve palsy (sensory testing should distinguish). The sign is common in, but not specific for, cervical pyramidal lesions—as the lesion becomes more severe, adjacent fingers also passively abduct.

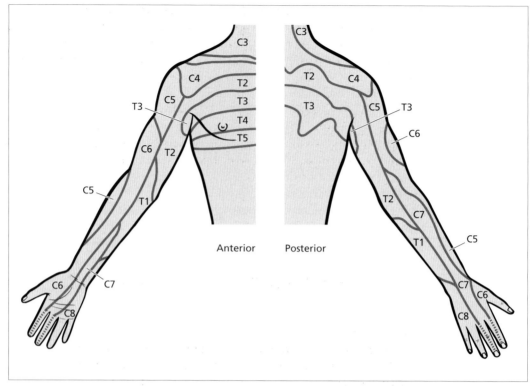

Figure B.2 Dermatomes in the upper limb (after Foerster, 1933, Oxford University Press, *Brain* **56**: 1). There is considerable variation and overlap between the cutaneous areas supplied by each spinal root so that an isolated root lesion results in a much smaller area of sensory impairment than the diagram indicates.

(b) 'Bend your elbow; stop me straightening it' (biceps — C5, 6),

(c) 'Push your arm out straight' — resist elbow extension (triceps — C7),

(d) 'Squeeze my fingers' — offer two fingers (C8, T1),*

(e) 'Hold your fingers out straight' (demonstrate); 'Stop me bending them' (if the patient can do this there is nothing wrong with motor C7 or the radial nerve),

(f) 'Spread your fingers apart' (demonstrate); 'Stop me pushing them together' (dorsal interossei — ulnar nerve),

(g) 'Hold this piece of paper between your fingers; stop me pulling it out' (palmar interossei — ulnar nerve),

(h) 'Point your thumb at the ceiling; stop me pushing it down' (abductor pollicus brevis — median nerve),

(i) 'Put your thumb and little finger together; stop me pulling them apart' (opponens pollicis — median nerve).

11 Test coordination

(a) 'Can you do this?' — demonstrate by flexing your elbows at right angles and then pronating and supinating your forearms as rapidly as possible,

(b) 'Tap quickly on the back of your hand' (demonstrate),

(c) 'Touch my finger; touch your nose; backwards and forwards quickly and neatly' (demonstrate if necessary — vary the target).

* See footnote, p. 51.

12 Check the biceps (C5, 6), triceps (C7), supinator (C5, 6) and finger (C8) **reflexes**.

13 Finally perform a **sensory screen** with *light touch* and *pinprick* bearing in mind the dermatomes shown in Fig. B.2 and the areas of sensation covered by the ulnar, median and radial nerves in the hand (see Fig B.4, p. 51). Finally, check *vibration* and *joint position* sense.

We leave you to consider where else you could look with each of the conditions given on the list in order to find additional information (see individual short cases). For example, you could look for nystagmus should you find cerebellar signs, or for Horner's syndrome should you suspect syringomyelia or Pancoast's syndrome.

For *checklist* see p. 528.

8 | 'Examine this patient's legs'

Stations 3 and 5
Variations of instruction in initial PACES survey (resultant diagnoses in brackets)

Examine this patient's legs (subarachnoid haemorrhage; hereditary sensory and motor neuropathy; mixed upper and lower motor neurone disorders)

Examine this lady's nervous system but concentrate on the legs (Charcot–Marie–Tooth disease)

This man is unable to walk. Examine his legs (?cauda equina lesion)

This 84-year-old lady has been having difficulty walking and with her balance. Would you examine her neurologically to find out why (peripheral neuropathy)

This lady has difficulty walking. Please examine her legs (?cervical myelopathy and diabetes)

Examine the legs but omit looking at the gait (subacute combined degeneration of the cord)

This patient has had weakness of the legs for 3 years. Please examine the legs and find out why (spastic paraparesis)

Examine this lady's lower limbs (Friedreich's ataxia)

Examine this foot (diabetic foot ulcer)

Look at, and examine, this man's legs (proximal myopathy secondary to polymyositis)

Please look at this patient's ankles and feet (Charcot's joint and foot ulcer)

This patient is diabetic. Please look at the feet (sensory loss, absent pulse and Charcot's joint)

Examine this man's legs (necrobiosis lipoidica diabeticorum).

Diagnoses from original, pre PACES, survey in order of frequency

Group 1 (spot, i.e. station 5)	Group 2 (neurological, i.e. station 3)
Paget's disease 13%	Spastic paraparesis 13%
Erythema nodosum 4%	Peripheral neuropathy 12%

Pretibial myxoedema 4%

Diabetic foot 3%

Necrobiosis lipoidica diabeticorum
 3%

Erythema ab igne 2%

Vasculitis 2%

Swollen knee 1%

Pemphigoid/pemphigus <1%

Deep venous thrombosis/ruptured
 Baker's cyst <1%

Multiple thigh abscesses <1%

Vasculitic leg ulcers <1%

Pyoderma gangrenosum <1%

Stigmata of sickle-cell disease <1%

Mycosis fungoides <1%

Diabetic ischaemia <1%

Ehlers–Danlos syndrome <1%

Bilateral below-knee amputation
 <1%.

Hemiplegia 5%

Cerebellar syndrome 4%

Cervical myelopathy 4%

Diabetic foot 3%

Motor neurone disease 3%

Old polio 3%

Absent leg reflexes and extensor plantars
 3%

Friedreich's ataxia 2%

Subacute combined degeneration of the
 cord 2%

Charcot–Marie–Tooth disease
 1%

Polymositis <1%

Lateral popliteal (common peroneal)
 nerve palsy <1%

Tabes <1%

Diabetic amyotrophy <1%.

Examination *routine*

An analysis of the conditions in our survey shows that they roughly fall into the two broad groups shown above:

Group 1: a spot diagnosis (i.e. station 5)

Group 2: a neurological diagnosis (i.e. station 3)

Either way initial clues may be gained by first performing a brief

1 *visual survey* of the patient as a whole. Look at the head and face for signs such as *enlargement* (Paget's disease), *asymmetry* (hemiparesis), *exophthalmos* with or without *myxoedematous facies* (pretibial myxoedema), or obvious *nystagmus* (cerebellar syndrome). Run your eyes over the patient for other significant signs such as thyroid *acropachy* (pretibial myxoedema), *rheumatoid hands* (swollen knee), nicotine-stained fingers (leg amputations), *wasted hands* (motor neurone disease, Charcot–Marie–Tooth disease, syringomyelia) and for muscle *fasciculation* (usually motor neurone disease).

Turning to the legs, look at the skin, joints and general shape and for any

2 **obvious lesion**, especially from the list of disorders in group 1. If such a lesion is visible a further full examination of the legs will not be required in most cases. You will be able to begin your description and/or diagnosis immediately (see individual short cases). If there is no obvious lesion look again specifically for

3 **bowing** of the tibia (see experience 72, vol. 2, p. 333), with or without enlargement of the skull. Though the changes of vascular insufficiency (absence of hair, shiny skin, cold pulseless feet, peripheral cyanosis, digital gangrene, painful ulcers) barely occurred in our survey, these should be *briefly* looked for (because they will direct you to examine the pulses, etc. rather than the neurological system).

Observing the legs from the neurological point of view note whether there is

4 **pes cavus** (Friedreich's ataxia, Charcot–Marie–Tooth disease) or

5 **one leg smaller** than the other (old polio, infantile hemiplegia). Next note

6 muscle bulk. Bear in mind that some generalized disuse atrophy may occur even in a limb with upper motor neurone weakness (e.g. severe spastic paraparesis—see experience 2, vol. 2, p. 326). There may be unilateral loss of muscle bulk (old polio), muscle wasting that stops part of the way up the leg (Charcot–Marie–Tooth disease), isolated anterior thigh wasting (e.g. diabetic amyotrophy) or generalized proximal muscle wasting (polymyositis) or muscle wasting confined to one peroneal region (lateral popliteal nerve palsy). Look specifically for

7 fasciculation (nearly always motor neurone disease).

8 Examine the **muscle tone** in each leg by passively moving it at the hip and knee joints (with the patient relaxed roll the leg sideways, backwards and forwards on the bed; lift the knee and let it drop, or bend the knee and partially straighten in an irregular and unexpected rhythm).

9 Test **power**:*
   (a) 'Lift your leg up; stop me pushing it down' (L1,2),
   (b) 'Bend your knee; don't let me straighten it' (L5, S1,2),
   (c) (Knee still bent) 'Push out straight against my hand' (L3,4),
   (d) 'Bend your foot down; push my hand away' (S1),
   (e) 'Cock up your foot; point your toes at the ceiling. Stop me pushing your foot down' (L4,5).

Moving smoothly into testing

10 coordination, take your hand off the foot and run your finger down the patient's shin below the knee saying
   (f) 'Put your heel just below your knee then run it smoothly down your shin; now up your shin, now down . . .' etc.†

11 Check the knee (L3,4) and ankle (S1,2) **jerks**‡ and by forced dorsiflexion with the leg held in slight knee flexion. Check for *ankle clonus* (and patellar clonus if there may be pyramidal disease).

12 Test the **plantar response** remembering that in slight pyramidal lesions an extensor plantar is more easily elicited on the outer part of the sole than the inner.§

13 Turning to **sensation**, dermatomes L2 to S1 on the leg (Fig. B.3, p. 36) are tested if you examine *light touch* (dab cotton wool lightly) and *pinprick* once each on the outer thigh (L2), inner thigh (L3), inner calf (L4), outer calf (L5), medial foot (L5) and lateral foot (S1). The most common sensory defect is a peripheral neuropathy with stocking distribution loss. Demonstrate this with light touch (usually the most sensitive indicator) and pinprick:

Test above the sensory level:
   'Does the pin feel sharp and prickly'—'Yes'.

---

* The screen of instructions from (a) to (e) will identify most legs in which there are abnormalities of motor function. You may wish to embellish these, where necessary, with instructions to test hip extension, hip adduction, hip abduction and hip rotation.

† If there is possible or definite cerebellar disease, you may wish to demonstrate dysdiadochokinesis in the foot by asking the patient to tap his foot quickly on your hand.

‡ One study has suggested that the plantar strike technique for examining ankle jerks may be more reliable than the better known tendon strike technique, especially in the elderly (*Lancet* 1994. **344**: 1619–20).

§ In slight pyramidal disease the extensor plantar is first elicited on the dorsilateral part of the foot (*Chaddock's manoeuvre*). As the degree of pyramidal involvement increases the area in which a *Babinski's sign* may be elicited increases first to cover the whole sole and then spreads beyond the foot until *Oppenheim's sign* (extensor response when the inner border of the tibia is pressed heavily—Fig. C3.18b, p. 237) or *Gordon's reflex* (extensor response on pinching the Achilles tendon) can be elicited. In such cases the big toe may be seen to go up as the patient takes his socks off.

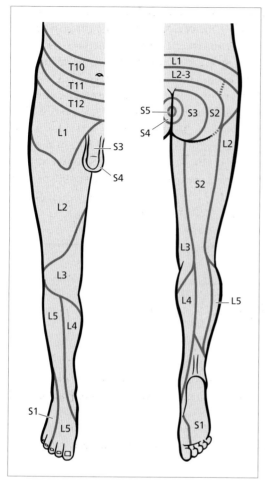

Figure B.3 Dermatomes in the lower limb (after Foerster, 1933, Oxford University Press, *Brain* **56**: 1). There is considerable variation and overlap between the cutaneous areas supplied by each spinal root so that an isolated root lesion results in a much smaller area of sensory impairment than the diagram indicates.

Test on the feet:

'Does the pin feel sharp and prickly' — 'No'.

'Tell me when it changes'.

Work up the leg to the sensory level and confirm afterwards by demonstrating the same level medially and laterally.* The level of the peripheral neuropathy may be different on the two legs. *Vibration* should be tested on the medial malleoli (and knee, iliac crest, etc., if it is impaired), and *joint position* sense in the great toes (remember to explain to the patient what you mean by 'up' and 'down' in his toes before you get him to close his eyes; whilst testing the position sense hold the toe by the lateral aspects).

---

*The same method can be used for rapid demonstration of a higher sensory level: normal sensation is demonstrated above the lesion, e.g. on the shoulder or chest. The pin is then rapidly moved up the whole body from the foot until the patient announces that the sensation is changing to normal. That area is then worked over rapidly to detect the actual sensory level.

Sometimes the examiner will stop you before you get this far. If the lesion is predominantly motor he may break in before you have tested sensation, and if predominantly sensory he may lead you to test sensation earlier or stop you at this point. You should, however, be sufficiently deft to perform the full examination described above quickly and efficiently, and be prepared to complete it by examining the patient's

14 gait (check the patient can walk by asking for either his or the examiner's permission to examine the gait). First, watch his *ordinary walk* to a defined point and back (see p. 203) and then watch him walk *heel-to-toe* (ataxia), on his *toes* and on his *heels* (footdrop). Finally perform

15 Romberg's test with the feet together and the arms outstretched. You must be ready to catch the patient if there is any possibility of ataxia. Romberg's test is only positive (sensory ataxia, e.g. subacute combined degeneration, tabes dorsalis) if the patient is more unsteady (tends to fall) with the eyes closed than open.

For *checklist* see p. 528.

9 | 'Examine this patient's legs and arms'

Station 3
Variations of instruction in initial PACES survey (resultant diagnoses in brackets)
This man has had a collapse—can you examine his limbs (left hemiplegia and atrial fibrillation).

Diagnoses from our original, pre PACES, survey in order of frequency
1   Motor neurone disease 29%
2   Cervical myelopathy 14%
3   Syringomyelia 14%
4   Friedreich's ataxia 14%
5   Parkinson's disease 7%.

Examination *routine*
As appropriate from 'Examine this patient's arms' (p. 29) and 'Examine this patient's legs' (p.33).

10 | 'Examine this patient's gait'

Mostly station 3, but also station 5
Variations of instruction in initial PACES survey (resultant diagnoses in brackets)
Examine this patient's gait (ankylosing spondylitis)
This man has difficulty walking and falls especially at night. Examine his gait and then his legs (cerebellar signs and sensory neuropathy)

This patient has difficulty in walking. Please examine him (cerebellar signs)
Examine the gait and anything else which is relevant (no diagnosis reached).

Diagnoses from our surveys in order of frequency

1 Ataxia 50%
2 Spastic paraparesis 20%
3 Parkinson's disease 10%
4 Charcot–Marie–Tooth disease 5%
5 Ankylosing spondylitis 5%
6 A nightmare (see p. 306) 5%.

Examination *routine*

As you approach the patient perform

1 a *quick **visual survey*** noting any *cerebellar signs* (nystagmus, intention tremor) or obvious signs of conditions such as *Parkinson's* disease (facies, tremor), *Charcot–Marie–Tooth* disease (peroneal wasting, pes cavus, etc.) or *ankylosing spondylitis*. Introduce yourself to the patient and ask him

2 **whether he can walk** without help (*cerebellar dysarthria* heard during his reply may be a useful clue). If he reports difficulty reassure him that you will stay with him in case of any problems.

3 **Ask him to walk** to a defined point and back whilst you look for any of the classic abnormal gaits (see p. 200), particularly ataxic (cerebellar or sensory), spastic, steppage (Charcot–Marie–Tooth) or parkinsonian (?pill–rolling tremor). As the patient walks make sure you note specifically

4 the **arm swing** (Parkinson's) and

5 any *clumsiness* on **the turns** (ataxia, Parkinson's) or 'sticky feet' with gait apraxia (slow, shuffling, short steps) or marche à petit pas (small, quick steps—also known as senile gait). Next test

6 **heel-to-toe** gait (demonstrate as you ask the patient to do this) which will *exacerbate* ataxia (note the side to which the patient tends to fall). Ask the patient to walk

7 **on his toes** (S1) and then

8 **on his heels** (L5; foot-drop —lateral popliteal nerve palsy, Charcot–Marie–Tooth disease). If he has a spastic gait or a hemiparesis he may find both these tests difficult to perform.

9 Now ask him to stand with his *feet together, arms out* in front; when you are satisfied with the degree of steadiness with the eyes open, ask him to *close his eyes* (you should be standing nearby to catch him if he shows a tendency to fall). **Romberg's test** is only positive (*sensory ataxia*) if the patient is more unsteady (tends to fall) with the eyes closed than with them open (dorsal column disease, e.g. subacute combined degeneration, tabes dorsalis, etc.).

10 If you suspect sensory ataxia a further test is to ask the patient to **close his eyes while walking** (he will become *more* ataxic). Again you should be ready to catch the patient should he fall. As always be ready to look for

11 **additional features** of the conditions on the list if appropriate (see individual short cases, and consider what you would do with each).

For *checklist* see p. 528.

11 | 'Ask this patient some questions'

Mostly stations 3 and 5, but also station 1
Variations of instruction from original, pre PACES, survey
Talk to this patient
Examine this patient's speech
Converse with this patient.

Diagnoses from original, pre PACES, survey in order of frequency
1 Dysphasia 24%
2 Cerebellar dysarthria 16%
3 Raynaud's 11%
4 Systemic sclerosis/CRST 8%
5 Pseudobulbar palsy 8%
6 Myxoedema 5%
7 Graves' disease 5%
8 Crohn's disease 5%
9 Ankle oedema due to nephrotic syndrome 5%
10 Senile dementia 5%
11 Parkinson's disease 3%.

Examination *routine*
Inspection of the list of cases in our survey which provoked this instruction reveals that they fall into four groups, each with a very different reason for the instruction:
Group 1: to spot the diagnosis and confirm it by eliciting *revealing answers* 39%
Group 2: to demonstrate and diagnose the type of a dysarthria 32%
Group 3: to diagnose a dysphasia 24%
Group 4: to assess higher mental function 5%.

With the group 1 patients you may have been given a lead such as 'Look at the hands' (Raynaud's) or 'Look at the face' (systemic sclerosis, myxoedema, etc.) before the instruction 'Ask this patient some questions'. At any rate you should start your examination as usual with

1 a ***visual survey*** of the patient from head to foot, particularly looking for evidence of: (i) the spot diagnosis in group 1 patients (Raynaud's, systemic sclerosis/CRST, hypo- or hyperthyroidism, Crohn's, nephrotic syndrome); (ii) a *hemiplegia* which may be associated with dysphasia; or (iii) any of the conditions associated with dysarthria (see p. 239) especially *nystagmus* or *intention tremor* (which may be revealed by even minor movements) in cerebellar disease, *pes cavus* in Friedreich's ataxia and the *facies/tremor* of Parkinson's disease.

In the group 1 patients once you are on to the diagnosis the sort of
2 **specific questions** the examiners are looking for (see also the individual short cases) are: *Raynaud's* (see also anecdote 15, vol. 2, p. 363):
'Do your fingers change colour in the cold?'
'What colour do they go?' ('Is there a particular sequence of colours?')

'How long have you had the trouble?'

'What is your job?' (vibrating tools, etc.)

and if there is any possibility of connective tissue disease:

'Do you have any difficulty with swallowing?' etc.

Systemic sclerosis:

'Do you have any difficulty with swallowing?'

'Do your fingers change colour in the cold?'

'Do you get short of breath?' (on hills? on flat? etc.)

We leave you to work out the straightforward questions you would ask the slow croaking patient with *myxoedematous facies*, the patient with *exophthalmos*, or the one who has *lid retraction* and is *fidgety*, or the patient who has *multiple scars* and *sinuses* on his abdomen. In the young patient who may have nephrotic syndrome you would be looking for the history of a sore throat.

If there are no features suggesting a group 1 patient, it is likely that the problem is either a dysarthria or dysphasia, and, as already mentioned, there may be clues pointing to one of these. You need to ask the patient

3 some **general questions** to get him *talking*:

'My names is . . . Please could you tell me your name?'

'What is your address?'

If you still need to hear a patient speak further ask

4 **more questions** which require *long answers* such as

'Please could you tell me all the things you ate for breakfast/lunch'.

To test

5 **articulation** ask the patient to repeat traditional words and phrases such as 'British Constitution', 'West Register Street', 'biblical criticism' and 'artillery'. As well as testing articulation such

6 **repetition** is useful for assessing speech when the patient only gives one-word answers to questions. If necessary ask the patient to repeat long sentences after you. Information gained from repetition may also be useful in your assessment of dysphasia (see below).

If the problem is *dysarthria*, it is really a spot diagnosis to test your ability to recognize and demonstrate the features of the different types (see p. 239). It is recommended that you find as many patients as possible with the conditions causing the various types of dysarthria and listen to them speak so that, as with murmurs, the diagnosis is a question of instant recognition. This is particularly true of the ataxic dysarthria of cerebellar disease. When you have heard enough to make the diagnosis, you should either describe the speech (see p. 239) and, with supporting signs seen on inspection, give the diagnosis, or proceed to look for

7 **additional signs** (in the same way as you might do after the 'What is the diagnosis' instruction).

If the patient has a *dysphasia* (see p. 240) you may wish to demonstrate that

8 **comprehension** is good (expressive dysphasia) or impaired (receptive dysphasia). Perform a few simple commands *without gesturing*, e.g.

'Please put your tongue out'.

'Shut your eyes'.

'Touch your nose', etc.

Assuming these are performed adequately proceed to look for expressive dysphasia by asking the patient to name some everyday items, e.g. a comb, pen, coins. If the patient is unable to name the objects test for

9 nominal dysphasia. Hold up your keys:

'What is this?' — patient does not answer.

'Is this a spoon' — 'No'.

'Is it a pen' — 'No'.

'Is it keys' — 'Yes'.

If the patient is able to name objects, test the ability to form sentences by asking the patient to describe something in more detail, e.g.

'Could you tell me where you live and how you would get home from here?'

'Could you tell me the name of as many objects in this room as possible?'

If there are expressive problems you should check to see if the problem is true expressive dysphasia or whether there is

10 orofacial dyspraxia.* Ask the patient to perform various orofacial movements (assuming there is no receptive dysphasia). These should be tested first by command *without gesture*, e.g.

'Please show me your teeth'.

'Move your tongue from side to side'.

Subsequently ask the patient to obey the same commands but *with gesture*, i.e. so the patient can mimic. This should give some idea as to whether the patient has either ideational or ideomotor dyspraxia.†

Our survey showed that it is extremely rare for candidates to be asked to assess

11 higher mental functions.‡ This is, however, an assessment which every Membership candidate should be equipped to make. The following is the 'abbreviated mental test' — more than four of the questions wrong suggests a well-established dementia:

1 Age

2 Time (to nearest hour)

3 Address for recall at end of test — this should be repeated by the patient to ensure it has been heard correctly: 42 West Street

4 Year

5 Name of this place

6 Recognition of two persons (doctor, nurse, etc.)

7 Date of birth (day and month sufficient)

8 Year of First World War

9 Name of present Monarch

10 Count backwards from 20 to 1.

Agnosia, apraxia, dyslexia, dysgraphia and dyscalculia are considered on p. 184.

For *checklist* see p. 529.

---

* It is important to make this distinction so that the type of speech therapy is appropriate — in orofacial dyspraxia the therapist needs to work on mouth movements rather than concentrating only on linguistic problems. It has recently been established that the lesion which leads to orofacial dyspraxia is in the operculum.

† Again it is relevant to therapy to establish if the patient can make movements when aided by gesture.

‡ Rare at the time of writing (see anecdote 38a, vol. 2, p. 365), though it is conceivable that any examiners who see this book will be given ideas as to the areas they are neglecting!

12 | 'Examine this patient's fundi'

Station 5

Variations of instruction in initial PACES survey (resultant diagnoses in brackets)

Examine this patient's fundi (diabetic retinopathy—many cases, all stages; unilateral optic atrophy and angioid streaks)

Look at the fundi (diabetic retinopathy—many cases, all stages)

Examine the eyes of this diabetic patient (pan-retinal photocoagulation and exudates near macula)

This patient feels as if he is walking on cotton wool and has had recurrent Bell's palsies. Please examine his eyes (it turned out to be preproliferative diabetic retinopathy)

This patient is blind. Examine his fundi (retinitis pigmentosa and cataracts)

This man had sudden onset blindness. Please look at the fundi and suggest why (glaucoma and retinal artery occlusion)

This patient has visual loss. Please examine the fundi (diabetic maculopathy)

Your house officer has examined this lady's fundi. She is a 23-year-old nurse. He is worried and has asked for your opinion (myelinated nerve fibres)

Examine this man's fundus (just the right one) (diabetic retinopathy)

Look at the fundi and describe what you find (cataracts and diabetic retinopathy)

This man has trouble with his vision. Examine the fundi (retinitis pigmentosa)

Examine the fundi. The patient has a central scotoma (retinitis pigmentosa and diabetic maculopathy)

This elderly man has had sudden onset of blindness in the right eye. Please examine him and tell me why (optic atrophy).

Diagnoses from survey in order of frequency

 1 Diabetic retinopathy 41%
 2 Retinitis pigmentosa 16%
 3 Optic atrophy 6%
 4 Papilloedema 4%
 5 Retinal vein thrombosis 2%
 6 Old choroiditis 2%
 7 Cataracts 2%
 8 Albinism 2%
 9 Myelinated nerve fibres 1%
10 Hypertensive retinopathy 1%
11 Glaucoma 1%
12 Laurence–Moon–Bardet–Biedl <1%
13 Asteroid hyalosis <1%
14 Retinal artery occlusion <1%
15 Drusen <1%
16 Cytomegalovirus choroidoretinitis (AIDS) <1%
17 Normal <1%.

Special note

It is the intention of the College that all candidates are tested with a fundus examination in station 5. In practice, our survey has shown that some centres have provided non-fundus eye cases (see p. 508). Nevertheless, you should assume you will be asked to examine the fundi. Though there are only a limited number of possibilities, it is clear from the survey that a lot of candidates experience more difficulty with a fundus than with any other short case. On our questionnaire a considerable number of candidates reported 'I said optic atrophy . . . ', or 'I said diabetic retinopathy . . . but I hadn't got a clue what it was' (see experiences 49–51, vol. 2, p. 331). Clearly there is not a lot that a book like this can do to help other than to warn you in advance of the problem, to provide you with a list of the likely conditions and to describe them (see individual short cases). Other than this the art of fundoscopy and fundal diagnoses can only be acquired with practise. With a moderate degree of clinical expertise and common sense most candidates ought to be able to overcome this hurdle.

Examination *routine*

Almost invariably if you are asked to look at the fundus the diagnosis must be in the fundus. However, it is a good practice to precede fundoscopy with

1 a **quick general look** at the patient (this will rarely help but the occasional diabetic in the examination may also have *foot ulcers* or *necrobiosis lipoidica* or may be wearing a *medic-alert* bracelet or neck chain), at his eyes (*arcus lipidus* at an inappropriately young age may suggest diabetes), and at his pupils (usually, but not always, dilated for the examination).

Turning to ophthalmoscopy, it may be your practice to focus immediately on the fundus and, in the vast majority of cases, this will provide the diagnosis. However, it would be preferable to cultivate the habit (if you can gain sufficient expertise to do it quickly and efficiently) of looking first at

2 the structures in front of the fundus, particularly the **lens** (diabetics will often reward you with early *cataract* formation; your examiner will sometimes not have noticed it, but as long as you are right when he checks you may score points). Adjust the lenses of the ophthalmoscope so that you move down through

3 the **vitreous** noting any *opacities* (e.g. asteroid hyalinosis, p. 502), *haemorrhages, fibrous tissue* or *new vessel formation* (diabetes) until you get to

4 the **fundus**. Localize the disc and examine it and its margins for *optic atrophy,** *papillitis* (p. 480) or *papilloedema* (p. 488) and for *myelinated nerve fibres* (p. 495). Trace the

5 **arterioles** and **venules** out from the disc noting particularly their calibre, light reflex (*silver wiring*) and AV crossing points (*AV nipping*, see p. 496).

6 Examine **each quadrant** of the fundus and especially the **macular area** and its temporal aspect.† You are looking particularly for *haemorrhages* (dot, blot, flame-shaped),

---

* There are normal variations in disc colour; in both infancy and old age it is naturally pale, as is the enlarged disc of a myopic eye. The advice of a well-known neurologist and experienced MRCP teacher to his MRCP candidates was: 'Don't diagnose optic atrophy unless it is a "barn door" optic atrophy'. It is well worth bearing this advice in mind (see experience 50. vol. 2, p. 331). Temporal pallor of the disc due to a lesion in the papillomacular bundle is often seen in multiple sclerosis. However, temporal pallor is not always pathological.

† The macula will come in to view if you ask the patient with a dilated pupil to look at the ophthalmoscopic light. Ideally, you should use the dot light for this, if it is available in your ophthalmoscope.

microaneurysms, exudates both hard (well-defined edges; increased light reflex) and soft (fluffy with ill-defined edges; *cotton-wool spots*). If hard exudates are present see if these form a ring (*circinates* in diabetes).

If you see haemorrhages you must look specifically for

(a) dot haemorrhages/microaneurysms,

(b) new vessel formation, and

(c) photocoagulation scars.

If you diagnose diabetic retinopathy your examiner will expect you to be able to comment on the presence or absence of all of these (see experience 51, vol. 2, p. 331). If you cannot find these diagnostic clues you may have noted the features that suggest hypertensive rather than diabetic retinopathy (silver wiring, AV nipping, more soft exudates than hard, haemorrhages which are mainly flame-shaped, early disc swelling with loss of venous pulsation* or frank papilloedema).

In the patient with diabetic retinopathy, it is of particular clinical significance to assess whether lesions (especially haemorrhages and hard exudates) involve or threaten (i.e. are near to) the macula.†

It would be useful if you knew that the patient was a diabetic (see experience 93 and quotation 42, vol. 2, pp. 338 and 370) but if you remain in doubt remember that diabetes and hypertension often coexist in a patient, and that it is more important that you have checked comprehensively for the above features, and report your findings honestly (mentioning the features in favour of one diagnosis or the other), than to guess or make up findings.‡ In PACES the College is keen that the instruction tells you the patient is diabetic if he/she is. In general, this does not help as many of the patients with different types of retinal pathologies in the exam have diabetes — because diabetic patients are the one group having regular fundal checks which may turn up pathologies other than diabetic retinopathy, e.g. drusen, old choroiditis, myelinated nerve fibres, etc. However, in the patient with haemorrhages and exudates it is of great value to know if the patient has diabetes.

We leave you to master the findings of the other fundal short cases and to ensure that you would recognize each (see individual short cases). The final point in this important *routine* is to

7 stay examining until you have finished and are **ready** to present your findings. Do not be put off by the impatient words or mumblings of your examiner; these will be forgotten when you present accurate findings and get the diagnosis right. Conversely, it is too late to go back and check if the examiner asks whether you saw a . . . and you are not sure (experiences 51, vol. 2, p. 331). You need to be able to give a clear and unequivocal 'Yes' or 'No'. Thus, the best tip we can offer as you look around the fundus is to stop at the disc, the macula, and in each quadrant of each eye and ask yourself the question: 'Are there any abnormalities? What are they?' before moving on to the next area.

For *checklist* see p. 529.

---

* Observation of venous pulsation is an expertise which comes with much practise of looking at normal as well as abnormal fundi. Though it could be useful if you have acquired this expertise before the examination, do not get bogged down studying the venous pulsation for too long if you are not used to it. See also p. 488.

† European diabetic retinopathy screening guidelines suggest that patients with haemorrhages or hard exudate within one disc diameter of the macula should be considered for referral to an ophthalmologist (p. 475).

‡ Making up findings is strictly inadvisable and can result in failure whereas missing one short case need not fail you.

13 | 'Examine this patient's eyes'

Stations 3 and 5

Variations of instruction in initial PACES survey (resultant diagnoses in brackets)

Examine this patient's eyes (retinitis pigmentosa; Graves' disease; complete IIIrd nerve palsy; IIIrd, IVth, VIth nerve palsy)

Examine the eyes and anything else appropriate (Graves' eye disease and signs of hyperthyroidism)

Look at this patient's eyes (exophthalmos; IIIrd nerve palsy)

This woman presents with painful eyes. Please examine her (chemosis and goitre)

Examine this lady's eye movements (partial IIIrd nerve palsy)

This lady has had neurosurgery. Please examine her eyes (right upper homonymous hemianopia)

This man is followed up in the eye clinic. Have a look at him and tell me why (exophthalmos and lid lag).

Diagnoses from our original, pre PACES, survey in order of frequency

1 Exophthalmos 27%
2 Ocular palsy 23%
3 Nystagmus 11%
4 Diabetic retinopathy 8%
5 Optic atrophy 7%
6 Myasthenia gravis 4%
7 Visual field defects 3%
8 Ptosis 3%
9 Retinitis pigmentosa 2%
10 Horner's syndrome 2%
11 Holmes–Adie pupil 1%
12 Argyll Robertson pupils 1%
13 Cataracts 1%
14 Papilloedema 1%.

Other diagnoses were: buphthalmos in a patient with Sturge–Weber syndrome (1%), normal eyes in a patient who was supposed to have internuclear ophthalmoplegia (1%) and retinal detachment (<1%).

Examination *routine*

A study of the above list maps out your examination steps when you hear this instruction. It is basically going to be a part of your cranial nerves *routine* (p. 26) but carried out in slightly more detail. It should be your habit to commence all examination *routines* by *scanning* the whole patient. The patient with nystagmus due to cerebellar disease (p. 186) may have an *intention tremor* which will occasionally be noticeable even with minor movements. The patient with exophthalmos may have *pretibial myxoedema* or *thyroid acropachy*. A number of other conditions with stigmata elsewhere on the body may cause eye signs. Though these conditions were not prominent in our survey, they should be borne in mind as you complete this *visual survey*: face and hands of acromegaly, foot ulcers in diabetes, pes cavus in Friedreich's ataxia, the long, lean look of myotonic dystrophy, etc. As you finish your *visual survey* briefly look again at

1 the **face** (e.g. myasthenic facies, tabetic facies, facial asymmetry in hemiparesis), and then concentrate on

2 the **eyes**. Ask yourself if there is

   (a) exophthalmos,

   (b) strabismus,

   (c) ptosis, or

   (d) other abnormalities such as xanthelasma or arcus senilis.

Look at

3 the **pupils** for inequality of size and shape; whether one or both are small (Argyll Robertson, Horner's) or large (Holmes–Adie, IIIrd nerve palsy). Remember it may be necessary to use subdued light to elicit anisocuria, particularly due to unilateral Horner's syndrome. Also check for iris abnormalities such as Lisch nodules in neurofibromatosis. Next, it is traditional to check

4 the **visual acuity** by asking the patient to read a newspaper or other print which you hold up, and by asking him to look at the clock on the wall (see p. 27); alternatively it would be preferable to pull out a pocket-sized Snellen's chart.* In the traditional *routine* you should next test

5 **visual fields** (see p. 25). However, in the majority of cases the important findings are on testing

6 **eye movements** (see p. 28). We leave you to decide if you wish to follow the traditional *routine* or check eye movements before acuity and visual fields (see experience 36 and quotation 51, vol. 2, pp. 330 and 371). You are looking for

   (a) ocular palsy (p. 203),

   (b) diplopia,

   (c) nystagmus, or

   (d) lid lag.

In order to test

7 the **pupillary light reflex**, take out your pen torch and shine the light twice (*direct* and *consensual*) in each eye. Then test

8 the **accommodation–convergence reflex** — hold your finger close to the patient's nose:

   'Look into the distance',

then suddenly

   'Now look at my finger'.†

Finally, examine

9 the **fundi**.

As usual, when you have the diagnosis, think what else you could look for (e.g. cerebellar signs in a patient with nystagmus; sympathectomy scar over the clavicle in

---

*We advise you to take a pocket-sized Snellen's chart (like the one provided in Appendix 3). It will enable you to put an approximate value on the patient's visual acuity while taking no extra time.

†Some neurologists believe that as this traditional method of examining the accommodation–convergence reflex may involve a change in optical axis and luminance, it is better to get the patient to follow a target down the optical axis over 2 m.

a patient with Horner's syndrome; absent limb reflexes in Holmes–Adie pupil) before shouting out the diagnosis even if it is obvious (e.g. exophthalmos).

For *checklist* see p. 529.

14 | 'Examine this patient's face'

Mostly stations 3 and 5, but also station 1
Variations of instruction in initial PACES survey (resultant diagnoses in brackets)
Look at the face (hereditary haemorrhagic telangiectasia)
Look at this patient's face (lupus pernio)
Look at this man's face and examine whatever else you think is necessary (?).

Diagnoses from our original, pre PACES, survey in order of frequency
 1 Lower motor neurone VIIth nerve lesion 12%
 2 Lupus pernio 8%
 3 Ptosis 7%
 4 Sturge–Weber syndrome 7%
 5 Hypothyroidism 7%
 6 Osler–Weber–Rendu syndrome 7%
 7 Myotonic dystrophy 4%
 8 Jaundice 4%
 9 Horner's syndrome 4%
10 Systemic sclerosis/CRST 3%
11 Peutz–Jeghers syndrome 3%
12 Upper motor neurone facial weakness 3%
13 Systemic lupus erythematosus 3%
14 Parkinson's disease 3%
15 Cushing's syndrome 2%
16 Neurofibromatosis 2%
17 Superior vena cava obstruction 2%
18 Plethora (polycythaemia rubra vera) 2%
19 Hypopituitarism 2%
20 Vitiligo and a goitre 2%
21 Cyanosis 2%
22 Paget's disease 1%
23 Bilateral parotid enlargement 1%
24 Exophthalmos 1%
25 Acromegaly 1%
26 Dermatomyositis (hands and face) 1%
27 Xanthelasma and arcus senilis 1%
28 Acne rosacea 1%
29 Dermatitis herpetiformis 1%
30 Malar flush 1%.

Examination *routine*

This instruction is really just a variation on the 'spot diagnosis' theme (see p. 62), only easier because you are told where the abnormalities lie. In a way similar to that described in the 'What is the diagnosis?' *routine*,

1 *survey* the patient from head to foot and then

2 **scan the face** and skull. The abnormality will usually be obvious (see above list) but if you find none then proceed to

3 **break down the parts** of the face into their constituents and scrutinize each, asking the question to yourself: 'Is it normal?' Thus if you have scanned the eyes and have not been struck by any obvious abnormality (e.g. ptosis or an abnormal pupil), you should look at all the structures such as the *eyelids* (mild degree of ptosis, heliotrope rash on the upper lid in dermatomyositis), *eyelashes* (sparse in alopecia*), *cornea* (arcus senilis, ground-glass appearance in congenital syphilis), *sclerae* (icteric, congested in superior vena cava obstruction and polycythaemia), *pupils* (small, large, irregular, dislocated lens in Marfan's, cataract in myotonic dystrophy) and *iris* ('muddy iris' in iritis)† on both sides. Look at the *face* for any erythema or infiltrates (lupus pernio, SLE, dermatomyositis, malar flush), around the *mouth* for tight, shiny, adherent skin (systemic sclerosis) or pigmented macules (Peutz–Jeghers) and, if indicated, in the mouth for telangiectases (Osler–Weber–Rendu), cyanosis or pigmentation (Addison's). The whole face can be rapidly covered in this manner. Having spotted the abnormality and, you hope, made the diagnosis you should, if appropriate, try to score extra points by demonstrating

4 **additional features** in the same way as described under 'What is the diagnosis?' Go through each diagnosis on the list and work out what additional features you would see elsewhere. Thus, if you find a lower motor neurone VIIth nerve lesion, demonstrate the weakness in the upper as well as the lower part of the face (see p. 211), then be seen to examine the ears for evidence of herpes zoster (Ramsay Hunt syndrome).

If despite carrying out the above routine there is still no apparent abnormality then examine the facial musculature (see 'Examine this patient's cranial nerves') for evidence of a VIIth nerve lesion which is not obvious.

For *checklist* see p. 529.

15 | 'Examine this patient's hands'

Mostly stations 3 and 5, but also station 1
Variations of instruction in initial PACES survey (resultant diagnoses in brackets)

Examine this patient's hands (rheumatoid hands and nodules; rheumatoid hands and cervical collar; osteoarthritis; psoriasis; rheumatoid arthritis)

Examine these hands (psoriasis; scleroderma; neurofibromatosis; deforming arthropathy, ?type)

---

* May be associated with the organ-specific autoimmune diseases (see pp. 293 and 306).

† Another uncommon but important sign which may occur in the iris is neovascularization in diabetes (rubeosis iridis). However, it is unlikely that this would occur in the context of 'Examine this patient's face' at the examination.

Please examine this patient's hands. He is a 15-year-old boy who presented with carpopedal spasm as a child (pseudohypoparathyroidism?)

This man has a painful knee. Please examine his hands and suggest why (gout)

This man has had painful hands. Please examine him (rheumatoid hands)

Look at this patient's hands (rheumatoid arthritis)

This is a lady of about 80 years. Please look at her hands (osteoarthritis and gout)

Examine the hands and any other relevant joints (CRST)

Examine these hands (chronic tophacious gout)

This patient has rheumatoid arthritis. Please check the functional status (rheumatoid arthritis)

Have a look at this lady's hand and talk me through your examination (rheumatoid hands).

Diagnoses from our original, pre PACES, survey in order of frequency

1 Rheumatoid hands 22%
2 Systemic sclerosis/CRST 13%
3 Wasting of the small muscles of the hand 12%
4 Psoriatic arthropathy/psoriasis 11%
5 Ulnar nerve palsy 9%
6 Clubbing 7%
7 Raynaud's 3%
8 Vasculitis 3%
9 Steroid changes (especially purpura) 3%
10 Acromegaly 2%
11 Motor neurone disease 2%
12 Xanthomata 2%
13 Cyanosis 2%
14 Chronic liver disease 2%
15 Thyroid acropachy 2%
16 Carpal tunnel syndrome 2%
17 Osteoarthrosis 2%
18 Osler–Weber–Rendu syndrome 1%
19 Tophaceous gout 1%.

Other diagnoses were: neurofibromatosis (<1%), systemic lupus erythematosus (<1%), cervical myelopathy (<1%), dermatomyositis ('examine hands and face'; <1%), nail–patella syndrome ('examine hands and knees', <1%), Charcot–Marie–Tooth disease (<1%), superior vena cava obstruction (<1%), facioscapulohumeral muscular dystrophy (<1%), Addison's disease (<1%) and Marfan's syndrome (<1%).

Examination *routine*

Analysis of the list given above suggests that when you hear this instruction, rheumatoid arthritis is likely to be present in about a quarter of the cases, and either scleroderma, wasting of the small muscles of the hand, psoriasis, ulnar nerve palsy or clubbing in about a further half. As you approach the patient you should bear this in mind and look specifically at

1 the **face** for typical expressionless facies, with adherent shiny skin, sometimes with telangiectasis (*systemic sclerosis*). It is clear from the survey list that a variety of other conditions may show signs in either the face or in the general appearance, particularly *cushingoid* facies (steroid changes in a patient with rheumatoid arthritis), *acromegalic* facies, *arcus senilis* or *xanthelasma* (xanthomata), *icterus* and *spider naevi* (chronic liver disease) or *exophthalmos* (thyroid acropachy). We leave you to consider the changes you may note as you approach the patient with any of the other conditions on the list (see individual short cases). Even if the diagnosis is not immediately clear on looking at the face it is likely that in many cases it will become rapidly apparent as you

2 **inspect the hands**. Run quickly through the six main conditions that make up 75% of cases:

(a) *rheumatoid arthritis* (proximal joint swelling, spindling of the fingers, ulnar deviation, nodules),

(b) *systemic sclerosis* (sclerodactyly with tapering of the fingers, sometimes with gangrene of the fingertips, tight, shiny, adherent skin, calcified nodules, etc.),

(c) generalized *wasting* of the small muscles of the hand, perhaps with dorsal guttering,

(d) *psoriasis* (pitting of the nails, terminal interphalangeal arthropathy, scaly rash),

(e) *ulnar nerve palsy* (may be a typical claw hand or may be muscle wasting which spares the thenar eminence; often this diagnosis will only become apparent when you have made a sensory examination), and

(f) *clubbing*.

The changes that you may see in the other conditions in the list are dealt with under the individual short cases, but if in these first few seconds you have not made a rapid spot diagnosis, study first the dorsal and then the palmar aspects of the hands, looking specifically at:

3 the **joints** for swelling, deformity or Heberden's nodes;

4 the **nails** for pitting, onycholysis, clubbing, nail-fold infarcts (vasculitis — usually rheumatoid) or splinter haemorrhages (unlikely);

5 the **skin** for *colour* (pigmentation, icterus, palmar erythema), for *consistency* (tight and shiny in scleroderma; papery thin, perhaps with purpuric patches in steroid therapy; thick in acromegaly), and for *lesions* (psoriasis, vasculitis, purpura, xanthomata, spider naevi, telangiectasis in Osler–Weber–Rendu and systemic sclerosis, tophi, neurofibromata, other rashes);

6 the **muscles** for isolated *wasting* of the thenar eminence (median nerve lesion), for generalized wasting especially of the first dorsal interosseous but sparing the thenar eminence (ulnar nerve lesion), for generalized wasting from a T1 lesion or other cause (p. 226) or for *fasciculation* which usually indicates motor neurone disease, though occasionally it can occur in other conditions such as syringomyelia, old polio or Charcot–Marie–Tooth disease.

Before leaving the inspection it is worth looking specifically for *skin crease pigmentation* (see experience 76, vol. 2, p. 334) before moving to

7 **palpation** of the hands for Dupuytren's contracture, nodules (may be palpable in the palms in rheumatoid arthritis), calcinosis (scleroderma/CRST), xanthomata, Heberden's nodes or tophi. In the vast majority of cases you will have, by now, some findings demanding either specific further action (see below) or a report with a diag-

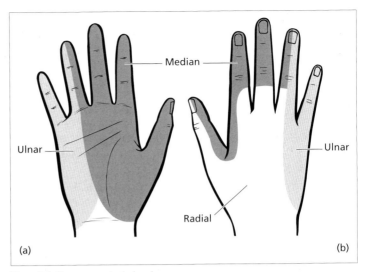

Figure B.4 Dermatomes in the hand.

nosis. Nonetheless, you should be prepared to continue with a full neurological examination of the hands to confirm a suspected neurological lesion, or if you have still made no diagnosis. If the hands appear normal it may be that there is a sensory defect. In these cases, it is more efficient, therefore, to commence the examination by testing

8 sensation. If you feel the examiners will not object, ask the patient if there has been any numbness or tingling in his hands and if so, when (?worse at night — carpal tunnel syndrome) and where. Bearing in mind the classic patterns of sensory defect in ulnar and median nerve lesions (Fig. B.4) and the dermatomes (see Fig. B.2, p. 32) seek and define an area of deficit to *pinprick* and *light touch* (dab cotton wool lightly), and check the *vibration* and *joint position* sense. With incomplete sensory loss due to either an ulnar or a median nerve defect, if you stroke the medial border of the little finger and the lateral border of the index finger with your fingers simultaneously, the patient may sense that the one side feels different from the other.

9 Check the **tone** of the muscles in the hand by flexing and extending all the joints including the wrist in a 'rolling wave' fashion.

10 The **motor** system of the hands can be tested with the instructions:

(a) 'Open your hands; now close them; now open and close them quickly' (myotonic dystrophy),*

(b) 'Squeeze my fingers' — offer two fingers (C8, T1),†

(c) 'Hold your fingers out straight' (demonstrate); 'stop me bending them' (C7),

(d) 'Spread your fingers apart' (demonstrate); 'stop me pushing them together' (dorsal‡ interossei — ulnar nerve),

(e) 'Hold this piece of paper between your fingers; stop me pulling it out' (palmar‡ interossei — ulnar nerve),

---

* Alternatively, you could miss this step out and go straight to step (b), but then issue the instruction 'Let go' and if there is any suspicion of myotonic dystrophy move to step (a).

† Some neurologists prefer to test the deep finger flexors by trying to extend flexed fingers, whilst steadying the wrist (flexor digitorum profundus, C8).

‡ Remember DAB and PAD: DAB = dorsal abduct, PAD = palmar adduct.

(f) 'Point your thumb at the ceiling; stop me pushing it down' (abductor pollicis brevis — median nerve),

(g) 'Put your thumb and little finger together; stop me pulling them apart' (opponens pollicis — median nerve).

Finally, for the sake of completeness, check the

11 radial pulses.

The action you take after finding an abnormality at any stage during the above *routine* will depend on what you find. Most commonly an abnormality found during the inspection will lead to most of the above being skipped in favour of a search for other evidence of the condition you suspect. It is worth emphasizing that there may be clues at

12 the elbows in several of the common conditions: rheumatoid arthritis (nodules), psoriatic arthropathy (psoriatic plaques), ulnar nerve palsy (scar, filling of the ulnar groove, restriction of range of movement at the elbow or evidence of fracture) and xanthomata. On the evidence of our survey you will need to examine the elbows in over 40% of cases (do not be put off by rolled-down sleeves). It is worth considering where else you would look, what for and what other tests you would do with the other conditions on the list (see individual short cases), but in particular remember to look for *tophi* on the ears if you suspect gout, and if you have diagnosed acromegaly seek an associated *carpal tunnel syndrome* (see experience 8a, vol. 2, p. 327). If on inspection you suspect a neurological deficit in the hand, you may wish to confirm it by performing only that part of the above *routine* relevant to that lesion, e.g. testing abduction and opposition of the thumb and seeking the classic sensory pattern if you see lone wasting of the thenar eminence and suspect carpal tunnel syndrome.

For *checklist* see p. 529.

16 | 'Examine this patient's skin'

Station 5
Variations of instruction in initial PACES survey (resultant diagnoses in brackets)

Examine this patient's skin (psoriasis; neurofibromatosis)
Look at this patient's skin (psoriasis)
Examine this lady's skin (neurofibromatosis)
This man has itchy skin. Please examine (eczema).

Diagnoses from our original, pre PACES, survey in order of frequency*

1 Psoriasis 15%
2 Vitiligo 10%
3 Systemic sclerosis/CRST 10%
4 Radiation burn on the chest 10%

---

* The instruction in the 'skin' subsection of station 5 may be 'Examine this patient's skin'. However, it may be 'Examine this patient's hands, face or rash' or just 'Look at this patient'. The figures here apply only to when the instruction was to examine the skin.

5 Epidermolysis bullosa dystrophica 10%
6 Purpura 5%
7 Pseudoxanthoma elasticum 5%
8 Localized scleroderma 5%.

Examination *routine*

This instruction is a rather more specific variation of the 'spot diagnosis' *routine* (p. 62). You should

1 perform a *visual survey* of the patient, from scalp to sole, with regard to the fact that most dermatological lesions have a predilection for certain areas. It is as well to remember some of the regional associations as you *survey* the patient:

Scalp	Psoriasis (look especially at the hairline for redness, scaling, etc.), alopecia,* ringworm (very uncommon)
Face	Systemic sclerosis (tight, shiny skin, pseudorhagades, beaked nose, telangiectasis), discoid lupus erythematosus (raised, red, scaly lesions with telangiectasis, scarring and altered pigmentation), xanthelasma, dermatomyositis (heliotrope colour to eyelids), Sturge–Weber, rodent ulcer (usually below the eye or on the side of the nose, raised lesion with central ulcer, the edges being rolled and having telangiectatic blood vessels)
Mouth	Osler–Weber–Rendu, Peutz–Jeghers, lichen planus (white lace-like network on mucosal surface), pemphigus, candidiasis (white exudate inside the mouth usually associated with a disease requiring multiple antimicrobial therapy, or an immunosuppressive disorder, e.g. leukaemia, AIDS, etc.), herpes simplex, Behçet's
Neck	Pseudoxanthoma elasticum, tuberculous adenitis with sinus formation (?ethnic origin)
Trunk	Radiotherapy stigmata, morphoea, neurofibromatosis, dermatitis herpetiformis (itching blisters over scapulae, buttocks, elbows, knees), herpes zoster along the intercostal nerves, pityriasis rosea, Addison's (areolar and scar pigmentation), pemphigus (trunk and limbs)
Axillae	Vitiligo, acanthosis nigricans (pigmentation and velvety thickening of axillary skin, perianal, areolar and lateral abdominal skin, 'tripe palms', mucous membranes involved, maybe underlying insulin resistance or malignancy)
Elbows	Psoriasis (extensor), pseudoxanthoma elasticum (flexor), xanthomata (extensor), rheumatoid nodules (extensor), atopic dermatitis (flexor), olecranon bursitis, gouty tophi
Hands	Systemic sclerosis (sclerodactyly, infarcts of finger pulps, prominent capillaries at nail folds), lichen planus (wrists), dermatomyositis (heliotrope lesions—Gottron's papules—on the joints of the dorsum of the fingers/hands, nail-fold capillary dilatation and infarction), Addison's (skin crease pigmentation), granuloma annulare, erythema multiforme (polymorphic eruption, 'target' lesions, mucous membrane involvement, macules, vesicles, bullae, etc.), SLE (erythematous patches over the dorsal surface of the phalanges), scabies (not in MRCP PACES!)

* Some causes of alopecia:
1 Diffuse—male pattern baldness, cytotoxic drugs, hypothyroidism, hyperthyroidism, iron deficiency

2 Patchy—alopecia areata, ringworm; with scarring—discoid lupus erythematosus, lichen planus.

Nails	Psoriasis (pitting, onycholysis), iron deficiency (koilonychia), fungal dystrophy, tuberous sclerosis (periungal fibromata)
Genitalia	Behçet's (iridocyclitis, uveitis, pyodermas, ulcers, etc.), lichen sclerosus (white plaques), candidiasis
Legs	Leg ulcer (diabetic, venous, ischaemic, pyoderma gangrenosum), necrobiosis lipoidica diabeticorum, pretibial myxoedema, erythema nodosum, Henoch–Schönlein purpura, tendon xanthomata in Achilles, erythema ab igne, pemphigoid (legs and arms), lipoatrophy
Feet	Pustular psoriasis, eczema, verrucae, keratoderma blenorrhagica (?eyes, joints, etc.).

During this *survey* you should consider

2 the **distribution** of the lesions (psoriasis on extensor areas, lichen planus in flexor areas, candidiasis in mucous membranes, tuberous sclerosis on nails and face, necrobiosis lipoidica diabeticorum usually bilateral, gouty tophi in the joints of hands, elbows and on the ears, etc.). Then after the *survey* (which should take a few seconds)

3 examine the **lesions** (see 'Examine this patient's rash') looking in particular for the *characteristic* features, e.g. scaling in psoriasis, shiny purple polygonal papules with Wickham's striae in lichen planus, etc. If you have made a diagnosis consider whether you need to look for any

4 associated lesions (arthropathy and nail changes with psoriasis, evidence of associated autoimmune disease with vitiligo, etc.). Go through the skin conditions which our survey has suggested occur in the exam and make sure that you would recognize each, would know what else to look for, and what to say in your presentation.

For *checklist* see p. 529.

17 | 'Examine this patient's rash'

Station 5
Variations of instruction in initial PACES survey (resultant diagnoses in brackets)
Take a look at this lady's rash (?examiners didn't know either)
This lady has a rash. Examine it (mixed connective tissue disease).

Diagnoses from our original, pre PACES, survey in order of frequency*
1 Psoriasis 20%
2 Purpura 10%
3 Vasculitis 10%

* See footnote, p. 52. The same sentiment applies here.

4 Neurofibromatosis 10%

5 Juvenile chronic arthritis (Still's disease) 10%

6 Xanthomata 5%

7 Necrobiosis lipoidica diabeticorum 5%

8 Radiation burn on the chest 5%.

Examination *routine*

This *routine* is generally the same as that discussed under 'Examine this patient's skin'.

1 You should quickly conduct a *visual survey* as described under 'skin' and note if there are any similar or related lesions elsewhere. Look at the

2 **distribution** of the lesions, whether confined to a single area (morphoea, erythema nodosum, rodent ulcer, melanoma, alopecia areata, etc.) or present in other areas such as psoriasis, neurofibromatosis, acanthosis nigricans, dermatomyositis, etc. While concentrating on the lesion in question, it is important to look at the

3 **surrounding skin** for any helpful clues such as *scratch marks* as evidence of itching,[*] *radiotherapy field markings* on the skin in the vicinity of a radiation burn, or *paper-thin skin* with purpura (corticosteroid therapy), etc. You should now

4 **examine the lesion** in detail. To determine the *extent* of the lesion you may have to ask the patient to undress, a procedure which will provide you with a little more time to survey other areas. Decide if the rash is *pleomorphic* or *monomorphic* (all the lesions are similar). If so examine one typical lesion carefully in terms of:

(a) *colour*, e.g. erythematous or pigmented,

(b) *size*,

(c) *shape*, e.g. oval, circular, annular, etc.,

(d) *surface*, e.g. scaling or eroded,

(e) *character*, e.g. macule, papule, vesicle, pustule, ulcer, etc.,

(f) *secondary features*, e.g. crusting, lichenification, etc.

It is advisable to be familiar with the correct use of the terms to describe rashes (especially if you do not recognize the lesion!). To say 'skin lesion' or 'skin rash' conveys no diagnostic meaning. In your presentation you should be able to describe the lesion with respect to the above six features, especially if you do not know the diagnosis. The following are some of the useful terms employed in describing skin lesions:

Macules: flat, circumscribed lesions, not raised above the skin — size and shape varies

Papules: raised, circumscribed, firm lesions up to 1 cm in size

Nodules: like papules but larger; usually lie deeper in skin

Tumours: larger than nodules, elevated or very deeply placed in the skin

Weals: circumscribed elevations associated with itching and tingling

Vesicles: small well-defined collections of fluid

Bullae: large vesicles

Pustules: circumscribed elevations containing purulent fluid which may, in some cases, be sterile (e.g. Behçet's)

---

[*] Some causes of itching:
1 Dermatological — scabies, dermatitis herpetiformis, lichen planus, eczema

2 Medical — cholestasis, chronic renal failure, lymphoma, polycythaemia rubra vera.

Scales: dead tissue from the horny layer which may be dry (e.g. psoriasis) or greasy (e.g. seborrhoeic dermatitis)

Crusts: these consist of dried exudate

Ulcers: excavations in the skin of irregular shape; remember that every ulcer has a shape, an edge, a floor, a base and a secretion, and it forms a scar on healing

Scars: the result of healing of a damaged dermis.

5 Finally, if indicated, look for **additional features** (arthropathy in psoriasis or Still's disease, cushingoid facies if purpura is due to steroids, clubbing with radiation burns on the chest, etc.).

For *checklist* see p. 530.

18 | 'Examine this patient's neck'

Mostly station 5, but also stations 1 and 3

Variations of instruction in initial PACES survey (resultant diagnoses in brackets)

Examine this patient's neck (goitre; pseudoxanthoma elasticum; multinodular goitre)

This patient has noticed a swelling in his neck — please examine (goitre)

This patient has a goitre. Please examine her (exophthalmos and non-nodular goitre).

Diagnoses from our original, pre PACES, survey in order of frequency

1 Goitre 46%
2 Generalized lymphadenopathy 17%
3 Graves' disease 12%
4 Jugular vein pulse abnormality 6%
5 Bilateral parotid enlargement/Mikulicz's syndrome 4%
6 Supraclavicular mass with Horner's syndrome 4%
7 Facioscapulohumeral muscular dystrophy 4%
8 Ankylosing spondylitis 2%
9 Hypothroidism 2%
10 Acanthosis nigricans <1%.

Examination *routine*

As usual, the first step is to

1 *survey* the patient quickly from head to foot (exophthalmos, myxoedematous facies, ankle oedema, etc.) and then to

2 **look at the neck.** According to the survey the reason for the instruction in half of the cases will be a *goitre*. If another abnormality is visible your further action will be dictated by what you see and we suggest you go through the list and establish a sequence of actions for each abnormality (e.g. if you see giant *v* waves you would wish to examine the heart and liver — see p. 162). If you do see a goitre, offer a drink to the patient:

'Take a sip of water and hold it in your mouth';

look at the neck:

'Now swallow'.

Watch the movement of the goitre, or the *appearance* of a *nodule* not visible before swallowing (behind sternomastoid—see Fig. C5.64c2, p. 436). Next ask the patient's permission to feel the neck, and then approach him from behind. If there has been no evidence of a goitre so far you may wish to palpate the neck for lymph nodes *before* feeling for a goitre. Otherwise

3 **palpate** the thyroid. With the right index and middle fingers feel below the thyroid cartilage where the isthmus of the thyroid gland lies over the trachea. Then palpate the two lobes of the thyroid gland which extend laterally behind the sternomastoid muscle. Ask the patient to swallow again while you continue to palpate the thyroid, ensuring that the neck is slightly flexed to ease palpation. Remember that if there is a goitre, when you give your presentation you are going to want to comment on its *size*, whether it is *soft*, or *firm*, whether it is *nodular* or *diffusely enlarged*, whether it *moves* readily on swallowing, whether there are *lymph nodes* (see below) and whether there is a vascular *murmur* (see below). Extend palpation upwards along the medial edge of the sternomastoid muscle on either side to look for a *pyramidal lobe* which may be present. Apologize for any discomfort you may cause because the deep palpation necessary to feel the thyroid gland causes pain,* particularly in patients with Graves' disease. *Percussion* over the upper sternum is used to assess any retrosternal extension of goitre. Next palpate laterally to examine

4 for **lymph nodes.** If you find lymph node enlargement check not only in the *supraclavicular fossae* and right up the neck but also in the *submandibular*, *postauricular* and *suboccipital* areas, ensuring that the head is slightly flexed on the side under palpation to allow access and scrutiny of slightly enlarged lymph nodes. Ascertain whether the lymph nodes are *separate* (reactive hyperplasia, infectious mononucleosis, lymphoma, etc.) or *matted* together (neoplastic, tuberculous), *mobile* or *fixed* to the skin or deep tissues (neoplastic), or whether they are *soft*, *fleshy, rubbery* (Hodgkin's disease) or *hard* (neoplastic). Particularly if you find lymph nodes without a goitre, examine for lymph nodes in the axillae and groins (lymphoma, chronic lymphatic leukaemia, etc.) and, if allowed, feel for the spleen.

5 **Auscultate** over the thyroid for evidence of increased vascularity. You may need to occlude venous return to rule out a venous hum, and listen over the aortic area to ensure that the thyroid bruit you hear is not, in fact, an outflow obstruction murmur conducted to the root of the neck.

6 If there is any evidence of thyroid disease consider beginning an assessment of **thyroid status** (see 'Examine this patient's thyroid status') by feeling and counting the pulse (NB do not miss *atrial fibrillation*, whether slow or fast). The examiner will soon stop you if he wishes to hear your description of a multinodular goitre in a euthyroid patient.

For *checklist* see p. 530.

---

* In viral thyroiditis (rare) the patient may complain of a painful
thyroid and the thyroid may be overtly tender on light palpation.

19 | 'Assess this patient's thyroid status'

Station 5
Variations of instruction in initial PACES survey (resultant diagnoses in brackets)
Examine this lady's thyroid status (euthyroid)
This lady has had previous problems with her thyroid. Examine her to determine her thyroid status (euthyroid).

Diagnoses from original pre PACES survey in order of frequency
1 Euthyroid Graves' disease 42%
2 Hyperthyroidism 17%
3 Euthyroid simple goitre 8%

Examination *routine*

Although the patient usually has signs of thyroid disease (exophthalmos, goitre), you are not being asked to examine these, but rather to assess whether the patient is clinically hypo-, eu- or hyperthyroid. Perform a speedy

1 *visual survey* looking specifically for *signs of thyroid disease* (exophthalmos, goitre, thyroid acropachy, pretibial myxoedema — all can occur in association with *any* thyroid status), and ask yourself if the facies are in any way myxoedematous. Observe the patient's

2 **composure**, whether *hyperactive, fidgety* and *restless* (hyperthyroid); normal, composed demeanour (euthyroid); or if she is somewhat *immobile* and *uninterested* in the people around her (hypothyroid).

3 **Take the pulse** and *count* it for 15 seconds, noting the presence or absence of *atrial fibrillation* (slow, normal rate, or fast). If the pulse is slow (less than 60), or if you suspect hypothyroidism, proceed immediately to test

4 for **slow relaxation** of the ankle,* supinator or other jerks. To test the reflexes you will require the patient's cooperation and the ensuing conversation may provide you with helpful clues (slow hesitant speech, slow movements, etc.). Otherwise

5 feel the **palms**, whether *warm* and *sweaty* or cold and sweaty (anxiety) and then

6 ask the patient to stretch out his hands to full extension of the wrist and elbow. If the **tremor** is not obvious, place your palm against his outstretched fingers to feel for it. Alternatively, you can place a piece of paper on the dorsum of his out-stretched hands — it will oscillate if a fine tremor is present.

7 Look at the **eyes**, noting exophthalmos (sclera visible above the lower lid — a sign not related to thyroid status) but looking specifically for *lid retraction* (sclera visible above the cornea). Test for lid lag (lid lag and retraction may diminish as the hyperthyroid patient becomes euthyroid).

---

* The slow relaxing ankle jerk in hypothyroidism is best demonstrated with the patient kneeling on a chair or bed with the feet hanging over the edge, and the examiner standing behind the patient. This manoeuvre is useful for the dressed patient in the out-patient department and may be useful in the PACES exam if the patient is dressed and sitting on a chair.

8 Examine the **thyroid** as described under 'Examine this patient's neck', remembering the steps are (i) look, (ii) palpate and (iii) auscultate.*

Putting the above findings together it should be possible to provide a definite conclusion about thyroid status; this is considered a very basic skill and it will not be taken lightly if, in your state of nerves, you make fundamental errors. Though the examiner may put you under pressure to test your confidence, keep calm and be particularly wary of being led to diagnose hypo- or hyperthyroidism in the presence of a normal pulse rate (see experience 81, vol. 2, p. 334).

9 Be prepared with the **standard questions** for assessment of thyroid status (temperature preference, weight change, appetite, bowel habits, palpitations, change of temper, etc.—see pp. 432 and 438) should the examiner wish you to question the patient. Indeed, if there is any doubt about the thyroid status after the above examination, offer to ask the patient these questions.

For *checklist* see p. 530.

20 | 'Examine this patient's knee'

Station 5
Possible diagnoses
Rheumatoid arthritis
Seronegative spondyloarthropathy
   Psoriatic arthritis
   Ankylosing spondylitis
   Inflammatory bowel disease
   Reactive arthritis
Gout
Pseudogout
Septic arthritis
Osteoarthritis
Haemarthrosis
Prepatellar bursitis
Baker's cyst
Charcot's joint.

Examination *routine*

If asked to examine a patient's knees you should bear the following in mind:

   (a) is it an *inflammatory* or *non-inflammatory* problem?

   (b) is it *a monoarthritis* or part of a more widespread arthropathy (*oligo-* or *polyarthropathy* or *spondyloarthropathy*)?

* A thyroid bruit is good evidence of thyroid overactivity; if present it can be heard over the isthmus and lateral lobe of the thyroid; it will not be obliterated by occluding the internal jugular vein (venous hum) or by rotation of the head and it will not be influenced by pressure of the stethoscope (use light pressure to avoid causing non-thyroid bruits).

(c) is the pain (if any) referred from elsewhere (i.e. hip)?

(d) are there any extra articular features?

(e) what is the functional impairment?

1 On approaching the patient **observe** for any other obvious features of joint disease (e.g. symmetrical deforming polyarthritis in the hands of *rheumatoid*, an asymmetrical arthritis and skin plaques of *psoriatic arthritis*, or podagra of the first MTP joint as seen in gout).

2 **Ask** the patient if they have any pain and expose the leg from the upper thigh to the foot.

3 **Inspect** the leg. Is there any obvious deformity (*valgus* or *varus* deformity or *flexion* deformity)? Are there any scars or wounds to suggest entry for infection? Is there any muscle wasting (*quadriceps*)? Is the knee swollen or erythematous? Look for loss of the medial and lateral dimples around the knees to suggest the presence of an effusion. Compare one side with the other as you progress through the examination.

4 **Palpate** the joint. Is it warm? Place your whole hand gently over the patient's knee and rest it there for a few seconds. Compare the temperature of this knee with the mid calf and mid thigh on the same side as well as the opposite knee. Do not be too quick to move your hands as you may miss subtle differences in temperature. Watch the patient's face for any sign that you are causing him/her discomfort. Ask if the knee is tender on palpation.

By this stage you should have an idea of whether this is an inflammatory or non-inflammatory problem and how active it is.

5 Examine for an **effusion**. For a small effusion look for the *bulge sign*. With your index finger, firmly wipe any fluid from the medial joint recess (moving from distal to proximal) into the lateral joint recess. Now apply a similar wiping motion from distal to proximal in the lateral joint recess. A distinct bulge will be seen to appear back in the medial compartment as the fluid moves back to this side of the joint. For larger effusions the bulge sign is absent and the presence of fluid needs to be assessed by the *patellar tap*. Firm pressure is applied over the suprapatellar pouch with the flat of one hand, using the thumb and index finger to push any fluid from the medial and lateral joint compartments into the retropatellar space. With the index finger or thumb of the other hand apply a short jerky movement to the patellar. The presence of significant fluid is indicated by a spongy feel followed by a 'tap' as the patellar hits the anterior aspect of the lower end of the femur.

6 Assess **movement**. Ask the patient to flex the knee as far as possible. Observe the degree of flexion (and any discomfort). Normal flexion is 135°.

7 Palpate for any **crepitus** over the joint as flexion occurs and feel behind the knee for a

8 **Baker's cyst.**

9 Assess for joint **instability**. Examine for *cruciate* instability (anterior and posterior draw test) and medial and lateral ligament instability. *McMurray's sign* can be used to examine for cartilage tears. The knee is fully flexed and then internally rotated before being straightened by the examiner. Pain or a clunking feeling over the knee joint suggests a cartilage tear. The test is repeated with external rotation of the knee.

10 Ask to examine the **other joints**. Do not forget to ask about examining the other knee and spine (for associated inflammatory spondylitis). Are there any features of *psoriasis, inflammatory bowel disease, reactive arthritis* (enthesitis, keratoderma blenorrhagica, conjunctivitis, balanitis) or tophi to suggest *gout*?

Finally, think of relevant *investigations* such as X-rays for changes of rheumatoid arthritis, osteoarthritis or pseudogout; synovial fluid analysis for crystals (negative or positive birefringence on polarized microscopy, gram stain and culture for infection).

For *checklist* see p. 530.

21 | 'Examine this patient's hip'

Station 5

Possible diagnoses

Osteoarthritis
Rheumatoid arthritis
Seronegative spondyloarthritis
   Ankylosing spondylitis
   Psoriatic arthritis
   Inflammatory bowel disease
   Reactive arthritis (chronic)
Septic arthritis
Avascular necrosis
Paget's
Iliopsoas bursitis
Sciatica.

Examination *routine*

1 **Inspect** the leg. Is the hip held in a flexed position? Is there any shortening of the leg? Is the leg externally rotated? Look for any scars. Are there any other obvious stigmata of rheumatic disease? Look for any walking aids.

2 **Ask** the patient if they have any pain. Ask them to show the location of the pain. Pain into the groin is more suggestive of hip disease.

3 Assess **movement**. With the patient lying flat and with their knee bent, ask them to flex their hip to the chest. Then, assess the degree of internal and external rotation. With both the knee and hip flexed to 90° rotate the hip joint internally and externally using the foot as a pointer and the knee as a pivot. Estimate the degree of rotation. Next, assess hip abduction and adduction by placing one hand on the opposite iliac crest (to keep the pelvis stationary) then, place your other hand under the ankle of the leg being examined and abduct and adduct the hip. The normal range of movement is flexion 120°, internal rotation 30°, external rotation 45°, abduction 60°, adduction 30°. A hip flexion deformity may be masked by an increased spinal lordosis. Flex the opposite hip (with knee bent) to flatten out the lumber lordosis (feel with your hand under the patient's spine). Any fixed flexion deformity of the opposite hip will be brought out by the flattening of the lumbar spine (*Thomas's test*).

4 If no abnormality is detected then consider whether the pain may be coming from the patient's spine. Carry out a **straight leg raise**. Slowly raise the patient's leg by taking

hold of their heel and lifting the leg slowly. Stop if pain occurs. Pain in the leg to the foot is indicative of pain originating in the *spine*—nerve root entrapment. You may need to undertake a *neurological assessment* to test for abnormalities in muscle strength (particularly of ankle plantar flexion), sensation or reflexes (be prepared to differentiate a nerve root from a peripheral nerve lesion).

5 Check for **tenderness** over the greater trochanter (trochanteric bursitis).

6 You may need to check for **leg length** inequality* (measure from the anterior superior iliac crest to the medial malleolus on the same side, compare with other leg).

7 Ask the patient to **walk**. An antalgic gait occurs when there is pain in one hip and the patient leans to the other side to avoid putting weight on the affected side. A waddling gait is indicative of hip muscle weakness (e.g. osteomalacia, myositis).

You would be interested to see X-rays of the pelvis. Consider what other investigations you would request for the conditions on the list above.

For *checklist* see p. 530.

22 | 'What is the diagnosis?'

Mostly station 5, but also stations 1 and 3
Variations of instruction in initial PACES survey (resultant diagnoses in brackets)
What is the diagnosis? (psoriasis)
This lady has had multiple fractures. What is your diagnosis? (?Turner's syndrome)
Examine this gentleman. What do you notice? (cushingoid due to steroids)
Examine this patient (peripheral and central cyanosis)
Look at this patient (acromegaly; scleroderma; drug eruption)
This woman has glycosuria. Look at her and examine anything that is relevant (acromegaly and xanthelasma)
This patient is tired all the time. Why is that? (koilonychia)
Examine this patient's spine (ankylosing spondylitis and aortic incompetence)
This lady has been having headaches. Please examine the appropriate systems (acromegaly)
Describe this lady's abnormalities (systemic sclerosis)
Look at this man and examine the patient as you feel appropriate (acromegaly)
This lady has had headaches. Please examine her (acromegaly)
You must know the diagnosis of this patient (neurofibromatosis)

---

* The reasons to examine for a shorter leg are: (i) for protrusio acetabulum, which occurs mainly in rheumatoid arthritis when the femoral head migrates through the acetabulum because of regional osteoporosis. (ii) Where there has been a fracture which has gone undetected at the neck of femur. (iii) When a patient has had a joint replacement (mainly hip, but knee also) where there has been a need to shorten the bone a bit more than the prosthesis allows. (iv) Where a Girdlestone procedure is carried out—when no hip joint prosthesis is placed (or removed) because of sepsis or patient's general health does not allow a major operation and, basically, the neck of the femur and femoral head are excised and the femur is held in place by the joint capsule, but migrates upwards. (v) Where there is apparent leg shortening which occurs due to pelvic tilt secondary to spinal disease—in this case the leg is not actually shortened hence the need to measure both leg lengths.

This lady complains of some abnormalities in her gums. Please examine her (lichen planus)

This lady has uncontrolled hypertension. Please examine her (pit tumour)

This middle-aged man complains of headaches. Would you like to assess him and tell me why? (acromegaly)

Have a look at this lady who presented to the A & E department with acute shortness of breath and tell me why (spontaneous pneumothorax due to tuberous sclerosis)

Look at the hands, look at the face and give the diagnosis (hypertrophic pulmonary osteoarthropathy)

What do you think of this lady? (cushingoid due to steroids).

Diagnoses from our original, pre PACES, survey in order of frequency

1 Acromegaly 11%
2 Parkinson's disease 5%
3 Hemiplegia 5%
4 Goitre 5%
5 Jaundice 5%
6 Myotonic dystrophy 4%
7 Pigmentation 4%
8 Graves' disease 4%
9 Exophthalmos 4%
10 Paget's disease 3%
11 Ptosis 3%
12 Choreoathetosis 3%
13 Drug-induced parkinsonism 3%
14 Breathlessness 2%
15 Purpura 2%
16 Hypopituitarism 2%
17 Addison's/Nelson's 2%
18 Cushing's syndrome 2%
19 Psoriasis 2%
20 Hypothyroidism 2%
21 Systemic sclerosis/CRST 2%
22 Sturge–Weber syndrome 2%
23 Spider naevi and ascites 1%
24 Marfan's syndrome 1%
25 Neurofibromatosis 1%
26 Cyanotic congenital heart disease 1%
27 Pretibial myxoedema 1%
28 Uraemia and dialysis scars 1%
29 Horner's syndrome 1%
30 Cachexia 1%
31 Osler–Weber–Rendu syndrome 1%
32 Ankylosing spondylitis 1%
33 Ulnar nerve palsy 1%
34 Turner's syndrome 1%
35 Down's syndrome 1%

36 Bilateral parotid enlargement/Mikulicz's syndrome 1%

37 Old rickets 1%

38 Torticollis 1%

39 Congenital syphilis 1%

40 Syringomyelia <1%

41 Herpes zoster <1%

42 Pemphigoid/pemphigus <1%

43 Bell's palsy <1%

44 Necrobiosis lipoidica diabeticorum <1%

45 Primary biliary cirrhosis <1%.

Examination *routine*

Advice commonly given by the candidates in our survey as a result of their Membership experiences was to 'keep calm'. When you stand before a patient with a condition from the above list and hear the instruction under consideration you are being asked to do what you do every day of your medical life. There are two differences, however, between everyday medical life and the examination: (i) the patients in the examination usually have classic, often florid, signs and should be easier to diagnose than most patients seen in the clinic; and (ii) in the examination, you may be overwhelmed by nerves and as a result make the most fundamental errors. You must indeed try to keep calm and remind yourself that this is likely to be an easy case, and that you will not only make a diagnosis (as you would with ease in the clinic), but will also find a way of scoring some extra marks. Unlike some of the instructions requiring long examination *routines*, the 'spot diagnosis' may be solved in seconds leaving time for something extra which you may be able to dictate, rather than leaving it to the examiner to lead. You should start with

1 *a visual survey* of the patient, running your eyes from the head via the neck, trunk, arms and legs to the feet, seeking the areas of abnormality, and thereby the diagnosis. We would suggest that you rehearse presenting the *records* for the various possibilities on the list (see individual short cases). If you are well prepared with the features of these short cases, then in the majority of instances you should be able to make a diagnosis, or likely diagnosis, which you can confirm or highlight by demonstrating additional features (see below). If you have scanned the patient briefly and not found any obvious abnormality, then

2 retrace the same ground scrutinizing each part more thoroughly and asking yourself at each stage, 'Is the head normal?', 'Is the face normal?', etc. If it is not normal describe the abnormality to yourself in the mind trying to match it up with one of the short case *records*. In this way cover the

(a) head (think especially of *Paget's* and *myotonic dystrophy* with frontal balding),

(b) face (think especially of *acromegaly*, *Parkinson's*, the facial asymmetry of *hemiplegia*, the long lean look of myotonic dystrophy, tardive dyskinesia, hypopituitarism, Cushing's, hypothyroidism, systemic sclerosis),

(c) eyes (*jaundice, exophthalmos*, ptosis, Horner's, xanthelasma),

(d) neck (*goitre*, Turner's, ankylosing spondylitis, torticollis),

(e) trunk (pigmentation, ascites, purpuric spots, spider naevi, wasting, pemphigus, etc.),

(f) arms (choreoathetosis, psoriasis, Addison's, spider naevi, syringomyelia),

(g) hands (acromegaly, *tremor*, clubbing, sclerodactyly, arachnodactyly, claw hand, etc.),

(h) legs (bowing, purpura, pretibial myxoedema, necrobiosis, lipoidica diabeticorum), and

(i) feet (pes cavus).

If you still do not have the diagnosis

3 specifically consider **abnormal colouring** such as *pigmentation, icterus* or pallor, and then cover the same ground again but in even more detail

4 **breaking down each part into its constituents**, scrutinizing them, and continually asking yourself the question: 'Is it normal?' This procedure is most profitable on the face (see p. 47).

Once you have the diagnosis, the natural impulse for most people is to give it in one word, and then stand back and wait for the applause. However, it is worth remembering that the majority of the candidates, who have all worked hard and prepared for the examination, are likely to 'spot' the diagnosis and yet only a few end up with the diploma. Do not let this opportunity pass you by; try to make more of the case yourself by proceeding to

5 look for **additional** and **associated features**, and then by making your presentation more elaborate. Describe the findings in detail (see individual short cases) and highlight the key features to support your diagnosis (lenticular abnormalities in myotonic dystrophy and Marfan's; thyroid bruit in Graves' disease; webbed neck in Turner's syndrome, and so on). It is worth going through the diagnoses on the list yourself, and considering what additional features you would look for, and how you could really go to town on an easy case. For example, if you diagnose acromegaly you could demonstrate the massive sweaty palms, commenting on the increased skin thickening and on the presence or absence of thenar wasting (carpal tunnel syndrome — see experience 8a, vol. 2, p. 327), and then proceed to test the visual fields. If you suspect Parkinson's disease, take the hands and test for cog-wheel rigidity at the wrist, demonstrate the glabellar tap sign (despite its unreliability) and then ask the patient to walk. If you diagnose hemiplegia, confirm that any facial weakness is upper motor neurone (see p. 184), and then check for atrial fibrillation. If you see a goitre, examine it and then assess the thyroid status.

For *checklist* see p. 530.

Section C
Short Case *Records*

*'Be professional in presentation. I agree it's an easy exam—it's easy to fail'.**

* Vol. 2, quotation 9, p. 369.

In this section we present aides-mémoire (clinical descriptions for presentation to the examiner) for over 200 short cases. We have called these aides-mémoire *records*. They are divided into the eight station subsections of the three clinical stations of PACES. The order in each subsection has been determined by the frequency with which, according to our surveys, these short cases have appeared in the PACES examination for that station. Thus short case no. 1 in a particular station subsection occurred most commonly, followed by short case no. 2 and so on. The percentages given represent our best estimate of your chance of meeting a particular short case in that station subsection in any one attempt at the MRCP PACES examination. Because our initial PACES survey has been relatively small, not all the short cases picked in our previous MRCP surveys have been picked up in that survey. We have in these cases extrapolated from the data in our previous, larger surveys to give an estimate of the likely chance of meeting the short case concerned. For most of the cases we are fairly confident that our estimates are in the right ballpark.

Nevertheless there is no doubt that the change to the PACES format has had an impact on the likelihood of meeting a small number of cases. For example, indeed the most extreme example, Paget's disease used to be a common short case in the old format and we estimated that if it occurred as commonly as it did previously and appeared in station 5, locomotor, it would be the second commonest in that station appearing with a frequency of 23% of attempts. Yet in our small PACES survey it did not occur at all. We suspect that this is because when examination centres are considering cases under the heading 'station 5, locomotor', they do not think immediately of Paget's disease as a possibility, i.e. Paget's disease does not have such an obvious home under the new PACES headings as it did in the short cases exam without headings. By contrast systemic sclerosis and psoriasis have obvious homes in both station 5, skin, *and* station 5, locomotor. It ends up that whereas in the old short cases exam there was an 11% chance of meeting systemic sclerosis in any one sitting this has now increased to 27% with PACES, and whereas there was an 11% chance of meeting psoriasis in any one sitting of the old short cases exam this has now increased to 23% with PACES. Our estimates range from diabetic retinopathy (41%) to pyoderma gangrenosum (0.2%) which means that on average you will see a diabetic fundus in two out of every five attempts at the MRCP PACES, but you may have to go through 500 attempts before you meet pyoderma gangrenosum!

Sometimes in the survey a particular short case was an additional feature of another short case. For example, a case of Graves' disease could also have a goitre, exophthalmos or pretibial myxoedema. With each short case we have pinpointed what the main focus was of that case. In the previous example, if the examiner asked for examination of the eyes, and all the attention was on the eyes, the main focus would be exophthalmos. If additional features (e.g. in this case goitre and pretibial myxoedema) were present, these were counted separately and the percentages for them are also given.* It cannot be overstressed that the first short cases we have dealt with in each station subsection occurred very commonly and the last very rarely, with all grades in between. The

* We believe that candidates did not always mention all the additional features in their reports to us. As an extreme example, not every candidate who reported meeting a case of mitral stenosis mentioned whether or not the pulse was irregular. Thus our appraisal of when 'irregular pulse' was an additional feature is likely to be an underestimate of its real frequency. Similarly ptosis was not always mentioned as being present in cases of Horner's syndrome or in association with a IIIrd nerve palsy. Consequently we believe that these 'additional features' figures tend to be underestimates.

implications for your priorities are obvious. There are those tempted to ignore the less common cases and, indeed a good case can be put — but it is a risky business (see footnote, p. 273).

It was the intention of the College that the headings of station 5 could be used loosely such that any short case, which could not readily find a home somewhere else, could be put in station 5. At the inception of PACES the College was keen that there should not be conditions previously tested in MRCP that would no longer be tested simply because they did not fall under the strict station 5 headings. We were told in a personal communication from the leading light in the establishment of PACES, Eric Beck, that the blue sclera of osteogenesis imperfecta might continue to appear in MRCP, by appearing in station 5. Thus we have included a small section, 'station 5, other', which incorporates some short cases which do not fit strictly under the four main station 5 headings.

It was very much the intention of the College in setting up station 5, eyes, that the eyes case would involve examining the fundus in all cases. It is clear from our survey that some centres have used eye cases without a fundus examination. There was even one candidate who was given two eye cases* and a total of five cases in the station (experience 19, vol. 2, p. 309). Whether the College will detect and clamp down on this remains to be seen but for now we have presented in this section the cases shown in our survey to occur and it is clear at present that you should be prepared to tackle any type of eye case in station 5, including all those covered under station 3, central nervous system.

In this section, the style of each *record* imagines you to be in the examination situation with the patient displaying the typical features of a particular condition; you are 'churning out' these to the examiner along with the answers to various anticipated questions. Thus, you play the *record* of the condition to the examiner. Of course the cases in the actual examination will only have some of the features (the *record* tends to describe the 'full house' case) and it is hoped that by becoming familiar with the whole *record* you will be well equipped:

1 to pick up all the features present in the cases you meet on the day by scanning through the *records* in your mind; and

2 to adapt the *record* for the purpose of presenting those features which are present.

To facilitate quick revision, the main points of each short case are highlighted in italics. The small print is a mixed bag of additional features and facts, lists of differential diagnoses and answers to some of the questions that might be asked. With the lists of differential diagnoses we have tended to put the most important ones (which you should consider first) in large print with longer lists in the small print. The lists are not necessarily meant to be comprehensive. Next to the diagnoses on these lists we have used brackets to give some of the features of the conditions concerned, or perhaps one or two features you could look for (indicated by?). The question mark is put there as a cue for you to look for important diagnostic features. We make no apology for repeating some of the features often, in the hope that by constant reinforcement they will become more firmly embedded in your memory. When unilateral signs could affect either side we have not usually specified the side in the *record* but have indicated this by R/L. In these cases, however, each R/L in the *record* refers to the

---

* See also experience 3, vol. 2, p. 287 — two skin cases!

same side. Also, . . . is occasionally used for a sign in the lung fields or retina which could occur in any zone or to indicate the size of an organ or sign where the size is unspecified.

Presentation to the examiner

Becoming familiar with the short case *records* will arm you for the examination, though obviously it will not always be necessary, or desirable, for you to use them. Sometimes it may be appropriate just to give the diagnosis — even so it may still be possible to enrich it with some of the well-known features from the *record*. If the examiner's question is: '*What is the diagnosis?*' you could answer 'Mitral stenosis' and await his reaction. On the other hand, if you are certain of your diagnosis, it would be better to say: 'The diagnosis is mitral stenosis because there is a rough, rumbling mid-diastolic murmur localized to the apex of the heart, there is a sharp opening snap and a loud first heart sound, a tapping impulse, an impalpable left ventricular apex, a left parasternal heave and a small volume pulse. Furthermore, the chaotic rhythm suggests atrial fibrillation and the patient has a malar flush.'

If you enlarge your response to 'What is the diagnosis?' by giving the features in this way, it is best to give the evidence in order of its importance to the diagnosis (as shown in the example). However, if the question is: '*What are your findings?*' it is best to give them in the order they are elicited: 'The patient has a malar flush and is slightly breathless at rest. The pulse is irregular in rate and volume. The jugular venous pressure is not elevated and the cardiac apex is not palpable but there is a tapping impulse parasternally on the left side and there is a left parasternal heave. The first heart sound is loud and there is an opening snap followed closely by a mid-diastolic rumble which is localized to the apex. These signs suggest that the patient has mitral stenosis.'

Remember, if you are talking in front of the patient, to avoid using words like 'cancer', 'motor neurone disease' and 'multiple sclerosis'. Use euphemisms such as 'neoplastic disease', 'anterior horn cell disease' and 'demyelinating disease'.

Remember that you can influence any discussion that follows by what you say. For example, the words: 'The diagnosis is aortic incompetence' may produce an interrogation by the examiner about anything he would like to ask you. However, if you say: 'He has aortic incompetence for which there are several causes', this invites the examiner to ask you the causes. It is, therefore, a good answer — as long as you know them!

Station 1
Respiratory

1 Interstitial lung disease (fibrosing alveolitis)
2 Pneumonectomy/lobectomy
3 Bronchiectasis
4 Dullness at the lung base
5 Chronic bronchitis and emphysema
6 Rheumatoid lung
7 Carcinoma of the bronchus
8 Old tuberculosis
9 Stridor
10 Kartagener's syndrome

11 Marfan's syndrome
12 Lung transplant
13 Chest infection/consolidation/pneumonia
14 Superior vena cava obstruction
15 Cor pulmonale
16 Obesity/pickwickian syndrome
17 Tuberculosis/apical consolidation
18 Pneumothorax
19 Cystic fibrosis
20 Normal chest

Case 1 | Interstitial lung disease (fibrosing alveolitis)

Frequency in survey: main focus of a short case in 21% of attempts at PACES station 1, respiratory. Additional feature in a further 2%.

Record

The patient is breathless on minimal exertion (and may be on long-term oxygen therapy). There is bilateral *clubbing* of the fingers. There is evidence of steroid purpura peripherally, (may be) *cyanosis*, reduced but symmetrical expansion of the chest (there may be dullness to percussion at the bases) and *fine inspiratory crackles* at the bases.

The likely diagnosis is diffuse interstitial lung fibrosis.

Causes of diffuse interstitial lung disease

Acute (less likely in the exam)
Vasculitis/haemorrhage (haemoptysis, falling haemoglobin)
Eosinophilic lung disease (drugs, fungi/parasites/ABPA)
Infection (immunosuppression)
ARDS (complicating acute severe illness often with septicaemia).

Chronic (more likely in the exam)
Cryptogenic fibrosing alveolitis* (most common cause is UIP (histological diagnosis) with insidious onset, dyspnoea and cough)
Rheumatoid lung disease (?hands, nodules)
Systemic sclerosis (?mask-like facies, telangiectasia, sclerodactyly—p. 280)
Systemic lupus erythematosus (?typical rash—p. 416)
Polymyositis (?proximal muscle weakness and tenderness—p. 415)
Dermatomyositis (?heliotrophic rash on eyes/hands and polymyositis—p. 288)
Sjögren's syndrome (?dry eyes and mouth)
Mixed connective tissue disease
Ankylosing spondylitis (?male with fixed kyphosis and stooped 'question mark' posture—p. 401)
Sarcoidosis (?extrapulmonary features, e.g. lupus pernio—p. 316)
Extrinsic allergic alveolitis (acute pulmonary and systemic symptoms occur 6 hours following inhaled allergen—?farmer, pigeon racer, etc.)
Asbestosis (?occupational history—lagger, etc.)
Silicosis (?occupational history—slate worker or granite quarrier, etc.)
Drug induced (e.g. bleomycin, busulphan, nitrofurantoin, amiodarone)
Radiation fibrosis
Chemical inhalation (e.g. beryllium, mercury)
Poison ingestion (e.g. paraquat)
ARDS.

---

*In the absence of an identifiable causal agent the fibrosing alveolitis is termed 'cryptogenic'. Occupational exposure to metal or wood dust is commoner in CFA patients than controls.

Case 2 | **Pneumonectomy/lobectomy**

Frequency in survey: main focus of a short case in 16% of attempts at PACES station 1, respiratory. Additional feature in a further 1%.

Survey note: some candidates had to discuss the chest X-ray of their pneumonectomy short case. It would usually show a 'white out' on one side, deviated trachea and compensatory hyperinflation on the other.

Record 1

There is a deformity of the chest with *flattening* on the R/L and a *thoracotomy scar* on that side. The trachea is *deviated* to the R/L and the apex beat is *displaced* in the same direction. On the R/L *expansion* is reduced, the percussion note is *dull* and the *breath sounds* are *diminished*. There is an area of bronchial breathing in the R/L upper zone (over the grossly deviated trachea).

These findings suggest a R/L pneumonectomy.

In the patient with lobectomy, as opposed to total pneumonectomy, the signs will be more confined. For example see *record* 2.

Record 2

There is a *deformity* of the chest with the left lower ribs *pulled in* and a left-sided *thoracotomy scar*. The *trachea* is central (may be displaced) but the *apex beat* is displaced to the left. The *percussion note is dull* over the left lower zone and *breath sounds* are *diminished* in this area.

These signs suggest a left lower lobectomy.

Surgical resection and the lung

Surgery has little role in the management of *small cell* carcinoma. In others, after a full assessment which includes clinical examination, lung function tests, bone and liver biochemistry, isotope bone scan, ultrasound or CT scan of the liver, mediastinal CT scan and, if necessary, mediastinoscopy, 25% of *non-small cell* lung cancers will be suitable for attempted surgical resection. The operative mortality for lobectomy is about 2–4% and this rises to about 6% for total pneumonectomy, which may be required if the tumour involves both divisions of a main bronchus or more than one lobe.

Surgical resection is often required for *solitary pulmonary nodules* of uncertain cause. The possibility

of undiagnosed small cell cancer in this instance is not necessarily a reason for avoiding thoracotomy; resection of small cell lung cancer presenting as a solitary pulmonary nodule may have a 5-year survival comparable to that of other forms of nodular bronchogenic carcinoma treated surgically (approximately 25%).

Surgical resection is indicated in the treatment of *bronchiectasis* (p. 75) when other forms of treatment have failed to control symptoms, particularly if it is localized and if recurrent haemoptysis is present.

In the days before antituberculous chemotherapy, tuberculosis was sometimes treated surgically—p. 83.

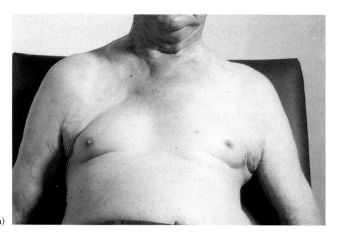

(a)

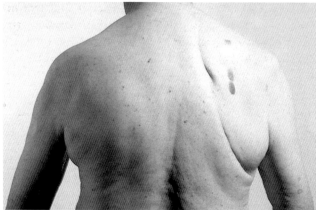

(b)

Figure C1.1 (a) Deformity of the right chest with flattening. (b) Right-sided thoracotomy scar on the back.

Case 3 | Bronchiectasis

Frequency in survey: main focus of a short case in 12% of attempts at PACES station 1, respiratory. Additional feature in a further 3%.

Record

This patient (who may be rather *underweight, breathless* and *cyanosed*) has *clubbing* of the fingers (not always present) and a frequent *productive cough* (the patient may cough in your presence;* there may be a *sputum pot* by the bed). There are (may be) *inspiratory clicks* heard with the unaided ear. There are *crepitations* over the . . . zone(s) (the area(s) where the bronchiectasis is) and (may be) widespread *rhonchi*.

The diagnosis could well be bronchiectasis. The frequent productive cough and inspiratory clicks are in favour of this. Other possibilities (clubbing and crepitations) are:

1 Carcinoma of the lung (?heavy nicotine staining, lymph nodes, etc.)
2 Fibrosing alveolitis* (marked sputum production and clicks are against this)
3 Lung abscess.

Possible causes of bronchiectasis

Respiratory infection in childhood (especially whooping cough, measles, TB)

Cystic fibrosis (young, thin patient, may have malabsorption and steatorrhoea, p. 101)

Bronchial obstruction due to foreign body, carcinoma, granuloma (tuberculosis, sarcoidosis) or lymph nodes (e.g. tuberculosis)

Fibrosis (complicating tuberculosis, unresolved or suppurative pneumonia with lung abscess, mycotic infections or sarcoidosis)

Hypogammaglobulinaemia (congenital and acquired)

Allergic bronchopulmonary aspergillosis (proximal airway bronchiectasis)

Marfan's syndrome (?tall, long extremities, high arched palate, p. 156)

Yellow nail syndrome (?excessively curled yellow nails with bulbous fingertips; lymphoedema of extremities, p. 304)

Congenital disorders such as sequestrated lung segments, bronchial atresia and Kartagener's syndrome†

Associated with smoking-related chronic obstructive pulmonary disease (COPD).‡

---

* It is worth asking the patient to 'give a cough' as it may help you differentiate brochiectasis from fibrosing alveolitis.

† The features of Kartagener's syndrome are dextrocardia, situs inversus, infertility, dysplasia of frontal sinuses, sinusitis and otitis media. Patients have ciliary immotility.

‡ The majority of bronchiectasis patients seen in chest clinics nowadays have no obvious cause but also have COPD from smoking. One study showed that a distinct proportion of COPD patients (up to 30%) also have bronchiectasis (as confirmed by CT).

Case 4 | Dullness at the lung base

Frequency in survey: main focus of a short case in 10% of attempts at PACES station 1, respiratory. Additional feature in a further 3%.

Record
The pulse is regular and the venous pressure is not elevated. The trachea is central,* the expansion is normal, but the percussion note is *stony dull* at the R/L base(s), with *diminished* tactile *fremitus* and vocal *resonance*, and *diminished breath sounds*. There is (may be) an area of bronchial breathing above the area of dullness.

The diagnosis is R/L pleural effusion.†

Causes of pleural effusion
Exudate (protein content >30 g l⁻¹)‡

Bronchial carcinoma (?evidence staining, clubbing, radiation burns on chest, lymph nodes)

Secondary malignancy (?evidence of primary especially breast, lymph nodes, radiation burns)

Pulmonary embolus and infarction (?DVT; blood-stained fluid will be found at aspiration)

Pneumonia (bronchial breathing/crepitations, fever, etc.)

Tuberculosis

Mesothelioma (asbestos worker, ?clubbing)

Rheumatoid arthritis (?hands and nodules)

Systemic lupus erythematosus (?typical rash)

Lymphoma (?nodes and spleen).

Transudate (protein content <30 g l⁻¹)

Cardiac failure (?JVP ↑, ankle and sacral oedema, large heart, tachycardia, S_3 or signs of a valvular lesion)

Nephrotic syndrome (?generalized oedema, patient may be young — p. 131)

Cirrhosis (?ascites, generalized oedema, signs of chronic liver disease — p. 106)

Other causes of pleural effusion
Meigs' syndrome (ovarian fibroma)

Subphrenic abscess (?recent abdominal disease or surgery)

Peritoneal dialysis

Hypothyroidism (?facies, pulse, ankle jerks)

Pancreatitis (more common on the left; fluid has high amylase)

---

* The trachea may be deviated if the effusion is very large. A large effusion without any mediastinal shift (clinically and on chest X-ray) raises the possibility of collapse as well as effusion.

† On your initial inspection there may be biopsy or aspiration needle marks, or the marks of a sticking plaster removed by the invigilator at the beginning of the day, as a clue that you are going to find a pleural effusion.

‡ Although the protein content >30 g l⁻¹ is not necessarily 100% sensitive and specific, it is still the most simple way of dividing exudate from transudate. Also, in exudates, the fluid to serum protein ratio is usually greater than 0.5, with a LDH of >200 IU and a fluid to serum LDH ratio of >0.6.

Dressler's syndrome (recent myocardial infarction, ?pericardial friction rub)

Trauma

Asbestos exposure

Yellow nail syndrome (yellowish-brown beaked nails usually associated with lymphatic hypoplasia, see p. 304)

Chylothorax (trauma or blockage of a major intra-thoracic lymphatic — usually by a neoplastic process).

Other causes of dullness at a lung base

Raised hemidiaphragm (e.g. hepatomegaly, phrenic nerve palsy)

Basal collapse

Collapse/consolidation (if the airway is blocked by, for example, a carcinoma there may be no bronchial breathing)

Pleural thickening (e.g. old TB or old empyema or asbestos induced with or without mesothelioma)

Pleural biopsy

Biopsy is carried out using an 'Abram's biopsy needle'. The specificity for detecting TB and malignancy is better with a pleural biopsy than with a pleural aspiration on its own. Remember that any biopsies for TB cultures should be placed in normal saline and not formalin.

Thoracoscopy

This is a technique involving visual inspection of the pleural cavity for diagnostic and therapeutic purposes (e.g. pleurodesis).

Case 5 | Chronic bronchitis and emphysema*

Frequency in survey: main focus of a short case in 8% of attempts at PACES station 1, respiratory. Additional feature in a further 2%.

Survey note: usually the patients in the examination fall between the extremes of the classical *records* below.

Record 1

This thin man (with an anxious, drawn expression) presents the classic 'pink puffer' appearance. He has *nicotine staining* of the fingers. He is tachypnoeic at rest with *lip pursing* during expiration, which is *prolonged*. The suprasternal notch to cricoid distance is reduced (a sign of hyperinflation; normally >3 finger breadths). His chest is *hyperinflated, expansion* is mainly *vertical* and there is a *tracheal tug*. He uses his *accessory muscles* of respiration at rest and there is *indrawing* of the *lower ribs* on inspiration (due to a flattened diaphragm). The percussion note is hyper-resonant, obliterating cardiac and hepatic dullness, and the breath sounds are quiet (this is so in classic pure emphysema—frequently, though, wheezes are heard due to associated bronchial disease).

These are the physical findings of a patient with emphysema (inspiratory drive often intact).†

Record 2

This (male) patient (who smokes, lives in a foggy city, works amid dust and fumes, and has probably had frequent respiratory infections) presents the classic 'blue bloater' appearance. He has *nicotine staining* on the fingers. He is stocky and *centrally cyanosed* with suffused conjunctivae. His chest is *hyperinflated*, he uses his *accessory muscles* of respiration; there is *indrawing* of the *intercostal muscles* on inspiration and there is a *tracheal tug* (both signs of hyperinflation). His pulse is 80/min, the venous pressure is not elevated (may be raised with ankle oedema and hepatomegaly if cor pulmonale is present), the trachea is central, but the suprasternal notch to cricoid distance is reduced. *Expansion* is equal but *reduced* to 2 cm and the percussion note is resonant; on auscultation the expiratory phase is prolonged and he has widespread *expiratory rhonchi* and (may be) coarse inspiratory crepitations. (His forced expiratory time—p. 20—is 8 seconds.) There is no flapping tremor of the hands (unless he is in severe hypercapnoeic respiratory failure in which case ask to examine the fundi—?papilloedema).

These are the physical findings of advanced chronic bronchitis‡ (inspiratory drive often reduced) producing chronic small airways obstruction (and, if ankle oedema, etc., right heart failure due to cor pulmonale).

---

* Chronic obstructive pulmonary disease (COPD), which encompasses both chronic bronchitis and emphysema, includes the criteria of an obstructive spirometry (i.e. one can have chronic bronchitis only without an obstructive spirometry and hence such a person technically does not have COPD but only chronic bronchitis).

† Emphysema is, however, a pathological diagnosis.
‡ Chronic bronchitis, though, is defined as sputum production (not due to specific disease such as bronchiectasis or TB) on most days for 3 months of the year on 2 consecutive years.

Causes of emphysema

Smoking (usually associated with chronic bronchitis; mixed centrilobular and panacinar)

Alpha-1 antitrypsin deficiency (?young patient; lower zone emphysema, panacinar in type; ?icterus, hepatomegaly, etc. of hepatitis or cirrhosis)

Coal dust (centrilobular emphysema—simple coal worker's pneumoconiosis—only minor abnormalities of gas exchange)

Macleod's (Swyer–James) syndrome—rare (unilateral emphysema following childhood bronchitis and bronchiolitis with subsequent impairment of alveolar growth; breath sounds diminished on affected side—more likely to meet this in the 'pictures' section of MRCP Part 2 written examination).

Record 1 (continuation)

The decreased breath sounds over the . . . zone of the R/L lung of this patient with emphysema raises the possibility of an emphysematous bulla.

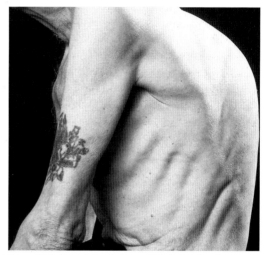

Figure C1.2 Hyperinflated rib cage. Note indrawing of intercostal muscles.

Case 6 | Rheumatoid lung

Frequency in survey: main focus of a short case in 8% of attempts at PACES station 1, respiratory.

Record

There is (maybe) cyanosis (there may also be dyspnoea) and the principal finding in the chest is of *fine inspiratory crackles* (or crepitations — whichever term you prefer) on auscultation at both bases.

In view of the *rheumatoid* changes (p. 384) in the *hands* (there may also be clubbing), the likely diagnosis is fibrosing alveolitis associated with rheumatoid disease (rheumatoid lung).

Classic fibrosing alveolitis develops in 2%* of patients with rheumatoid arthritis and has a poor prognosis. It may progress to a honeycomb appearance on chest X-ray, bronchiectasis, chronic cough and progressive dyspnoea. Pulmonary function tests show reduced diffusion capacity, diminished compliance and a restrictive ventilatory pattern.

Gold, used in the therapy of rheumatoid arthritis, can also induce interstitial lung disease; it is indistinguishable from rheumatoid fibrosing alveolitis except that the gold-induced disease may reverse when the drug is discontinued.

Other pulmonary manifestations of rheumatoid disease

Pleural disease† Though frequently found at autopsy, rheumatoid pleural disease is usually asymptomatic. The rheumatoid patient may have a pleural rub or pleural effusion but only occasionally would the latter be of sufficient size to cause respiratory limitation. The pleural fluid at diagnostic aspiration is never blood stained and often contains immune complexes and rheumatoid factor; it is high in protein (exudate) and LDH and low in glucose, C3 and C4. The white count in the pleural fluid is variable but usually < 5000/μl.

Intrapulmonary nodules. Single or multiple radiological nodules may be seen in the lung parenchyma before or after the onset of arthritis. They are usually asymptomatic but may become infected and cavitate. As they have a predilection for the upper lobes and can cause haemoptysis, they can resemble tuberculosis or even carcinoma. They can rupture into the pleural space causing a pneumothorax. Massive confluent pulmonary nodules may be seen in rheumatoid lungs in association with pneumoconiosis (*Caplan's syndrome*).

Obliterative bronchiolitis. Rarely, small airways obstruction may develop into a necrotizing bronchiolitis, classically associated with dyspnoea, hyperinflation and a high-pitched expiratory wheeze or 'squawk' on auscultation. This complication may also result from therapy with gold or penicillamine.

Two other manifestations are *pulmonary arteritis* (reminiscent of polyarteritis nodosa) and *apical fibrobullous disease.*

---

* Though fibrosing alveolitis becomes overt in only 2% of patients, 25% of patients with rheumatoid arthritis show interstitial changes on chest X-ray and 50% have reduced diffusion capacity, suggesting that subclinical fibrosing alveolitis is common. There is no relationship between the extent of lung disease and the titre of rheumatoid factor.

† Though our surveys have not thrown up a case of pleural effusion and rheumatoid hands, it would nevertheless be worth a glance at the hands of a patient with a pleural effusion for possible rheumatoid changes as well as for the clubbing.

Case 7· | **Carcinoma of the bronchus**

Frequency in survey: did not occur in the initial small survey of PACES station 1, respiratory.

Predicted frequency from older, more extensive MRCP short case surveys: main focus of a short case in 8% of attempts at PACES station 1, respiratory. Additional feature in a further 6%.

Survey note: candidates reported a variety of signs. The three *records* given are typical.

Record 1

There is *clubbing* of the fingers which are *nicotine-stained*. There is a hard *lymph node* in the R/L supraclavicular fossa. The pulse is 80/min and regular, and the venous pressure is not raised. The trachea is central, chest expansion normal, but the percussion note is *stony dull* at the R/L base and *tactile fremitus, vocal resonance* and *breath sounds* are all *diminished* over the area of dullness.

 The likely diagnosis is carcinoma of the bronchus causing a *pleural effusion*.

Record 2

The patient is *cachectic*. There is a *radiation burn* on the R/L upper chest wall. There is *clubbing* of the fingers which are *nicotine-stained*. The pulse is 80/min, venous pressure is not elevated and there are no lymph nodes. The *trachea* is *deviated* to the R/L and *expansion* of the R/L upper chest is *diminished*. *Tactile vocal fremitus* and *resonance* are *increased* over the upper chest where the *percussion note* is *dull* and there is an area of *bronchial breathing*.

 It is likely that this patient has had radiotherapy for carcinoma of the bronchus which is causing *collapse* and *consolidation of the R/L upper lung*.

Record 3

There is a *radiation burn* on the chest. There are *lymph nodes* palpable in the R/L axilla. The trachea is central. I did not detect any abnormality in expansion, vocal fremitus, vocal resonance or breath sounds, but there is *wasting* of the *small muscles* of the R/L *hand*, and *sensory loss* (plus pain) over the T1*dermatome. There is a R/L *Horner's syndrome* (p.232).

 The diagnosis is *Pancoast's syndrome* (due to an apical carcinoma of the lung involving the lower brachial plexus and the cervical sympathetic nerves).

Other complications of carcinoma of the bronchus

1 Other local effects such as:

Superior vena cava obstruction (?oedema of the face and upper extremities, suffusion of eyes, fixed engorgement of neck veins and dilatation of superficial veins, etc. — p. 90)

Stridor (often associated with superior vena cava obstruction; dysphagia may occur)

2 Metastases and their effects (pain, ?hepatomegaly, neurological signs, etc.)

*The weakness, sensory loss and especially pain may be more widespread (C8,T1,2).

3 Non-metastatic effects such as:

Hypertrophic pulmonary osteoarthropathy (?clubbing plus pain and swelling of wrists and/or ankles — subperiosteal new bone formation on X-ray)

Neuropathy (peripheral neuropathy — sensory, motor or mixed; cerebellar degeneration and encephalopathy; proximal myopathy, polymyositis, dermatomyositis, reversed myasthenia — Eaton–Lambert syndrome)

Endocrine (inappropriate antidiuretic hormone, ectopic ACTH, ectopic parathormone or para-thormone-related peptide,* carcinoid)

Gynaecomastia (if rapidly progressive and painful may be due to a HCG-secreting tumour)

Thrombophlebitis migrans (?DVT)

Non-bacterial thrombotic endocarditis

Anaemia (usually normoblastic; occasionally leucoery-throblastic from bone marrow involvement)

Pruritus

Herpes zoster (p. 342)

Acanthosis nigricans (grey–brown/dark brown areas in the axillae and limb flexures, in which skin becomes thickened, rugose and velvety with warts — p. 374)

Erythema gyratum repens (irregular wavy bands with a serpiginous outline and marginal desquamation on the trunk, neck and extremities).

Record 4 (lobectomy)

There is a R/L *thoracotomy scar*. The *trachea* is *deviated* to the R/L. On the R/L side *chest expansion* is *diminished*, percussion note more resonant and breath sounds are harsher. The patient has had a R/L lobectomy to remove a tumour, resistant lung abscess or localized area of bronchiectasis.

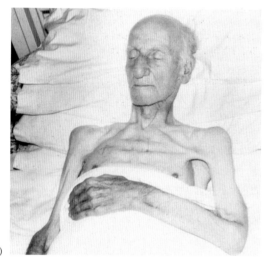

(a)

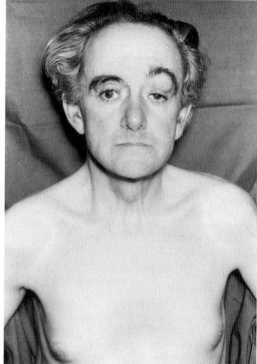

(b)

Figure C1.3 (a) Cachexia due to carcinoma of the bronchus (note radiotherapy ink marks). (b) Pancoast's tumour (note gynaecomastia and left Horner's syndrome).

* Hypercalcaemia may also be due to bone secondaries.

Case 8 | **Old tuberculosis**

Frequency in survey: main focus of a short case in 6% of attempts at PACES station 1, respiratory.

Record 1

The trachea is *deviated* to the R/L. The R/L upper chest shows *deformity* with *decreased expansion, dull percussion* note, *bronchial breathing* and *crepitations*. The apex beat is (may be) *displaced* to the R/L. There is a *thoracotomy scar* posteriorly with evidence of rib resections.

The patient has had a R/L thoracoplasty for treatment of tuberculosis before the days of chemotherapy.

Record 2

The tracheal deviation to the R/L and the diminished expansion and crackles at the R/L apex suggest R/L apical fibrosis.

Old tuberculosis is the likely cause.

Record 3

Expansion is diminished on the R/L with dullness and reduced/absent breath sounds at the R/L lung base. There is a R/L supraclavicular scar (there may also be crepitations).

The patient has had a phrenic nerve crush for TB before the days of chemotherapy.

Case 9 | **Stridor**

Frequency in survey: main focus of a short case in 4% of attempts at PACES station 1, respiratory.

Record

The patient is comfortable at rest. From the *bedside* I can hear a noisy, *high pitched sound* with each inspiration. Her respiratory rate is 12/min. Chest expansion is normal, resonance is normal and auscultation reveals *normal vesicular breath sounds* and no added sounds. There is (maybe) a *healed tracheostomy scar* present.

In view of the tracheostomy scar it is likely that the inspiratory stridor is due to tracheal stenosis following prolonged ventilatory support via a tracheostomy.

Inspiratory stridor usually implies upper airways obstruction and tracheal narrowing (extrathoracic).

Causes of inspiratory stridor

1 Acute (infective epiglottitis, croup)
2 Trauma (foreign body, smoke inhalation)
3 Chronic (neoplastic, tracheal stenosis).

Expiratory stridor is usually found with lower intrathoracic obstruction.

Causes of expiratory stridor

1 Foreign body
2 Intraluminal mass/neoplasm
3 Lower tracheal stenosis
4 Bronchial stenosis.

Causes of tracheal stenosis

1 Congenital (webs, tracheomalacia), *or*
2 Acquired (tracheostomy or intubation)
3 Post trauma, *or*
4 Post infections (e.g. TB)
5 Neoplastia.

Management would include referral to thoracic surgeon who would consider rigid bronchoscopy with possible dilatation and/or stent insertion. Primary reconstruction may be considered as definitive treatment.

Case 10 | Kartagener's syndrome

Frequency in survey: main focus of a short case in 2% of attempts at PACES station 1, respiratory.

Record

This patient (who may be rather *underweight, breathless* and *cyanosed*) has *clubbing* of the fingers (not always present) and a frequent *productive cough* (the patient may cough in your presence;* there may be a *sputum pot* by the bed). There are (may be) *inspiratory clicks* heard with the unaided ear. There are *crepitations* over the . . . zone(s) (the area(s) where the bronchiectasis is) and (may be) widespread *rhonchi*.

The apex beat is *not palpable on the left side*, and the heart sounds can barely be heard there but can be heard instead on the *right* side. The patient has dextrocardia.†

The findings in the chest are in keeping with bronchiectasis and this in association with dextrocardia suggests that the diagnosis is Kartagener's syndrome.

Features of Kartagener's syndrome

1 Dextrocardia
2 Bronchiectasis
3 Situs inversus
4 Infertility
5 Dysplasia of frontal sinuses
6 Sinusitis
7 Otitis media.

Patients with Kartagener's syndrome have ciliary immmotility.

---

* It is worth asking the patient to 'give a cough' as it may help you differentiate bronchiectasis from fibrosing alveolitis.
† Consider the possibility of this diagnosis if you cannot feel the apex beat and then have difficulty hearing the heart sounds. As you gradually move the stethoscope towards the right side of the chest, they get louder.

Case 11 | **Marfan's syndrome**

Frequency in survey: main focus of a short case in 2% of attempts at PACES station 1, respiratory.

Survey note: see experience 10, vol. 2, p. 298.

Marfan's syndrome is dealt with on p. 407.

Case 12 | Lung transplant

Frequency in survey: main focus of a short case in 2% of attempts at PACES station 1, respiratory.

Record 1

This *young* man (who has had a *major operative procedure* for a *severe chronic respiratory problem*) is not breathless at rest. His respiratory rate is 12/min. He is bilaterally clubbed. He has a *mid-sternotomy scar*. Expansion is equal and normal both sides. Percussion is normal and *breath sounds* are *vesicular* with no added sounds in both lungs.

In view of his age I suspect that the chronic respiratory problem requiring a surgical procedure was cystic fibrosis and I suspect that he has had a double lung transplantation that has been successful.

Record 2

This middle-aged man (who had a right lung transplant and has been increasingly breathless in recent months) has an *increased respiratory rate* of 18/min. He is taking *oxygen* $2 \, \text{l min}^{-1}$ via nasal cannulae. He is bilaterally clubbed. He has features of *Cushing's* syndrome. There is a *right thoracotomy scar*. He has reduced expansion in both lungs. The left base is dull to percussion. There are fine inspiratory crackles to the mid-zones in the left lung and a few scattered *inspiratory squeaks* in the right lung.

The findings in the left lung suggest that the lung transplant was for pulmonary fibrosis. It may be that he has had recurrent episodes of acute rejection during recent months and has now developed bronchiolitis obliterans syndrome (BOS) for which he takes large doses of steroids and is on continuous oxygen therapy. (He will have a spirometry recording book to demonstrate the fall in FEV_1 and FVC over the last 12 months and may be on the active retransplant list — look for the bleeper.)

Indications for lung transplantation

1 Pulmonary vascular: primary pulmonary hypertension, pulmonary hypertension secondary to systemic disease and Eisenmenger's syndrome
2 Restrictive pulmonary diseases: idiopathic pulmonary fibrosis, fibrosis secondary to connective tissue disease, sarcoidosis and chronic allergic alveolitis
3 Obstructive diseases: emphysema with or without α_1-antitrypsin deficiency, Langerhan's cell granulomatosis and lymphangioleiomyomatosis
4 Suppurative disease including cystic fibrosis and bronchiectasis.

Complications of lung transplantation

1 Perioperative, e.g. dehiscence of graft
2 Infection: viral, especially cytomegalovirus, but also herpes simplex; bacterial; fungal — *Candida*, *Aspergillus*; other opportunistic infections, e.g. pneumocystis
3 Rejection: may be hyperacute (within hours) or acute — most patients experience one or two episodes during the first 6 months. *Bronchiolitis obliterans syndrome* is progressive airways obstruction with rapid progression and poor survival. Acute rejection

is a major prognostic factor. It is characterized by non-productive cough, dyspnoea and malaise. Pulmonary function shows irreversible airflow obstruction, reduced total lung capacity and gas transfer. No effective treatment is available. A regimen of immunosuppressives is commonly employed. Retransplantation may be considered.

4 Side effects of drugs, e.g. azathioprine, cyclosporin, corticosteroids.

Case 13 | Chest infection/consolidation/pneumonia

Frequency in survey: main focus of a short case in 1% of attempts at PACES station 1, respiratory. Additional feature in many others (carcinoma of the bronchus and old tuberculosis—pp. 81 and 83).

Record

There is reduced movement of the R/L side of the chest. There is *dullness* to percussion over . . . (describe where) with *bronchial breathing, coarse crepitations, whispering pectoriloquy* and a *pleural friction rub.*

These features suggest consolidation (say where).

Commonest causes of consolidation

Bacterial pneumonia (pyrexia, purulent sputum, haemoptysis, breathlessness)

Carcinoma (with infection behind the tumour; ?clubbing, wasting, etc.—p. 81)

Pulmonary infarction (fever less prominent, sputum mucoid, occasionally haemoptysis and blood-stained pleural effusion).

Causes of community acquired pneumonia

Streptococcus pneumoniae
Haemophilus influenzae
Mycoplasma pneumoniae
Influenza A
Chlamydia pneumoniae
Legionella species
Other viruses.

Case 14 | Superior vena cava obstruction

Frequency in survey: did not occur in the initial small survey of PACES station 1, respiratory.

Predicted frequency from older, more extensive MRCP short case surveys: main focus of a short case in 3% of attempts at PACES station 1, respiratory.

Record

There is stridor. The face and upper extremities are *oedematous* (puffy) and *cyanosed*, and the eyes are *suffused*. The *superficial veins* over these areas are *dilated* and there is *fixed engorgement* of the *neck veins*. The undersurface of the tongue is covered with multiple venous angiomata. There is (may be) a radiation burn on the chest wall.

The diagnosis is superior vena cava obstruction, most likely due to carcinoma* of the bronchus, particularly small cell carcinoma (?lymph nodes, chest signs, clubbing, etc. — p. 81). It has been treated by radiotherapy.†

The patient may complain of headaches (may be severe on coughing), difficulty in breathing, dysphagia, dizziness or blackouts. Physical signs are frequently absent or minimal.

Other causes of superior vena cava obstruction

Lymphoma
Aortic aneurysm
Mediastinal fibrosis
Mediastinal goitre.

---

* The compression may either be by the tumour or by involved lymph nodes.

† Radiotherapy, or chemotherapy, is required urgently in this condition. A stent can sometimes be placed in the superior vena cava as a palliative procedure. Dexamethasone is also used.

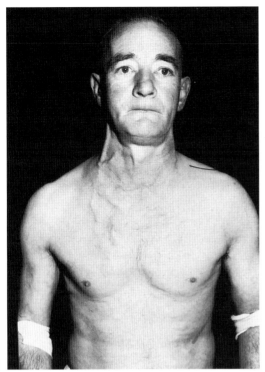

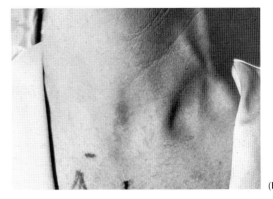

(a)

(b)

Figure C1.4 (a, b) Superior vena cava obstruction. Note the radiotherapy ink marks in (b).

Case 15 | **Cor pulmonale**

Frequency in survey: did not occur in the initial small survey of PACES station 1, respiratory.

Predicted frequency from older, more extensive MRCP short case surveys: main focus of a short case in 2% of attempts at PACES station 1, respiratory.

Record

The patient's fingers are *nicotine-stained* and there is *central cyanosis*. There is (may be) *finger clubbing* (if associated with pulmonary fibrosis). The pulse is regular, the *venous pressure is raised* (give height) with prominent small *a* waves and giant *v* waves (if there is secondary tricuspid incompetence), and there is *ankle* and *sacral oedema*. *Expiration is prolonged and noisy*. The *accessory muscles* of respiration are in use at rest, and there is a *tracheal tug*. The trachea is central, expansion is equal, the percussion note is resonant, and tactile fremitus and vocal resonance are normal. There is a *left parasternal heave* and a palpable second heart sound* (?pansystolic murmur of tricuspid incompetence (rare)). The heart sounds are often difficult to hear due to hyperexpansion of the lungs. There are (may be) widespread *expiratory rhonchi* and coarse inspiratory crepitations and the forced expiratory time (see p. 20) is 8 seconds. (There is no *flapping tremor* of the hands—if there were you would want to examine the fundi for papilloedema.)

These findings suggest cor pulmonale due to chronic bronchitis and emphysema. (Right heart failure is often precipitated by acute infection.)

The auscultatory cardiac signs of pulmonary hypertension, some of which may be audible,* are:

Loud pulmonary second sound

Pulmonary early systolic ejection click

Right ventricular fourth heart sound

Pansystolic murmur of functional tricuspid incompetence (giant *v* waves)

Early diastolic murmur of functional pulmonary incompetence (Graham Steell murmur).

Causes of pulmonary hypertension

COPD (with or without emphysema; by far the commonest cause—p. 78)

Recurrent pulmonary emboli (signs of pulmonary hypertension without clinical evidence of other lung disease; ?DVT)

Primary pulmonary hypertension (signs of pulmonary hypertension without clinical evidence of other lung disease; usually a female)

Non-pulmonary causes of alveolar hypoventilation (kyphoscoliosis, obesity (p. 94), neuromuscular weakness).

Lung diseases which only occasionally result in cor pulmonale including:

Progressive massive fibrosis (?coal dust tattoos on the skin; chronic bronchitis is the commonest cause of cor pulmonale in miners)

Bronchiectasis (especially cystic fibrosis; ?clubbing,

---

* These findings, which may be prominent in cor pulmonale due to other causes, may be difficult to elicit in cor pulmonale where a barrel-shaped chest and hyperinflation are present, and the heart is enfolded by overinflated lungs.

cyanosis, full sputum pot, productive cough, crepitations — p. 75)

Cryptogenic fibrosing alveolitis (?clubbing, cyanosis, basal crackles — p. 72)

Systemic sclerosis (hands, facies — p. 280)

Sarcoidosis (?lupus pernio — p. 316)

Asthma (severe and chronic; may be missed if the reversibiliy is not checked in chronic small airways obstruction).

Case 16 | Obesity/Pickwickian syndrome

Frequency in survey: did not occur in the initial small survey of PACES station 1, respiratory.

Predicted frequency from older, more extensive MRCP short case surveys: main focus of a short case in 1% of attempts at PACES station 1, respiratory.

Survey note: most cases revolved around features of the Pickwickian syndrome, though there was one case with an apronectomy scar and small testes in which Klinefelter's was suggested.

Record

The patient is *massively obese* and *cyanosed*. He has rapid and shallow breathing, his *venous pressure is elevated* and there is *ankle oedema*.

These features suggest *cor pulmonale* secondary to the extreme obesity—the pickwickian syndrome.*

Respiratory problems associated with obesity

Severe obesity leads to increased demand for ventilation, increased breathing workload, respiratory muscle inefficiency, decreased functional reserve capacity and expiratory reserve volume. There is alveolar hypoventilation and reduced ventilatory sensitivity to CO_2. Peripheral lung units can close, resulting in a ventilation–perfusion mismatch. The overall result is chronic hypoxaemia with cyanosis and hypercapnia; the end-stage is the *Pickwickian syndrome* in which nocturnal obstructive apnoea† and hypoventilation are so marked that the patient can only have undisturbed sleep when upright (more usually sitting than standing as in the original description!*), often in the daytime.

Pulmonary hypertension occurs, there are usually morning headaches and impotence and there may be polycythaemia. Eventually cardiac failure supervenes.

Sleep apnoea is very common in the severely obese. The most obese are not necessarily the most severely affected. It may be obstructive or central.† Daytime somnolence is common and is partly due to the hypoxia and partly from the continual disturbance of sleep at night—the patient tends to wake after each episode of sleep apnoea (cessation of breathing for 10 seconds or longer).

Body mass index (BMI) = weight (kg)/height (m)^2. As a rule of thumb, health risks increase as BMI increases above 25; however, BMI normally increases with age and one study found that the BMI associated with the lowest mortality was approximately: 19.5 at age 20, 21 at age 30, 22.5 at age 40, 24.5 at age 50, nearly 26 at age 60 and 27.5 at age 70.

---

* The term is derived from the character in Charles Dickens' *Pickwick Papers* and was first applied by Osler. The character, Joe, kept beating the door even after hearing a response from inside the room, because if he stopped, he would fall asleep standing on his feet! (See *American Journal of Medicine* 1956, **21**: 811—18 to read Dickens' wonderful description.)

† *Obstructive sleep apnoea*—the upper pharyngeal cavity collapses due to the negative intrathoracic pressure and the process is aided by a short neck and large accumulations of fat often in combination with micrognathia and enlarged tonsils. There are vigorous thoracoabdominal movements but no air entry into the lungs. The obstruction leads to hypoventilation and hypoxia which somehow trigger apnoeic episodes making the hypoxia and hypercapnia worse. Weight loss and sometimes surgical removal of the obstructive tissues may help.

Central sleep apnoea—cessation of ventilatory drive from the brain centres so that diaphragmatic excursions stop for periods of 10–30 seconds. There are no thoracoabdominal movements and there is no activity. It is not known why the obese are prone to this.

Body fat can be estimated by measuring skinfold thickness with callipers at the biceps, triceps, subscapular and suprailiac regions.

Adipocytes increase in size and then number as necessary to accommodate excess nutrient calories; but once formed, though they can decrease in size with weight loss, their total number does not decrease (the 'ratchet effect'). *Lipoprotein lipase* (LPL) generates free fatty acids (FFA) from circulating chylomicrons and VLDL and the FFA can then enter adipocytes. LPL activity is high in obese people and rises with initial weight loss and this may be a factor in the accelerated weight regain of many patients. Maintained weight loss, however, is associated with a decrease in LPL activity. Fat cells from the upper body are probably different in responsiveness to testosterone and oestrogens than lower body fat cells leading to:

Android fatness: fat distributed in upper body above the waist

Gynaecoid fatness: fat predominantly in lower body—lower abdomen, buttocks, hips, thighs.

Android fatness carries a greater risk for hypertension, cardiovascular disease, hyperinsulinaemia, diabetes, gallbladder disease, stroke and a higher mortality than does gynaecoid fatness. A waist:hip (circumference) ratio greater than 0.85 for women and 1.0 for men is abnormal.

Other clinical manifestations of obesity

Insulin resistance (enlarged adipocytes less sensitive to the antipolytic and lipogenic actions of insulin; decreased number of insulin receptors as well as postreceptor defects; liver and muscle also less sensitive to insulin; basal and stimulated hyperinsulinaemia results*)

Diabetes mellitus (NIDDM approximately three times higher in the overweight; 85% of NIDDM patients in the USA are obese; though the development of NIDDM requires the appropriate genetic legacy, obesity by enhancing insulin resistance tends to unmask and exacerbate the underlying propensity)

Hypertension* (prevalence three times higher in the obese; mechanism is uncertain—hyperinsulinaemia* leading to increased tubular reabsorption of sodium may be a factor; weight loss by dieting lowers blood pressure even without dietary salt restriction)

Cardiovascular disease (in obesity increased blood volume, stroke volume, left ventricular end-diastolic volume, and filling pressure result in high cardiac output; this leads to left ventricular hypertrophy and dilatation, the former being exacerbated by hypertension; the result is greater risk of congestive heart failure and sudden death)

Lipid abnormalities (obesity is associated with low HDL cholesterol;* LDL may be elevated; hypertriglyceridaemia* is more prevalent, possibly because the insulin resistance and hyperinsulinaemia* cause increased hepatic production of triglycerides; the hypertriglyceridaemia tends to improve with weight loss; if a true genetic lipoprotein disorder coexists, more intensive therapy may be required)

Venous circulatory disease (severe obesity is often associated with varicose veins and venous stasis; congestive cardiac failure adds to the dependent oedema; increased propensity for thrombophlebitis and thromboembolism)

Cancer (obese women have a higher incidence of endometrial cancer, postmenopausal breast cancer, and cancer of the gallbladder and the biliary system; obese men have a higher mortality from cancer of the colon, rectum and prostate for unknown reasons)

Gastrointestinal disease (cholesterol gallstones leading to cholecystitis; obesity may be associated with fatty liver with modest abnormalities of liver function tests)

Arthritis (osteoarthritis due to excess stress placed on the joints of the lower extremities and back; multifactorial elevation in uric acid levels in the obese)

Skin (intertrigo in redundant folds of skin; fungal and yeast infections; *acanthosis nigricans*, which should always be looked for in obese patients, may be associated with severe insulin resistance—p. 374)

Increased mortality (obesity itself may make an independent contribution to mortality, though the effect generally occurs through linkage with factors such as hypertension, diabetes and hyperlipidaemia.*

Endocrine causes of obesity

(<1% of obese patients)

Hypothyroidism (thickened and coarse facial features, dry skin, non-pitting swelling of subcutaneous tissues, hoarse voice, thinning hair, slow pulse, slow relaxing ankle jerks—p. 438)

Polycystic ovarian syndrome (hirsutism, oligo- or

* NB syndrome X (Reaven's syndrome). This refers to the clustering of insulin insensitivity, hyperinsulinaemia, varying degrees of glucose intolerance, hypertension, increased triglycerides and de-

creased HDL; a clustering which may predispose to vascular disease, in particular coronary artery disease. It is postulated that insulin insensitivity/hyperinsulinaemia is the underlying factor.

amenorrhoea, excess androgen production of ovarian origin, ultrasound scan may show polycystic ovaries; patients with polycystic ovaries are often obese and insulin resistant)

Hypothalamic disease (damage to hypothalamic appetite systems and tracts by surgery, trauma, inflammation, craniopharyngioma or other tumours may lead to hyperphagic obesity)

Cushing's (truncal obesity, moon face, purple striae, proximal muscle weakness—p. 441).

Rare genetic diseases associated with obesity include

Prader–Willi syndrome (obesity may be massive, almond-shaped eyes, acromicria, mental retardation, diabetes, hypogonadism—p. 459)

Laurence–Moon–Bardet–Biedl syndrome (?retinitis pigmentosa, hypogonadism, dwarfism, mental retardation, polydactyly—p. 504)

Alström syndrome (see p. 504)

Cohen's syndrome (microcephaly, mental retardation, short stature, facial abnormalities and obesity)

Carpenter's syndrome (see p. 504)

Blount's disease (bowed legs, tibial torsion, obesity).

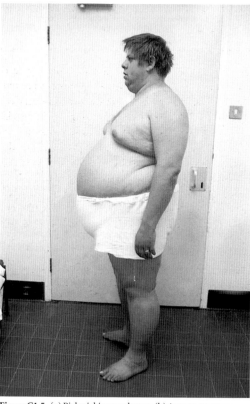

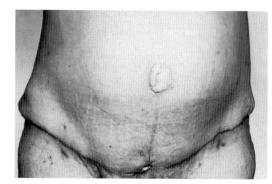

(b)

(a)

Figure C1.5 (a) Pickwickian syndrome. (b) Apronectomy scar.

Case 17 | Tuberculosis/apical consolidation

Frequency in survey: did not occur in the initial small survey of PACES station 1, respiratory.

Predicted frequency from older, more extensive MRCP short case surveys: main focus of a short case in 1% of attempts at PACES station 1, respiratory.

Record

The trachea in this Asian patient is central (may be deviated*) and the expansion is normal (may be reduced at the apex*). The percussion note is *dull* at the R/L apex with *diminished tactile fremitus*. There is *bronchial breathing* with *inspiratory crackles* over the area of dullness.

The diagnosis is R/L apical consolidation, with tuberculosis being a serious contender as the underlying cause.†

Principal varieties of tuberculosis

Primary pulmonary tuberculosis. The first infection with the tubercle bacillus (primary TB) usually includes involvement of the draining lymph node (the Ghon focus). All other TB lesions are regarded as postprimary and are not accompanied by major involvement of the draining lymph nodes (in Europeans), though sometimes in immigrants gross enlargement of the lymph nodes may be seen. *Erythema nodosum, phlyctenular conjunctivitis* and *pleural effusion* may accompany primary pulmonary tuberculosis.

Miliary tuberculosis. Acute dissemination of tubercle bacilli via the blood stream may occur if the initial infection is an overwhelming one or the patient's defences are poor due to malnutrition, corticosteroid or immunosuppressive drug therapy, HIV or intercurrent disease. This condition should be borne in mind in at-risk groups (see below)

Tuberculous meningitis. May occur at any age but is particularly common in small children as a complication of the primary infection.

Postprimary pulmonary tuberculosis. This form may arise either as direct progression of a primary lesion, re-

activation of an old lesion, haematogenous spread or from contact with a patient with *open* (sputum-positive) TB. The predisposing factors for reactivation are malnutrition, poor and overcrowded housing conditions, silicosis and other occupational diseases, alcoholism and cigarette smoking, immunosuppressive drugs, and diseases associated with impaired cellular immunity (e.g. Hodgkin's disease, leukaemia, lymphoma, AIDS). Complications of postprimary pulmonary TB include *empyema, laryngitis, aspergillomata* (colonization of a cavity), *amyloidosis, TB of the organs* and *adult respiratory syndrome*.

Bone and joint tuberculosis. There is a high rate in immigrants of Asian origin. Usually of haematogenous origin. The commonest site for skeletal TB is the spine followed by the weight-bearing joints. AFB may be obtained from synovial fluid or bone but diagnostic exploration may have to be undertaken. Patients with TB can also have a reactive arthritis known as *Poncet's disease*; this usually settles with control of the TB.

Urinary tract tuberculosis. Results from haematogenous spread to the kidney with subsequent spread down

---

* In the examination setting there are usually elicitable signs, even though in clinical practice one often encounters patients with pulmonary TB, sometimes with excessive radiological changes, who have no physical signs. The patient may have signs of fibrosis (e.g. deviated trachea), as seen in advanced cases, but the candidate

should consider the diagnosis of pulmonary TB when there is only a dull percussion note, or a few crepitations at the apex of the lung.
† The differential diagnosis should include *carcinoma of the bronchus,* atypical pneumonia especially due to *Klebsiella pneumoniae,* pulmonary infarction and fungal infection.

the ureteric tract. The patient may present with dysuria, nocturia, loin pain or may have painless haematuria, though many patients with positive urine cultures are asymptomatic. A history of recurrent urinary tract infection or *pyuria with negative bacterial cultures* should be regarded with suspicion for urinary tract TB.

Genital tuberculosis. A large majority of patients have evidence of tuberculosis at extragenital sites. Females present with infertility, pelvic inflammatory disease or amenorrhoea. Adnexal masses are palpable on pelvic examination in about half the cases.

Tuberculous peritonitis. Usually haematogenous. Often associated with weight loss, abdominal pain and gross ascites. Diagnosis can be made at laparoscopy when the peritoneum studded with whitish granulomata can be seen. Peritoneal fluid is rarely positive for AFB by stained smear and even by culture is positive in somewhat less than 50% of cases. May occur in the alcoholic with cirrhosis (see footnote, p. 116).

Tuberculous lymphadenitis. Mostly seen in patients of Afro-Asian origin. The patient may present with painless swelling of cervical lymph glands, or sometimes with pyrexia and lymphadenopathy. Untreated swelling may form a 'cold' abscess or sinus.

Cutaneous tuberculosis. This may present in one of many ways including a *primary complex* (an ulcerating papule on the face), *miliary* TB (particularly in immuno-compromised children), *verrucous* TB (warty lesions as an occupational hazard in patients working with infected material), *scrofuloderma* (breakdown of skin over a tuberculous focus) and *lupus vulgaris* (see p. 354).

At-risk groups

Contacts—should be screened by tuberculin testing and chest X-ray

Immigrants from the Asian subcontinent have a high notification rate

Inhabitants of some institutions—prisons, lodging houses, hostel dwellers and mental institutions

Nursing homes—outbreaks of TB among the elderly in nursing homes have been reported

Medical laboratory workers—the incidence is high among staff in hospital pathology departments

Other groups—doctors, dentists, hospital employees, schoolteachers and those carers who work with children are potentially exposed to the risks for contracting TB.

Treatment

Most patients can be treated at home. Segregation is required only for those patients who have smear positive disease; they should be kept in hospital for the first 2 weeks of treatment. Treatment regimens should last for 6 months except in those who have tuberculous meningitis; they should be treated for 12 months.

Drug therapy should be given as combination tablets to aid compliance. The initial phase of 2 months should include three drugs (isoniazid, rifampicin and pyrazinamide). Ethambutol should be added if there is a risk of drug resistance. Treatment should be continued for 4 more months with rifampicin and isoniazid. Regular checks by nurses and health visitors are necessary to ensure compliance. The rifampicin in the combination tablets produces a pink/orange discoloration of the urine which will aid these checks.

Case 18 | Pneumothorax

Frequency in survey: did not occur in the initial small survey of PACES station 1, respiratory.

Predicted frequency from older, more extensive MRCP short case surveys: main focus of a short case in 0.5% of attempts at PACES station 1, respiratory.

Record

The R/L *side* of the chest (of this tall, thin, young adult male — old patients are usually bronchitic) *expands poorly* compared with the other side. Though the *percussion note* on the R/L side is *hyper-resonant*, the tactile fremitus, vocal resonance and *breath sounds* are all *diminished* (large pneumothorax of one side may push the *trachea* and apex beat to the opposite side).

These findings suggest a pneumothorax of the R/L side.

Male to female ratio is 6:1.

A 'crunching' sound in keeping with the heart beat may be heard when the pneumothorax is small.

Treatment is not required in a healthy individual with a small pneumothorax (i.e. if only a quarter of one side is affected). Drainage is indicated for:

Larger pneumothorax associated with dyspnoea, increasing in size or not resolving after 1 week

Tension pneumothorax

Pneumothorax complicating underlying severe chronic bronchitis with emphysema

Pneumothorax exacerbating acute severe asthma (hence a chest X-ray is mandatory in acute severe asthma).

When drainage is indicated, simple aspiration (with a plastic cannula, syringe and three-way tap so that aspirated air can be voided) should usually be attempted before resorting to intercostal drainage via a tube attached to an underwater seal. Tension pneumothorax should be released urgently by stabbing an intravenous cannula through the chest wall at the second intercostal space, mid-clavicular line, pending the insertion of an intercostal drain.

Recurrent spontaneous pneumothorax is treated by obliteration of the pleural space (pleurectomy; application of irritating substances into the pleural cavity; scarification of the pleura followed by intrapleural suction).

Causes of pneumothorax
Traumatic
Penetrating chest wounds

Iatrogenic (chest aspiration, intercostal nerve block, subclavian cannulation, transbronchial biopsy, needle aspiration lung biopsy, positive pressure ventilation)

Chest compression injury (including external cardiac massage).

Spontaneous
Primary (a common cause in young men*)

Secondary
   chronic obstructive pulmonary disease
   asthma
   congenital cysts and bullae
   pleural malignancy
   rheumatoid lung disease (p. 80)
   bacterial pneumonia (p. 76)
   tuberculosis
   cystic fibrosis (p. 101)
   tuberous sclerosis (p. 297)

---

* The risk of a second pneumothorax in a young adult following the first episode is of the order of 25%. After a second episode, the risk increases to the order of 50%.

endometriosis of the pleura
Marfan's syndrome (p. 156)
sarcoidosis
histiocytosis X

whooping cough
oesophageal rupture
Pneumocystis carinii pneumonia.

Case 19 | Cystic fibrosis

Frequency in survey: did not occur in the initial small survey of PACES station 1, respiratory.

Predicted frequency from older, more extensive MRCP short case surveys: main focus of a short case in 0.5% of attempts at PACES station 1, respiratory.

Record

This young patient (who is usually *underweight*, of *short stature* and rather pale, but may also be *breathless* and *cyanosed*) has *clubbing* of the fingers (often present) and a *productive cough* (there may be a *sputum pot* by the bed). There are (may be) *inspiratory clicks* and *expiratory wheeze* (heard with the unaided ear). There are *crepitations* over . . . (the area of bronchiectasis—state where). There is (may be) widespread *polyphonic expiratory wheeze*.

These features suggest *bronchiectasis* (p. 75) and as this is a young patient this suggests that the underlying disorder is cystic fibrosis. If so the patient is also likely to have *pancreatic insufficiency* and *malabsorption*.* The diagnosis can be confirmed by the *sweat sodium test*.†

Some patients have well-developed *cor pulmonale* with *cyanosis, ankle oedema* and *right heart failure*.

Cystic fibrosis is a genetic disorder (autosomal recessive) and a child born to two heterozygote carriers has a 25% chance of having the disease. The disorder usually occurs in Caucasians; Africans and Asians are seldom affected.

---

* In most cases there is a history of frequent large foul stools which are difficult to flush down. These patients are underachievers in weight and height for their age; they have a good appetite, steatorrhoea and a protuberant abdomen. Hepatic symptoms are relatively uncommon but there may be *jaundice*. Sometimes there may be *portal hypertension*, glycosuria, biliary cirrhosis, cholelithiasis, intussusception and aspermia.

† A history of recurrent respiratory infections and of gastrointestinal symptoms, especially recurrent abdominal pain and faecal impaction, are highly suggestive of cystic fibrosis. The sodium and chloride levels are in excess of $70\,mmol\,l^{-1}$ in the sweat, and these levels do not fall after the administration of aldosterone $(0.1\,mg\,kg^{-1})$ for a week.

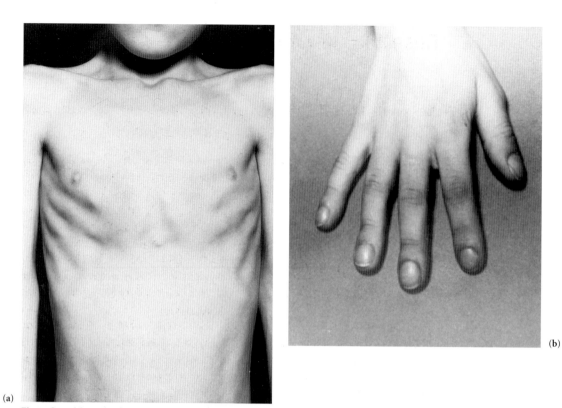

Figure C1.6 (a) Hyperinflated rib cage with rib recession in an undernourished patient. (b) Clubbing of cyanosed fingers.

Case 20 | **Normal chest**

Frequency in survey: did not occur in the initial small survey of PACES station 1, respiratory.

The College have made it clear that 'normal' is an option in stations 1, 3 and 5 of PACES. Because of the change in the structure of the exam compared to the old short cases format, it is likely to occur more frequently than it did before. This is because in order for PACES to proceed there must be a chest case in station 1, respiratory. If, at the last minute, neither of the scheduled chest cases turn up on the day; or if in the middle of a carousel the only one who did turn up decides not to continue or is too ill to continue, a substitute case has to be found at short notice. In the old, pre PACES, days the exam would have proceeded without a chest case whilst the wards were searched and one was found. In the case of PACES, if there is not time for this, one option is to proceed with a patient with a chest which is normal and make up an appropriate scenario. One simply has to imagine oneself as the invigilating registrar to think what that might be. One would first look amongst any surplus cases in the other stations for a patient with something relating to the chest. Failing that one might look for someone who is a smoker or a member of the nursing, portering or other support staff who smokes and come up with a scenario such as:

'You have been asked to see this . . . -year-old smoker for insurance purposes. Please examine the chest . . .'

There may be a clue in the case scenario and the fact that the scenario has been hurriedly hand-scribbled. In the case of station 1, respiratory, this is possibly less likely to happen because there are at any one time so many chest cases in the hospital, and the case found at short notice is more likely to be one with COPD. Nevertheless, it could happen if time was short.

From our pre PACES surveys if was clear that the commonest reason for finding no abnormality is missing the physical signs that are present (probably the anecdote on p. 177, possibly anecdote 2, p. 135 and experience 49, vol. 2, p. 331). Other reasons for cases of 'normal' will be either because the physical signs are no longer present by the time the patient comes to the examination (see anecdote on p. 277), or that the examiners and candidate disagree with the selectors of the cases about the presence of physical signs (this may have happened in the anecdote on p. 508; see also experience 87b (p. 335) and anecdote 55 (p. 367), vol. 2).

Station 1
Abdominal

1 Chronic liver disease

2 Hepatosplenomegaly

3 Polycystic kidneys

4 Splenomegaly (without hepatomegaly)

5 Transplanted kidney

6 Hepatomegaly (without splenomegaly)

7 Ascites

8 Polycythaemia rubra vera

9 Generalized lymphadenopathy

10 Single palpable kidney

11 Primary biliary cirrhosis

12 Abdominal mass

13 Carcinoid syndrome

14 Crohn's disease

15 Idiopathic haemochromatosis

16 Nephrotic syndrome

17 Hereditary spherocytosis

18 Felty's syndrome

19 Normal abdomen

Case 1 | Chronic liver disease

Frequency in survey: main focus of a short case in 21% of attempts at PACES station 1, abdominal. Additional feature in a further 5%.

Record

The patient is *icteric, pigmented* and (rarely) *cyanosed* (due to pulmonary venous shunts). He has *clubbing, leuconychia, palmar erythema, Dupuytren's contracture** and there are several *spider naevi*. He has a flapping tremor of the hands (suggesting some portosystemic encephalopathy). There are scratch marks on the forearms and back, and there is purpura. There is *gynaecomastia, scanty body hair* and his *testes* are *small*. There is 5 cm *hepatomegaly* and 3 cm *splenomegaly*. He has *ascites* and *ankle oedema*, and there are *distended abdominal veins* in which the flow is away from the umbilicus.

The diagnosis is likely to be cirrhosis of the liver with portal hypertension.

Possible causes

1 Alcohol
2 Viral hepatitis
   (a) hepatitis B (?health or clinical laboratory worker)
   (b) hepatitis C† (the major cause of post-transfusion hepatitis; also transmitted between i.v. drug users)
   (c) hepatitis D (unusual; requires antecedent or simultaneous hepatitis B virus (HBV) infection)
3 Autoimmune chronic active hepatitis (pubertal or menopausal female, steroid responsive; associated with diabetes, inflammatory bowel disease, thyroiditis and pulmonary infiltrates; ?smooth muscle antibodies)
4 Primary biliary cirrhosis (middle-aged female, scratch marks, xanthelasma; ?antimitochondrial antibody—p. 121)
5 Haemochromatosis (male, slate-grey pigmentation—p. 129)
6 Cryptogenic.

Other causes

Cardiac failure (?JVP ↑, *v* waves, *S3* or a valvular lesion, tender pulsatile liver if tricuspid incompetence)

Constrictive pericarditis‡ (JVP raised, abrupt *x* and *y* descent, loud early *S3* ('pericardial knock'—a valuable sign but only present in <40% of cases) though heart

---

*Twenty signs which may be present in the hands of the patient with chronic liver disease are clubbing, Dupuytren's contracture, palmar erythema, spider naevi, flapping tremor, leuconychia, scratch marks, icterus, pallor, pigmentation, cyanosis, xanthomata, purpura, koilonychia, paronychia, abscesses, oedema, muscle wasting, tattoos (?HBsAg–positive), needle marks (intravenous drug abuse—more likely in antecubital fossa).

† In the management of *hepatitis C virus* (HCV), alcohol intake should be reduced as it hastens disease progression. Antiviral

therapy with ribavarin and interferon can be tried if the patient is viraemic with abnormal liver histology. The cirrhotic patient should be considered for liver transplantation. There is a high incidence of hepatoma with HCV and patients should be screened for this (α-fetoprotein and USS of abdomen).

‡ The spleen may be palpable. In the absence of evidence of *bacterial endocarditis* or *tricuspid valve disease*, the presence of splenomegaly in a patient with congestive heart failure should arouse suspicion of *constrictive pericarditis* or *pericardial effusion with tamponade*.

sounds often normal, slight 'paradoxical pulse', *no signs in lung fields*, chest X-ray may show calcified pericardium; rare but important cause of ascites as response to treatment may be dramatic)

Budd–Chiari syndrome (in the acute phase ascites develops rapidly with pain, there are no cutaneous signs of chronic liver disease and the liver is smoothly enlarged and tender; if the inferior vena cava is involved there is no hepatojugular reflux)

Biliary cholestasis (bile obstruction with or without infection), which leads to secondary biliary cirrhosis

Toxins and drugs (methotrexate, methyldopa, isoniazid, carbon tetrachloride, amiodarone, aspirin, phenytoin, propylthiouracil, sulphonamides)

Wilson's disease (?Kayser–Fleischer rings, tremor, rigidity, dysarthria)

Alpha-1 antitrypsin deficiency (?lower zone emphysema)

Other metabolic causes (galactosaemia, tyrosinaemia, type IV glycogenosis)

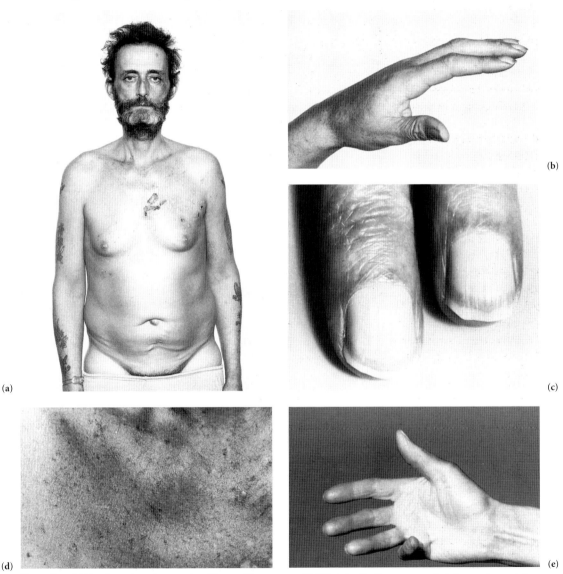

(a)

(b)

(c)

(d)

(e)

Figure C1.7 (a) Note from above downwards; spider naevi, herpes zoster (debilitated patient), gynaecomastia, tattoo marks, everted umbilicus, swelling of the flanks, abdominal wall veins and paucity of hair. (b) Clubbing of the fingers and leuconychia (same patient as (a)). (c) Leuconychia. (d) Spider naevi (close up). (e) Dupuytren's contracture.

Case 2 | Hepatosplenomegaly

Frequency in survey: main focus of a short case in 17% of attempts at PACES station 1, abdominal. Additional feature in a further 6%.

Record

There is hepatosplenomegaly, the *spleen* is enlarged . . . cm below the left costal margin. The *liver* is palpable at . . . cm below the right costal margin; it is non-tender, firm and smooth (now look for clinical *anaemia, lymphadenopathy* and signs of *chronic liver disease*).

Likely causes to be considered are:

No other signs or clinical anaemia only
1 Myeloproliferative disorders (p. 111)
2 Lymphoproliferative disorders (p. 111)
3 Cirrhosis of the liver with portal hypertension* (less likely if there are no other signs of chronic liver disease).

Hepatosplenomegaly plus palpable lymph nodes†
1 Chronic lymphatic leukaemia
2 Lymphoma.
Other conditions to be considered include infectious mononucleosis (?throat), infective hepatitis (?icterus) and sarcoidosis.

Signs of chronic liver disease
Cirrhosis of the liver with portal hypertension (p. 106).

Other causes of hepatosplenomegaly

Hepatitis B or C‡ (?icterus, tattoo marks, needle marks)
Brucellosis ('Examine this farmer's abdomen')
Weil's disease (?icterus, sewerage worker or fell into canal)
Toxoplasmosis (glandular fever-like illness)
Cytomegalovirus infection (glandular fever-like illness)

Pernicious anaemia and other megaloblastic anaemias (NB SACD—p. 223. NB associated organ-specific autoimmune disease—p. 293)
Storage disorders (e.g. Gaucher's—spleen is often huge; glycogen storage disease)
Amyloidosis (?underlying chronic disease)§
Other causes of portal hypertension (e.g. Budd–Chiari syndrome = hepatic vein thrombosis—see pp. 106 and 116)

---

* The cirrhotic liver is often small and impalpable. The exceptions are alcoholic liver disease, primary biliary cirrhosis and cirrhosis complicated by hepatoma (bruit).
† These conditions can also occur without palpable lymph nodes.
‡ NB Hepatitis serology heads the list of investigations of icterus of uncertain cause.
§ Though hepatosplenomegaly can occur in primary and myeloma-associated amyloidosis, it is commoner in the secondary

form. Other organs particularly involved in secondary amyloidosis are kidneys (nephrotic syndrome), adrenals (clinical adrenocortical failure may occur) and alimentary tract (rectal biopsy). Conditions associated with secondary amyloidosis include rheumatoid arthritis (including juvenile type), TB, leprosy, chronic sepsis, Crohn's disease, ulcerative colitis, ankylosing spondylitis, paraplegia (bedsores and urinary infection), malignant lymphoma and carcinoma. See also footnote on p. 180.

Infantile polycystic disease (in some variants of this, children have relatively mild renal involvement but hepatosplenomegaly and portal hypertension).

Common causes on a worldwide basis

Malaria

Kala-azar

Schistosomiasis

Tuberculosis.

Case 3 | **Polycystic kidneys**

Frequency in survey: main focus of a short case in 14% of attempts at PACES station 1, abdominal. Additional feature in a further 2%.

Record

There are *bilateral masses* in the *flanks* which are *bimanually ballotable.* I can *get above* them and the percussion note is *resonant* over them.* I suspect, therefore, that they are renal masses and a likely diagnosis is polycystic kidneys (*?uraemic facies*; the *blood pressure* may be raised). The *arteriovenous fistula/shunt* on his arm indicates that the patient is being treated with haemodialysis (about 50% develop renal failure†).

Other causes of bilateral renal enlargement include:
1   Bilateral hydronephrosis
2   Amyloidosis (?underlying chronic disease, hepatosplenomegaly, etc. — see p. 108)
3   Tuberous sclerosis (?adenoma sebaceum, p. 297)
4   Von Hippel–Lindau disease.‡

Polycystic disease of the liver in adults may cause a nodular liver enlargement (liver function may be normal despite massive hepatomegaly). About 50% have renal involvement. Cystic liver is a major feature of autosomal recessive polycystic kidney disease (ARPKD — previously called infantile polycystic disease), but a minor feature of autosomal dominant polycystic kidney disease (ADPKD — previously called adult polycystic disease).

Other features of ADPKD

Cysts may also occur in other organs — most important are sacular aneurysms (berry aneurysms) of the cerebral arteries§ which, in combination with the hypertension, leads to serious risk of intracranial haemorrhage (cause of death in 10% of cases according to some authorities). There may be focal defects

Mitral valve prolapse (p. 159) may occur in 25% as a further manifestation of the systemic collagen defect. Patients often have palpitations and atypical chest pain. Other valvular abnormalities are also more common and echocardiography should be undertaken if a murmur is detected

It may present with flank pains, bleeding, urinary tract infection, nephrolithiasis, obstructive uropathy or obstruction of the surrounding structures

Renal cell carcinoma is not more common than in the general population, but it can be difficult to diagnose — CT and MRI may be useful

Presymptomatic screening by USS criteria and gene identification†, is deferred to 20 years of age as it is not conclusive before this. The exceptions to this are if there is a family history of aneurysm or if hypertension or other signs of renal disease are present.

---

* Look for abdominal scars from previous peritoneal dialysis or cyst aspiration. The latter is performed to relieve obstruction of the outflow tract by the cyst, intractable pain or haematuria.

† There are at least three gene mutations that can lead to ADPKD; the commonest (85%), PKD1 (chromosome 16), is associated with a greater risk of renal failure than PKD2 (15% — chromosome 4). PKD3 is rare and has not been mapped.

‡ An autosomal dominant condition caused by a defective tumour suppressor gene and characterized by retinal angiomata, brain and spinal cord haemangiomata, renal cell carcinomata, endolymphatic sac tumours, phaeochromocyto-mata, papillary cystadenomata of the epididymis, angiomata of the liver and kidney, and cysts of the pancreas, kidney, liver and epididymis.

§ Five per cent of patients with ADPKD overall, but prevalence increases to 20% in individuals with a family history of brain aneurysm.

Case 4 | Splenomegaly (without hepatomegaly)

Frequency in survey: main focus of a short case in 13% of attempts at PACES station 1, abdominal. Additional feature in a further 2%.

Record

The spleen is palpable at . . . cm.

or

There is a *mass* in the *left hypochondrium*. On palpation I *cannot get above* the mass, it has a *notch*, and on inspiration moves diagonally across the abdomen. The *percussion note* is *dull* over the left lower lateral chest wall and over the mass.

I think this is the spleen enlarged at . . . cm. Likely causes* to be considered are:

Very large spleen†

1 Chronic myeloid leukaemia (Philadelphia (Ph) chromosome positive in 90%‡)
2 Myelofibrosis

and in other parts of the world

3 Chronic malaria
4 Kala-azar.

Spleen enlarged 4–8 cm (2–4 finger breadths)

1 Myeloproliferative disorders§ (e.g. CML and myelofibrosis)
2 Lymphoproliferative disorders¶ (e.g. lymphoma and chronic lymphatic leukaemia)
3 Cirrhosis of the liver with portal hypertension (spider naevi, icterus, etc.—p. 106).

---

* To help you remember some common causes to mention in the examination we have given the three or four most common causes of a spleen of a particular size. An alternative way of dividing up splenomegaly which can be found in many textbooks is:
1 Infectious and inflammatory splenomegaly (e.g. SBE, infectious mononucleosis, sarcoidosis)
2 Infiltrative splenomegaly
  (a) benign (e.g. Gaucher's, amyloidosis)
  (b) neoplastic (e.g. leukaemias, lymphoma)
3 Congestive splenomegaly (e.g. cirrhosis, hepatic vein thrombosis)
4 Splenomegaly due to reticuloendothelial hyperplasia (e.g. haemolytic anaemias).
† *Gaucher's* disease and *rapidly progressive lymphoma* (especially high-grade lymphoma) may also cause a huge spleen. *Chronic congestive splenomegaly* (Banti's syndrome = splenomegaly, pancytopenia, portal hypertension and gastrointestinal bleeding) may also cause massive splenomegaly. A huge spleen developing in a patient with *polycythaemia rubra vera* is usually due to the development of myelofibrosis.
‡ In Ph-positive CML, the Ph chromosome (9:22 translocation; first described in 1973) is present in all dividing cells of the myeloid

series and in some B lymphocytes. In the early 1980s, interferon α was shown to reduce WBC count and induce haematological remission in some patients, inducing Ph-negativity in about 10% and a 1–3-year longer survival than treatment with hydroxyurea. From 2002, a new drug, Glivec, which is a tyrosine kinase inhibitor, is likely to improve further the management and prognosis of CML. It is targeted at the molecular product of the Ph chromosome.
§ When listing the causes of splenomegaly or hepatosplenomegaly in the limited time of the examination, to use the term 'myeloproliferative disorders' in its broadest interpretation is a useful way of covering several conditions in one phrase. If asked to explain it (unlikely), one strict definition covers a group of related disorders of haemopoietic stem cell proliferation: CML, myelofibrosis, polycythaemia rubra vera and essential thrombocythaemia. The term can be used more broadly to cover acute myeloid leukaemia as well. A small spleen is more likely to be due to acute leukaemia than CML or myelofibrosis because splenic enlargement in the latter conditions is often already marked at the time of presentation.
¶ The lymphoproliferative disorders are chronic lymphatic leukaemia, lymphoma, myelomatosis, Waldenström's macro-

Spleen just tipped or enlarged 2–4 cm (1–2 finger breadths)

1 Myeloproliferative disorders§
2 Lymphoproliferative disorders¶ (?palpable lymph nodes)
3 Cirrhosis of the liver with portal hypertension
4 Infections such as:
   (a) glandular fever (?throat, lymph nodes)
   (b) infectious hepatitis (?icterus)
   (c) subacute bacterial endocarditis (?heart murmur, splinter haemorrhages, etc.).

Other causes of splenomegaly

Polycythaemia rubra vera (?plethoric, middle-aged man)

Brucellosis ('Examine this farmer's abdomen')

Sarcoidosis (?erythema nodosum or history of; lupus pernio; chest signs)

Haemolytic anaemia (?icterus)

Pernicious anaemia and other megaloblastic anaemias (?pallor; NB SACD—p. 223; NB associated organ-specific autoimmune diseases, especially autoimmune thyroid disease, diabetes, Addison's, vitiligo, hypo-parathyroidism—see p. 293)

Idiopathic thrombocytopenic purpura (?young female, purpura)

Felty's syndrome (?hands, nodules)

Amyloidosis (?underlying chronic disease, other organ involvement—see p. 108)

SLE (?typical rash)

Lipid storage disease (spleen may be enormous—e.g. Gaucher's)

Myelomatosis

Chronic iron deficiency anaemia

Thyrotoxicosis

Other infections (subacute septicaemia, typhoid, disseminated TB, trypanosomiasis, echinococcosis)

Other causes of congestive splenomegaly* (hepatic vein thrombosis, portal vein obstruction, schistosomiasis, congestive heart failure).

globulinaemia, acute lymphatic leukaemia and hairy cell leukaemia. Of these, the first two and Waldenström's macroglobulinaemia are usually associated with lymphadenopathy and hepatomegaly. Multiple myeloma seldom causes palpable spenomegaly.

Case 5 | Transplanted kidney

Frequency in survey: main focus of a short case in 9% of attempts at PACES station 1, abdominal.

Survey note: although in real life the majority of patients who have a renal transplant have other causes, it is noteworthy that our surveys suggested that all the cases who appeared as MRCP short cases had polycystic kidney disease.

Record

There is fullness in the flanks and an impression of a swelling under the scar in the right iliac fossa. On palpation there are bilateral masses in the flanks that are bimanually ballotable (there may be one ballotable mass and one nephrectomy scar) and suggestive of *polycystic kidneys*. There is also an easily palpable rounded *mass under the scar in the right iliac fossa* which feels like a kidney.

I suspect this patient has had a renal transplant for renal failure due to polycystic kidney disease (p. 110).

Three most common diseases leading to referral for transplantation*

Diabetes mellitus with renal failure (transplantation offered earlier than in other forms of renal disease — post-transplant rehabilitation is more satisfactory if the damage due to other diabetic complications is minimal)

Hypertensive renal disease (incidence of end-stage renal failure not decreasing despite 'better' treatment of hypertension — reason not clear; occurs more often in the Afro-Caribbean than in the Caucasian patient)

Glomerulonephritis.

Diseases in which renal transplantation is a particular problem

Haemolytic-uraemic syndrome (disease can recur and cyclosporin can increase the risk of this; rapid graft failure may ensue)

Sickle cell disease (increased incidence of sickle crises may result from the improved haematocrit)

Systemic sclerosis (post-transplant rehabilitation may be limited by the chronic vascular and gastrointestinal manifestations)

Focal glomerulosclerosis (recurrence within the graft is common)

Oxalosis (there may be severe recurrence of stone disease)

Cystinosis and Fabry's disease—p. 368 (continued disease activity).

Renal transplant outcomes

	5 year	10 year
HLA-identical living donor	88%	73%
Other living donor	74%	56%
HLA-matched cadaver	70%	56%

* These three causes of end-stage renal failure account for 75% of referrals for renal transplantation.

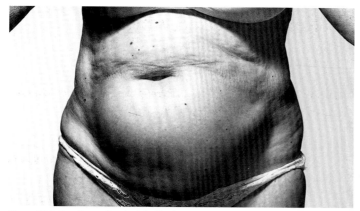

Figure C1.8 Renal transplant in right iliac fossa.

Case 6 | Hepatomegaly (without splenomegaly)

Frequency in survey: main focus of a short case in 5% of attempts at PACES station 1, abdominal. Additional feature in a further 4%.

Record

The liver is palpable at . . . cm below the right costal margin (*?icterus, ascites*, signs of *cirrhosis* (do not miss gynaecomastia), *pigmentation, lymph nodes*).

Common causes

Cirrhosis — usually alcoholic (?spider naevi, gynaecomastia, etc. — p. 106)

Secondary carcinoma (?hard and knobbly, cachexia, evidence of primary)

Congestive cardiac failure (?JVP↑, ankle oedema, *S3* or cardiac murmur; tender pulsatile liver with giant *v* waves in the JVP in tricuspid incompetence).

Other causes of hepatomegaly

Infections such as hepatitis A, glandular fever, Weil's disease and hepatitis B (remember hepatitis serology heads list of investigations in icterus of uncertain cause)

Primary tumours, both malignant (hepatoma may complicate cirrhosis) and benign (liver cell adenoma is associated with oral contraceptive use)

Lymphoproliferative disorders (?lymph nodes)

Primary biliary cirrhosis (?middle-aged female, scratch marks, xanthelasma, etc. — p. 121)

Haemochromatosis (?male, slate-grey pigmentation, etc. — p. 129)

Sarcoidosis (?erythema nodosum or history of, lupus pernio, chest signs)

Amyloidosis (?rheumatoid arthritis or other underlying chronic disease — see footnote, p. 108)

Hydatid cyst (?Welsh connection — NB patient's name)

Amoebic abscess (?tropical connection — name, appearance)

Budd–Chiari syndrome (?icterus, ascites, tender hepatomegaly)

Riedel's lobe

Emphysema (apparent hepatomegaly).

Hard and knobbly hepatomegaly — possible causes

Malignancy — primary or secondary

Polycystic liver disease (?kidneys — p. 110)

Macronodular cirrhosis (following hepatitis B with widespread necrosis)

Hydatid cysts (may be eosinophilia; rupture may be associated with anaphylaxis)

Syphilitic gummas (late benign syphilis; there is usually hepatosplenomegaly and anaemia; rapid response to penicillin).

Case 7 | **Ascites**

Frequency in survey: main focus of a short case in 4% of attempts at PACES station 1, abdominal. Additional feature in a further 6%.

Survey note: occurred in the examination: (i) as part of cirrhosis; (ii) on its own without a clearly defined underlying cause, in which case it was the main focus and possible causes were often discussed; and (iii) in association with an obvious mass or the irregular liver of malignancy.

Record

There is *generalized swelling* of the abdomen and the umbilicus is *everted*. The flanks are *stony dull* to percussion but the centre is resonant (floating, gas-filled bowel). The dullness is *shifting* and a *fluid thrill* can be demonstrated (in tense, large ascites).

This is ascites.

Usual causes

1 Cirrhosis with portal hypertension (?hepatomegaly, icterus, spider naevi, leuconychia, etc.—p. 106; treatment consists of diuretic therapy with spironolactone or amiloride and paracentesis if necessary)

2 Intra-abdominal malignancy (especially ovarian and gastrointestinal—?hard knobbly liver, mass, cachexia, nodes, e.g. Troisier's sign)

3 Congestive cardiac failure (?JVP↑, ankle and sacral oedema, hepatomegaly (pulsatile if tricuspid incompetence), large heart, tachycardia, *S3* or signs of the cardiac lesion).

Other causes

Nephrotic syndrome (?young, underlying diabetes (fundi), evidence of chronic disease underlying amyloid, evidence of collagen disease, etc.—p. 131)

Other causes of hypoalbuminaemia (e.g. malabsorption)

Tuberculous peritonitis* (?ethnic origin, chest signs)

Constrictive pericarditis (JVP raised, abrupt *x* and *y* descent, loud early *S3* ('pericardial knock'), though heart sounds often normal, slight 'paradoxical' pulse, *no signs in lung fields*; chest X-ray may show calcified pericardium; rare but important as response to treatment may be dramatic)

Budd–Chiari syndrome (ascites develops rapidly with pain, icterus but no signs of chronic liver disease, smoothly enlarged tender liver; causes include tumour infiltration, oral contraceptives, polycythaemia rubra vera, ulcerative colitis and severe dehydration)

Myxoedema (?facies, ankle jerks, etc.—very rare)

Meigs' syndrome (ovarian fibroma—important as easily correctable by surgery)

Pancreatic disease

Chylous ascites (due to lymphatic obstruction—milky fluid).

---

* NB Tuberculous peritonitis may attack debilitated alcoholics. Therefore it should always be considered when ascites is present in a cirrhotic. Fever or abdominal pain are suggestive but may not be present. Examination of the ascitic fluid may help—an exudative protein content (>25 g l⁻¹) with lymphocytes is also suggestive. Staining of the fluid for acid–fast bacilli (AFB) is rarely positive and culture is only positive in somewhat less than 50%. Diagnostic procedures include peritonoscopy (bowel adhesions may cause difficulty) and open peritoneal biopsy. Cirrhotic patients should also have ascites tapped to rule out spontaneous bacterial peritonitis as well as TB.

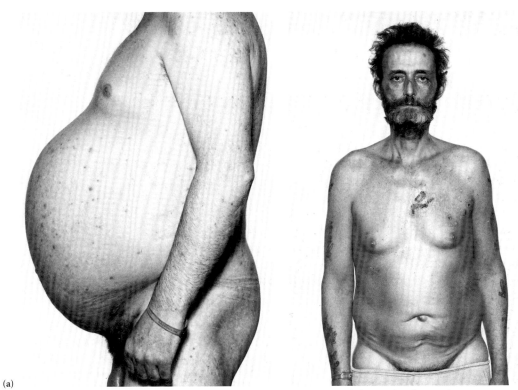

(a)

(b)

Figure C1.9 (a) Gross ascites. (b) Residual ascites in another patient on treatment with diuretics (see also p. 107).

Case 8 | Polycythaemia rubra vera

Frequency in survey: main focus of a short case in 4% of attempts at PACES station 1, abdominal.

Record

This patient has *facial plethora* and a *dusky cyanosis* of the face, hands, feet and (look at the lips and ask the patient to protrude his/her tongue) mucous membranes. There are (may be) ecchymoses (spontaneous bruising) and *scratch marks* (pruritus). (Ask the patient's permission to gently pull down the lower eyelids.) The conjunctival vessels are markedly engorged. (If allowed, look at the fundi for markedly dilated retinal veins, and ask to feel the abdomen for splenomegaly* and to take the blood pressure which may be raised.)

These features suggest a diagnosis of polycythaemia rubra vera.

The diagnosis of primary polycythaemia is based upon demonstration of raised red cell mass and exclusion of secondary causes of polycythaemia (see below). *Pseudopolycythaemia* (reduced plasma volume) is associated with diuretic use and dehydration.

In primary polycythaemia, the characteristic laboratory findings reveal the consequences of increased bone marrow activity. Typically, the red cell, white cell and platelet counts are elevated. The haemoglobin and the haematocrit are raised. The mean corpuscular volume is reduced suggestive of iron deficiency erythropoiesis. Being a primarily malignant disorder, red cell proliferation continues until the iron stores are exhausted giving an iron deficiency picture with a high haemoglobin level.

Causes of secondary polycythaemia

Physiologically appropriate increased erythropoietin production

Arterial hypoxaemia — chronic pulmonary disease, right-to-left shunt, pickwickian syndrome (p. 94), etc.

Abnormal release of oxygen from haemoglobin — congenitally decreased red cell 2,3-DPG; smokers — carboxyhaemoglobinaemia

Interference with tissue oxygen metabolism — cobalt poisoning.

Physiologically inappropriate erythropoietin production

Neoplasms — renal, adrenal, hepatocellular, ovarian, cerebellar, haemangioblastoma, phaeochromocytoma, etc.

Non-neoplastic renal disease — cysts, hydronephrosis.

---

* Splenomegaly occurs in over 70% of patients and hepatomegaly may be present in about 40% of patients.

Case 9 | Generalized lymphadenopathy

Frequency in survey: did not occur in the initial small survey of PACES station 1, abdominal.

Predicted frequency from older, more extensive MRCP short case surveys: main focus of a short case in 4% of attempts at PACES station 1, abdominal. Additional feature in a further 6%.

Record

There is generalized lymphadenopathy with/without . . . cm *splenomegaly* (or hepatosplenomegaly).

The likeliest causes would be a *lymphoreticular disorder* (Hodgkin's and non-Hodgkin's lymphoma, etc.) or *chronic lymphatic leukaemia.*

Other causes

Infectious mononucleosis* (?sore throat)
Sarcoidosis (?erythema nodosum or history of)
Tuberculosis (?ethnic origin, lung signs)
Brucellosis (?farm worker)
Toxoplasmosis* (glandular fever-like illness)
Cytomegalovirus* (glandular fever-like illness)
Thyrotoxicosis (?exophthalmos, goitre, tachycardia, etc. — p. 432)
Progressive generalized lymphadenopathy (HIV — p. 350).

Diagnosis and staging of non-Hodgkin's lymphoma

The precise histological subtype needs to be established according to the current WHO/REAL classification and the extent of the disease:

Lymph node biopsy—fine needle aspirate is not adequate for histological subtyping
CT scan—usually chest, abdomen and pelvis; occasionally neck
Bone marrow aspirate and trephine
Other less frequently used staging investigations— isotope bone scan (if bone involvement is suspected), LP, CT or MRI of the head (in certain subtypes, e.g. lymphoblastic lymphoma where the risk of CNS disease is high)
ENT examination of the postnasal space.

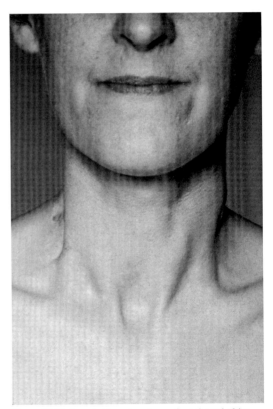

Figure C1.10 A cervical lymph node seen from the end of the bed.

---

* Lymph nodes likely to be tender in acute infectious cases.

Case 10 | Single palpable kidney

Frequency in survey: did not occur in the small initial survey of PACES station 1, abdominal.

Predicted frequency from older, more extensive MRCP short case surveys: main focus of a short case in 3% of attempts at PACES station 1, abdominal. Additional feature in a further 3%.

Record

There is a mass (describe consistency, edges, size, etc.) on the R/L side* of the abdomen in the midzone. It is *bimanually ballotable*, I can *get above it*, and the percussion note is *resonant* over it.

It is, therefore, likely to be renal in origin (check for the pale, brownish-yellow tinge of uraemia, dialysis fistula/shunt/scars, etc.).

Possible causes

1 Polycystic disease (p. 110) with only one kidney palpable
2 Carcinoma (?weight loss, evidence of secondaries, anaemia, polycythaemia, pyrexia)
3 Hydronephrosis
4 Hypertrophy of a single functioning kidney (unilateral renal agenesis (1 : 500–1000 births) may predispose in the long term to proteinuria, hypertension and glomerular sclerosis).

Features of renal cell carcinoma

Accounts for 2% of adult malignancies
Increased risk with smoking
Spreads to the aortic and paraortic nodes
Distant metastases may occur in the lung (50%), bone (49%), skin (11%), liver (8%) and brain (3%)
Haematuria is the most frequent presenting symptom. Pain and abdominal mass are also common but the classic triad of haematuria, pain and abdominal mass occur together in <10% of patients.
Treatment is with nephrectomy and immunotherapy—interferon α and interleukin 2.

---

* NB A palpable right kidney may be normal in a thin person.

Case 11 | **Primary biliary cirrhosis**

Frequency in survey: did not occur in the initial small survey of PACES station 1, abdominal.

Predicted frequency from older, more extensive MRCP short case surveys: main focus of a short case in 3% of attempts at PACES station 1, abdominal.

Record

This middle-aged lady is *icteric* (may not be) with *pigmentation* of the skin. There are *excoriations* (due to scratching) and she has *xanthelasma* (other xanthomata frequently occur over joints, skin folds and at sites of trauma). The liver is enlarged . . . cm (may be very large; there may be splenomegaly).

The clinical diagnosis is primary biliary cirrhosis (there may be *clubbing*). The scratch marks are due to *pruritus* (the predominant presenting symptom).

HLA phenotypes B8 and C4B2 = threefold increase in risk
Serum antimitochondrial antibody positive in 95–99%
Smooth muscle antibody positive in 50%
Antinuclear factor positive in 20%.

Impaired biliary excretion of copper occurs with excessive copper deposition in the liver. This may not be an important factor in the pathogenesis of the progressive liver disease, but it can be helpful in the diagnosis — sometimes differentiation from chronic active hepatitis (25% have antimitochondrial antibody) can be difficult (clinically and histologically) and the issue can be resolved by staining the biopsy specimen for copper. Kayser–Fleischer rings occasionally occur. Penicillamine (immunological, antifibrotic, as well as chelating effects) has been used in advanced disease but there is no evidence that it improves survival. Immunosuppressive agents (including corticosteroids, azathioprine, methotrexate and cyclosporin A) and antifibrotics (e.g. colchicine) may have a small effect. Ursodeoxycholic acid improves serum biochemistry, decreases the rate of referral for liver transplantation and reduces pruritis, but no effect on histology or survival has yet been convincingly demonstrated. Supplements of fat-soluble vitamins, calcium and phosphate are given in view of malabsorption. The pruritus often responds to cholestyramine (taken before and after meals), though phenobarbitone, rifampicin, opiate antagonists (e.g. naloxone) or pro-pofol may also help. Resistant pruritus responds to norethandrolone but this deepens jaundice. Physical intervention (bile diversion, haemoperfusion, charcoal column perfusion or plasmapheresis) may also help severe pruritus. Liver transplantation has been used successfully but there is some evidence that the disease may recur in the transplanted liver.

The patient is at risk of
Bleeding oesophageal varices
Steatorrhoea and malabsorption, leading to
Osteomalacia.

Associated conditions*
Sjögren's syndrome
Systemic sclerosis
CRST syndrome
Rheumatoid arthritis
Hashimoto's thyroiditis
Renal tubular acidosis
Coeliac disease
Dermatomyositis.

* The incidental finding of a raised alkaline phosphatase in patients with the conditions on this list should raise the suspicion of an associated primary biliary cirrhosis.

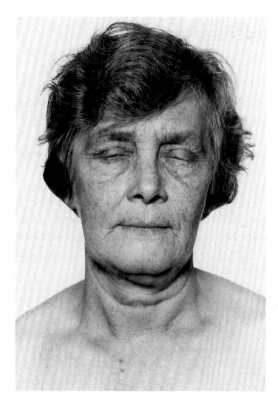

Figure C1.11 Note xanthelasma, pigmentation and spider naevi.

Case 12 | Abdominal mass

Frequency in survey: main focus of a short case in 2% of attempts at PACES station 1, abdominal. Additional feature in a further 1%.

Survey note: discussion usually concerned differentiation from/of enlarged organs (spleen, kidney, liver) or differential diagnosis.

Record 1

In this young (?somewhat pale-looking) adult patient there is a freely mobile 5×4 cm (measure) firm non-tender mass in the *right iliac fossa*. None of the abdominal organs is enlarged, and there are no fistulae.

The diagnosis could be Crohn's disease (p. 127).

Other causes of a mass in the right iliac fossa

1 Ileocaecal tuberculosis (?ethnic origin, chest signs)
2 Carcinoma of the caecum (?older person, non-tender and hard mass, lymph nodes; investigate with colonoscopy)
3 Amoebic abscess (?travelled abroad)
4 Lymphoma (?hepatosplenomegaly, lymph nodes elsewhere; investigate with CT scan)
5 Appendicular abscess (investigate with USS)
6 Neoplasm of the ovary (investigate with USS/CT scan)
7 Ileal carcinoid (rare).

Record 2

A freely mobile tender 6×5 cm mass is palpable in the *left iliac fossa* in this elderly patient. None of the other organs is palpable.

It is probably a diverticular abscess (usually tender; investigate with USS/CT scan).

Other causes of a mass in the left iliac fossa

1 Carcinoma of the colon (?non-tender, hepatomegaly; investigate with colonoscopy)
2 Neoplasm of the left ovary (investigate with USS/CT scan)
3 A faecal mass (no other signs)
4 Amoebic abscess.

Record 3

In this thin and pale patient there is a round, hard 8×6 cm non-tender mass with ill-defined edges in the *epigastrium*. It does not move with respiration. Neither the liver nor the spleen is enlarged (check neck for lymph nodes).

The probable diagnosis is a neoplasm such as:
1 Carcinoma of the stomach (?Troisier's sign; investigate with upper GI endoscopy)

2 Carcinoma of the pancreas (?icterus; NB Courvoisier's sign; investigate with CT scan)

3 Lymphoma (?generalized lymphadenopathy, spleen; investigate with CT scan).

Record 4

In this elderly patient there is a *pulsatile* (pulsating anteriorly as well as transversely), 6 × 4 cm firm mass* palpable 2 cm above the umbilicus and reaching the epigastrium. Both femoral pulses are palpable just before the radials (no evidence of dissection) and there are no bruits heard either over the mass or over the femorals. (Look for evidence of peripheral vascular insufficiency in the feet.)

This patient has an aneurysm of his abdominal aorta (the commonest cause is arteriosclerosis†).

If you find a mass in either upper quadrant you should define its:

Size

Shape

Consistency

Whether you can get above it

Whether it is bimanually ballotable

Whether it moves with respiration

Whether it is tender.

In either upper quadrant it has to be differentiated from a renal mass (p. 110); if in the left hypochondrium it has to be differentiated from a spleen (p. 111) and in the right hypochondrium from a liver (p. 115). Other causes of an upper quadrant mass include:

Carcinoma of the colon

Retroperitoneal sarcoma

Lymphoma (?generalized lymphadenopathy, spleen)

Diverticular abscess (?tender).

---

* Pulsations without a mass may be transmitted from a normal aorta. A mass from a neighbouring structure may overlie the aorta and transmit (only anterior) pulsations.

† Mycotic aneurysms (see anecdote 30, vol. 2, p. 364) are a major complication (2.5% of patients with valvular infections) of infective endocarditis and are most commonly associated with relatively non-invasive organisms such as *Streptococcus viridans*. They may occur at any age, either during the active phase or months (sometimes years) after the endocarditis has been successfully treated. More common sites of mycotic aneurysms are the brain (2–6% of all aneurysms in the brain), sinuses of Valsalva, and ligated ductus arteriosus. Clinical manifestations of abdominal aortic aneurysms (e.g. backache) appear after the lesions have started to leak slowly. Surgical treatment is almost always indicated.

Case 13 | Carcinoid syndrome

Frequency in survey: main focus of a short case in 2% of attempts at PACES station 1, abdominal.

Record

There is *cutaneous flushing*,* facial *telangiectasiae*, and the *liver is palpable* . . . cm below the right costal margin (may be irregular).

In view of the history of *diarrhoea*† these features are suggestive of the carcinoid syndrome.

Carcinoid tumours arise from enterochromaffin cells and are most commonly found in the appendix or rectum but these rarely give rise to the carcinoid syndrome. The actual carcinoid syndrome is produced by carcinoid tumours (usually ileal, but also from the stomach, bile duct, duodenum, pancreas, lung and gonads) which have metastasized to the liver, presumably because the metastatic tumour impedes hepatic clearance of mediators (including *serotonin* (*5-HT*), bradykinin, histamine and tachykinins, as well as prostaglandins) released from the tumour. The flush (head and upper thorax) is red initially but then becomes purple and commonly lasts only a few minutes but may continue for hours.* Frequent flushing may lead to telangiectasiae. During a flush the heart rate increases and the blood pressure falls.‡

Other features of carcinoid syndrome

Fibrotic lesions (probably due to chronic 5-HT excess):
 Right-sided endocardial fibrosis (33% of patients; heart failure due to *pulmonary stenosis*, tricuspid incompetence or both is less common but implies a poor prognosis)
 Pleural, peritoneal and retroperitoneal fibroses

Bronchoconstriction (20% of patients; wheezing occurs during episodes of flushing and is probably not due to 5-HT)
Abdominal pain,† weight loss and cachexia
Diagnosis confirmed by the finding of a very high urinary 5-HIAA
Somatostatin analogues, cyproheptadine (may ameliorate the diarrhoea) and leucocyte interferon may be beneficial in treatment. Surgical debulking may be required.

Ectopic humoral syndromes in histological carcinoid tumours§

Cushing's syndrome (ACTH in bronchial carcinoid)
Dilutional hyponatraemia (antidiuretic hormone in bronchial carcinoid)
Gynaecomastia (HCG in gastric carcinoid)
Acromegaly (GHRH in foregut carcinoid)
Hypoglycaemia (insulin in pancreatic carcinoid).

---

* Flushing tends to be more intense and longer lasting with bronchial carcinoids and more patchy (anywhere on the body) with gastric carcinoids. Headache commonly follows the flush. It may be precipitated by alcohol, food, stress, palpation of the liver, or it may follow administration of catecholamines, pentagastrin or reserpine. The mediator of the flush is uncertain and is probably not 5-HT. Conversely, the diarrhoea does seem to be mediated by 5-HT as it can be reduced by inhibition of 5-HT synthesis. Never-

theless the diarrhoea is typically exacerbated during episodes of flushing.
† This important clue may be in the written instruction. Diarrhoea (2–30 stools per day), frequently accompanied by abdominal cramping, is not usually disabling but can occasionally be voluminous with malabsorption and fluid and electrolyte imbalance.
‡ Cf. pallor and hypertension with phaeochromocytoma.
§ Typically such patients do not have carcinoid syndrome.

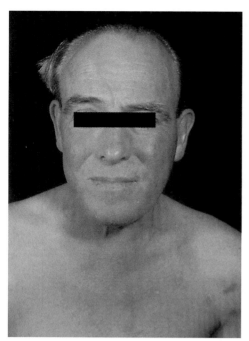

Figure C1.12 Cutaneous flush in the carcinoid syndrome.

Case 14 | Crohn's disease

Frequency in survey: main focus of a short case in 1% of attempts at PACES station 1, abdominal.

Survey note: there were several different presentations: as a right iliac fossa mass, as multiple scars and sinuses on the abdomen, as perianal Crohn's disease and as Crohn's disease of the lips. In one-third of cases the clue was given that the patient had diarrhoea.

Record 1

The *multiple laparotomy scars* suggest a chronic, relapsing, abdominal condition which has led to crises requiring surgical intervention on several occasions. In view of the associated *fistula* formation, Crohn's disease is likely.

Record 2

The chronically *swollen lips* (granulomatous infiltration) and history of chronic diarrhoea are suggestive of Crohn's disease (examine inside the *mouth* for *ulcers* which vary in size).

Record 3

There is a (characteristic) *dusky blue discoloration* of the perianal skin. There are *oedematous skin tags* (which look soft but are very firm), there is *fissuring, ulceration* and *fistula* formation.

The diagnosis is perianal Crohn's disease (may antedate disease elsewhere in the bowel).

Record 4
Right iliac fossa mass—see p. 123.

Other physical signs in Crohn's disease
Fever
Anaemia (malabsorption, chronic disease and GI blood
   loss)
Clubbing
Arthritis(including sacroiliitis)
Erythema nodosum (p. 324)
Pyoderma gangrenosum (p. 378)
Iritis
Ankle oedema (hypoproteinaemia).

Treatment of Crohn's disease
Remember that as well as the usual treatment with steroids and other immunosuppressive medication, anti-TNFα antibodies can cause closure to the fistulae in non-responsive Crohn's (majority relapse).

Other causes of anal fistulae (rare)
Simple fistula from an abscess of an anal gland
Tuberculosis
Ulcerative colitis
Carcinoma of the rectum.

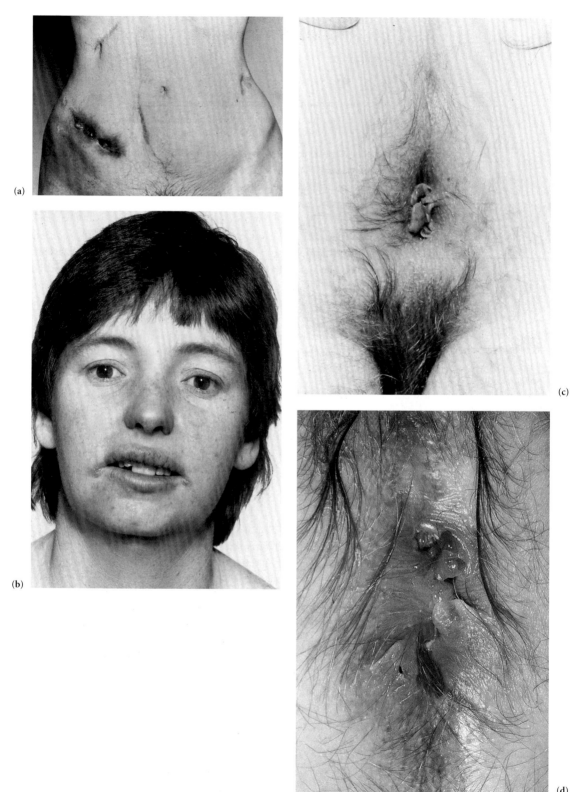

Figure C1.13 (a) Multiple scars and fistulae. (b) Crohn's lips. (c) Perianal lesions. (d) Anal Crohn's disease, note purplish discoloration of the perianal skin, oedematous skin tags, fissuring, ulceration and fistula formation.

Case 15 | Idiopathic haemochromatosis

Frequency in survey: did not occur in the initial small survey of PACES station 1, abdominal.

Predicted frequency from older, more extensive MRCP short case surveys: main focus of a short case in 1% of attempts at PACES station 1, abdominal.

Record

There is (in this thin patient) *slate-grey pigmentation,* decreased body hair and gynae-comastia* (and testicular atrophy* — iron deposition affecting hypothalamic–pituitary function). The *liver** is *enlarged* at . . . cm (in 95% of symptomatic patients; spleen is present in 50%).

The diagnosis is haemochromatosis.

Males > females.

In males it may present at any time in adult life. In females it usually presents after the menopause (physiological iron loss protects).

Autosomal recessive — association with HLA-A3. The HFE gene was identified in 1996 as the gene whose mutations give rise to genetic haemochromatosis. The gene is located on the short arm of chromosome 6 and the most important mutation is C282Y, in which a substitution of cysteine by tyrosine occurs at position 282 of the mature protein (others are H63D and S65C). Homozygous C282Y mutation is responsible for about 90% of genetic haemochromatosis in Northern Europe. Haemochromatosis is a common genetic disorder — the carrier rate is about 1/10 in populations of Northern European origin. Homozygote rates vary between 1/200 and 1/600.

Other features which may be present

Spider naevi

Palmar erythema

Ascites

Jaundice

Diabetes mellitus* (not entirely due to iron deposition in the pancreas because insulin levels may be normal and there is a higher incidence of diabetes in relatives with-

out iron overload; high incidence of insulin resistance and fat atrophy)

Arthropathy* (pseudogout — especially the second and third MCP joints, wrists, hips and knees)

Cardiac involvement* (large heart, dysrhythmias, congestive cardiac failure; it is the presenting manifestation in 15% — sometimes young adults; it may be *misdiagnosed* as idiopathic cardiomyopathy)

Hepatocellular carcinoma (develops in 33% of cirrhotic patients; it does not appear to occur if the disease is treated in the pre-cirrhotic stage; hence the importance of *family screening*)

Addison's disease, hypothyroidism and hypoparathyroidism are exceedingly rare.

Treatment

Weekly *phlebotomy* (500 ml) until the haemoglobin concentration falls below 11 g dl^{-1} and the patient is marginally iron deficient (serum ferritin < 10 µg l^{-1} — this usually takes 2–3 years), then maintenance phlebotomy to keep the serum iron and ferritin in the low normal range (about once every 3 months). When phlebotomy is initiated before cirrhosis develops, survival is normal. If anaemia and hypoproteinaemia preclude phlebotomy, *desferrioxamine* may be indicated. This is most practi-

---

* The association of hepatomegaly, skin pigmentation, diabetes mellitus, heart disease, arthritis and evidence of hypogonadism should always suggest haemochromatosis. These days the pre-cirrhotic condition is often diagnosed in young relatives by family screening. The diagnosis should be considered in any patient with

unexplained hepatomegaly, idiopathic cardiomyopathy, abnormal pigmentation or loss of libido (may antedate other clinical manifestations of the disease). Ninety per cent of patients show bronzing of the skin due to excess melanin. In half, haemosiderin is also present, giving the skin the classic slate-grey appearance.

cably administered by high dose subcutaneous infusion using a portable pump. *Ascorbic acid* given concurrently improves iron excretion.

NB Patients with alcoholic liver disease often have increased stainable iron on liver biopsy. These can be divided into two groups: (i) mild to moderate increase in stainable iron but relatively normal body iron stores (<3 g); and (ii) gross iron deposition and increased body iron stores. Phlebotomy may prolong survival in the latter (the majority of whom have idiopathic haemochromatosis) but not the former group.

Case 16 | Nephrotic syndrome

Frequency in survey: did not occur in the initial small survey of PACES station 1, abdominal.

Predicted frequency from older, more extensive MRCP short case surveys: main focus of a short case in 0.7% of attempts at PACES station 1, abdominal.

Record

There is *extensive oedema* affecting the ankles, lower legs and periorbital tissues (especially in the morning) of this (may be young*) patient. The skin is pale (oedema in the skin). There are (may be) white bands across the nails (from chronic hypoalbuminaemia). There are (may be) bilateral *pleural effusions* and *ascites*.

This patient's extensive oedema could be due to nephrotic syndrome.†

Commonest cause

Glomerulonephritis (77%—usually minimal change in childhood but membranous in adults).

Causes of nephrotic syndrome

1 *Minimal change disease*
  (a) Primary (idiopathic):
      with atopy HLA-B12
      without atopy
  (b) Secondary:
      lymphoma
      carcinoma (renal, lung, pancreas)
      IgA nephropathy
      diabetes mellitus
      AIDS
2 *Focal and segmental glomerulosclerosis*
  (a) Primary:
      idiopathic
      superimposed on minimal change
  (b) Secondary:
      infection—HIV
      drugs—heroin abuse, NSAIDs, analgesic abuse
      reduced renal cell mass—cortical necrosis, renal dysplasia
      normal renal cell mass—diabetes mellitus, hyper-

tension, Alport's syndrome, sickle cell disease, cystinosis, sarcoidosis
3 *Membranous glomerulonephritis*
  (a) Primary (idiopathic)
  (b) Secondary:
      infection—hepatitis B (75% of cases), hepatitis C, malaria, schistosomiasis
      multisystem—SLE, mixed connective tissue disease, dermatomyositis, Sjögren's syndrome
      neoplastic (lung, colon, stomach, breast), lymphoma
      drugs—gold, mercury, penicillamine
      familial—sickle cell disease
      miscellaneous—*de novo* in renal allograft, bullous pemphigoid, Fanconi's syndrome
4 *Mesangiocapillary glomerulonephritis*
  (a) Primary (idiopathic):
      type 1—subendothelial deposits
      type 2—dense deposit disease
  (b) Secondary—SLE, cryoglobulinaemia, scleroderma, light and heavy chain disease
5 *Fibrillary glomerulonephritis*
Amyloidosis, multiple myeloma, cryoglobulinaemia, lupus nephritis.

---

* The oedema of the acute poststreptococcal glomerulonephritis (proteinuria, haematuria, oliguria, oedema, hypertension, renal failure) which mainly affects children and young adults, is usually due to salt and water retention. Only in a small proportion does heavier proteinuria leading to nephrotic syndrome develop.

† Defined as proteinuria >3.5 g/1.75 m^2 of body surface per 24 hours, hypoalbuminaemia and oedema. Hypercholesterolaemia is often present.

Malaria due to *Plasmodium malariae* is an important cause in areas where it is endemic. There are about 70 rare causes.

Investigations for nephrotic syndrome

Urine microscopy (?red cells, casts, lipid deposits), 24-hour urinary protein

Urinary protein selectivity (clearance ratio of IgG to transferrin below 0.15 in minimal change disease, which carries a good prognosis)

Creatinine clearance (GFR)

Specific tests for the causal diseases (glucose, antinuclear factors, etc.)

Renal biopsy.

Complications

Thrombosis (deep venous, arterial, pulmonary, renal vein) — due to dehydration, immobility and a hyper-coagulable state (urinary loss of antithrombin and increased hepatic production of fibrinogen)

Malnutrition (normal protein diet unless marked uraemia)

Atheroma and ischaemic heart disease (hypercholesterolaemia*

Infection.

Treatment

General and supportive measures (low salt diet, diuretics and lipid-lowering agents) should be given to all patients. Specific therapy with corticosteroids in minimal change disease has a successful outcome, especially in children. Corticosteroids with cytotoxic therapy are also given to other varieties with variable outcomes. Prolonged anticoagulation is required if thromboembolic episodes occur.

---

* Most nephrotic patients have elevated total and LDL cholesterol levels with low or normal HDL cholesterol. Xanthelasmata accumulate rapidly in nephrotic syndrome.

Case 17 | Hereditary spherocytosis

Frequency in survey: did not occur in the initial small survey of PACES station 1, abdominal.

Predicted frequency from older, more extensive MRCP short case surveys: main focus of a short case in 0.3% of attempts at PACES station 1, abdominal.

Survey note: some candidates were shown a pale adult of about 30 years of age and asked to examine the abdomen.

Record

This patient has *splenomegaly* (sometimes there may also be hepatomegaly), *pale skin* and conjunctivae* and *icteric sclerae.** The spleen is enlarged (say by how much) below the left costal edge (there may be a splenectomy scar† instead).

The underlying cause of this triad of jaundice, anaemia and splenomegaly may be haemolytic anaemia.‡

Causes of haemolytic anaemias

Hereditary haemolytic anaemias:
  hereditary spherocytosis
  hereditary elliptocytosis
  thalassaemia
  sickle cell anaemia
Acquired haemolytic anaemia:
  acquired autoimmune haemolytic anaemia
  primary or idiopathic haemolytic anaemia

Secondary haemolytic anaemia:
  lymphoproliferative disorders
  SLE
  chronic inflammatory disease (e.g. ulcerative colitis)
    drugs (e.g. methyldopa)
  infections (e.g. brucellosis, infectious mononucleosis, etc.)
  non-lymphoid neoplasms (e.g. ovarian tumours).

---

* Jaundice may be barely detectable or absent in some cases but anaemia is a regular feature of hereditary spherocytosis.
† Splenectomy is advisable in severe cases of hereditary spherocytosis and in mild cases with complications such as gallstones. Splenectomy removes a protective blood filtering bed and renders patients, especially the young ones, more vulnerable to infections. This tendency can be minimized, but not completely eliminated, by immunization and careful attention to all infections. Recommendations for postsplenectomy prophylaxis include vaccinations for pneumococcus, haemophilus influenzae B and meningococcus C, annual flu vaccine and lifelong penicillin prophylaxis.
‡ The other contender for this triad is a group of systemic conditions (e.g. infective endocarditis, SLE, pernicious anaemia, infec-

tious mononucleosis, etc.). The absence of various stigmata of these and the presence of some for hereditary spherocytosis (e.g. leg ulcers), the hint of a family history (autosomal dominant) from the examiner, and a relatively young age may give you enough confidence to suggest the diagnosis. However, the definitive diagnosis of this condition cannot be made without laboratory help (low mean corpuscular volume, high mean corpuscular haemoglobin concentration, because the red cells tend to be dehydrated, spherocytosis on the blood film, increased osmotic fragility and, in most cases, a decreased spectrin content of the red cells). Anaemia, jaundice and splenomegaly are also present in other varieties of hereditary and acquired haemolytic anaemias. They may also, of course, occur together in chronic liver disease but then one would expect other diagnostic clues (p. 106).

Case 18 | Felty's syndrome

Frequency in survey: did not occur as the main focus of a short case. In the original, pre PACES, survey it was, however, considered to be present in a short case in 1% of attempts at MRCP short cases.

Record

There is a *symmetrical deforming arthropathy* with *spindling* and *ulnar deviation* of the fingers, and *nodules* at the elbows. The *spleen* is enlarged at . . . cm. (Check for anaemia.)

If *neutropenia** is present (?evidence of secondary infection) this, in combination with rheumatoid arthritis and splenomegaly, would constitute Felty's syndrome.

Occurs in older patients with long-standing rheumatoid disease (5%).

Other signs and features of Felty's syndrome

Lymphadenopathy
Skin pigmentation
Vasculitic leg ulceration

Keratoconjunctivitis sicca
Thrombocytopenia
Haemolytic anaemia
Lack of relationship between the degree of haematological abnormality and the size of spleen
Tests for antinuclear factor are often positive as well as rheumatoid factor which is invariably positive.

---

* Splenectomy may correct the neutropenia and prevent further infections in some patients, but many do not improve.

Case 19 | Normal abdomen

Frequency in survey: did not occur in the initial small survey of PACES station 1, abdominal.

The College have made it clear that 'normal' is an option in stations 1, 3 and 5 of PACES. Because of the change in the structure of the exam compared to the old short cases format, it is likely to occur more frequently than it did before. This is because in order for PACES to proceed there must be an abdomen case in station 1, abdominal. If, at the last minute, neither of the scheduled abdomen cases turn up on the day; or if in the middle of a carousel the only one who did turn up decides not to continue or is too ill to continue, a substitute case has to be found at short notice. In the old, pre PACES, days the exam would have proceeded without an abdomen case whilst the wards were searched and one was found. In the case of PACES, if there is not time for this, one option is to proceed with a patient with an abdomen that is normal and make up an appropriate scenario. One simply has to imagine oneself as the invigilating registrar. One would first look amongst any surplus cases in the other stations for a volunteer or one might ask a member of the nursing, portering or other support staff. At the planning meetings for PACES, the College came up with the following scenario as an example of one that might be used:

'This . . . -year-old patient presented with haematemesis. Please examine the abdomen . . .'

There may thus be a clue in the case scenario and the fact that the scenario has been hurriedly hand-scribbled.

From the pre PACES surveys it was clear that the commonest reason for finding no abnormality is missing the physical signs that are present (probably the anecdote on p. 177; possibly anecdote 2, below; see also experience 49, vol. 2, p. 331). Other reasons for cases of 'normal' will be either because the physical signs are no longer present by the time the patient comes to the examination (see the anecdote on p. 277), or that the examiners and candidate disagree with the selectors of the cases about the presence of physical signs (may have happened in the anecdote on p. 508; see also experience 87b, p. 335, and anecdote 55, vol. 2, p. 367). The following anecdotes are from the original, pre PACES, surveys.

Anecdote 1
A candidate was asked to examine the abdomen. She could find no abnormality and told the examiner she thought the abdomen was normal. She was asked to demonstrate the 'tests' for splenic enlargement. She passed the examination and in retrospect she still feels that it was a normal abdomen.

Anecdote 2
A candidate was asked to examine a man's abdomen. He could find no abnormality and diagnosed a normal abdomen. In retrospect he is not sure if he missed something. Though he failed the clinical he felt he had passed the short case section.

Station 3
Cardiovascular

1 Prosthetic valves
2 Mitral incompetence (lone)
3 Mixed aortic valve disease
4 Mixed mitral valve disease
5 Other combinations of mitral and aortic valve disease
6 Mitral stenosis (lone)
7 Aortic stenosis (lone)
8 Aortic incompetence (lone)
9 Ventricular septal defect
10 Irregular pulse
11 Hypertrophic cardiomyopathy
12 Marfan's syndrome
13 Eisenmenger's syndrome

14 Mitral valve prolapse
15 Patent ductus arteriosus
16 Tricuspid incompetence
17 Fallot's tetralology with a Blalock shunt
18 Raised jugular venous pressure
19 Coarctation of the aorta
20 Slow pulse
21 Dextrocardia
22 Pulmonary stenosis
23 Cannon waves
24 Pulmonary incompetence
25 Infective endocarditis
26 Atrial septal defect
27 Normal heart

Case 1 | Prosthetic valves

Frequency in survey: main focus of a short case in 17% of attempts at PACES station 3, cardiovascular. Additional feature in some others.

Survey note: both mitral and aortic prostheses occurred (often leaking). There may also be murmurs from the unreplaced valve.

Record 1

There is a *midline sternotomy scar*. There is a *click at the first heart sound* (closing of the mitral prosthesis) and an *opening click** in diastole (this may occasionally be followed by a mid-diastolic flow murmur, particularly with the older ball and cage valves).

These clicks represent the opening and closing of a *mitral valve prosthesis*. (The pansystolic murmur ± signs of heart failure suggest it is leaking.†)

Record 2

There is a *midline sternotomy scar*. The first heart sound is normal (unless there is accompanying mitral stenosis), and is followed by an *ejection click** (opening of the prosthesis), an *ejection systolic murmur* and a *click at* (as part of) *the second sound* (closing of the prosthesis).

These clicks suggest an *aortic valve prosthesis*. (The early diastolic murmur and collapsing pulse (?wide pulse pressure) suggest it is leaking.†)

Complications of prosthetic valves

Thromboembolic disease (anticoagulants or antiplatelet agents reduce but do not abolish)

Haemorrhage due to inadvertent overanticoagulation

Infective endocarditis (always consider when leakage develops)

Leakage due to wear of the valve

Leakage due to inadequacy or infection (bacterial endocarditis) of valve siting

Near total or even total dehiscence of the valve from its siting (the valve will be seen to rock on X-ray screening when there is serious leakage)

Ball embolus (the ball of the Starr–Edwards valve)

Valve obstruction from thrombosis/fibrosis clogging up the valve mechanics — usually older mitral valve replacements

Haemolysis (aortic valve).

NB Porcine heterografts and cadavaric homografts do not cause clicks. They last on average 8–10 years and are therefore only used nowadays in the elderly or are seen in adult survivors of congenital heart disease (where they are often calcified, producing signs of valve/conduit obstruction).

---

* Clicks can be audible without a stethoscope. Their cessation or diminution can be a harbinger of serious valve dysfunction, and should always be taken seriously if reported by the patient or a relative.

† Transoesophageal echocardiography (TOE) is usually required to assess the function of prosthetic valves in detail — particularly if malfunction is suspected (the metal causes artefactual echos which can be a serious problem when dealing with the limited echo windows available to the transthoracic echocardiographer; multiple views are available with TOE).

Case 2 | Mitral incompetence (lone)

Frequency in survey: main focus of a short case in 13% of attempts at PACES station 3, cardiovascular.

Record

The pulse is regular (give rate). The venous pressure is not raised and there is no ankle or sacral oedema (unless in cardiac failure). The apex beat is *thrusting* (volume over-load) in the sixth intercostal space in the anterior axillary line, and there is (may be) a systolic thrill. There is a left *parasternal heave*. The *first heart sound* is *soft*, and there is a *third heart sound* (both suggest severe mitral incompetence). There is a loud *pansystolic murmur* at the apex, *radiating* to the *axilla*.

The diagnosis is mitral incompetence with signs of pulmonary hypertension.

Causes of mitral incompetence*

1 Degenerative mitral valve disease
2 Rheumatic heart disease (affects males more commonly than females; contrast with mitral stenosis which affects females more commonly than males)
3 Severe left ventricular dilatation (due to any cause—lateral displacement of the papillary muscles and sometimes possibly dilatation of the mitral annulus† interfere with coaptation of the valve leaflets)
4 Mitral valve prolapse (p. 159)
5 Papillary muscle dysfunction (ischaemia, infarction or other degenerative disease of the chordae tendinae)
6 Previous mitral valvotomy for mitral stenosis (left thoracotomy scar).

Other physical signs (which may occur in severe mitral incompetence)
Mid-diastolic rumbling murmur‡ (brief and rare)
Sharp and abbreviated peripheral pulse (lack of sustained forward stroke volume because of the regurgitant leak)
Wide splitting of the second sound (early closure of the aortic valve because the regurgitant loss shortens the left ventricular ejection time)

Fourth heart sound (acute severe regurgitation with sinus rhythm).

Other causes of mitral incompetence*
Infective endocarditis (fever, splenomegaly, petechiae, splinter haemorrhages, clubbing, Osler's nodes, Janeway lesions, Roth's spots, etc.)
Annular calcification (especially in the elderly female)
Hypertrophic cardiomyopathy (see p. 155)

* Regardless of the aetiology, mitral incompetence is a condition which gradually worsens spontaneously ('mitral incompetence begets mitral incompetence')—enlargement of the left atrium and left ventricle both worsen the incompetence and a vicious circle is set up.
† Left ventricular dilatation is common but the frequency of dilatation of the mitral valve annulus is an uncertain and contro-versial point. The mitral valve ring is a thick fibrous structure, so that if significant dilatation does occur, it probably indicates severe left ventricular disease.

‡ A short mid-diastolic murmur in the context of mitral incom-petence could indicate associated mitral stenosis, or it could repre-sent a flow (left atrium to left ventricle) murmur. The presence of an opening snap in such cases indicates mitral stenosis. In the absence of an opening snap the mid-diastolic murmur has two possible causes: (i) severe mitral incompetence with an increased flow murmur; or (ii) associated mitral stenosis and a calcified mitral valve. In the former there is often a third heart sound. In the latter the murmur is usually longer.

Rupture of the chordae tendinae* (usually causes acute severe mitral incompetence; causes include infective endocarditis, rheumatic mitral valve disease, mitral valve prolapse, trauma)

Connective tissue disorders:

(a) SLE (Libman–Sachs endocarditis — p. 416)

(b) rheumatoid arthritis (?hands, ?nodules)

(c) ankylosing spondylitis (?male with fixed kyphosis and stooped posture; aortic valve more commonly affected — p. 401)

Congenital with or without other abnormalities:

(a) Marfan's syndrome (?tall with long extremities, arachnodactyly, high-arched palate, etc. — p. 156)

(b) Ehlers–Danlos syndrome (?hyperextensible skin and joints, thin scars, etc. — p. 334)

(c) pseudoxanthoma elasticum (?loose skin or 'chicken skin' appearance in antecubital fossae, inguinal regions, neck, etc. — p. 299)

(d) osteogenesis imperfecta (?blue sclerae, deformity from old fractures, etc. — p. 516)

(e) ostium primum atrial septal defect (p. 175)

Endomyocardial fibrosis (10% of cardiac admissions in East Africa; also occurs in West Africa, Southern India and Sri Lanka; the aetiology is unknown).

Indications for surgery

Improvements in surgical techniques, particularly valve repair, and the reduction in operative mortality, have reduced the threshold of physicians for considering surgery in moderately disabled patients (i.e. breathlessness caused by normal activity) — particularly if cardiomegaly and an elevated end-systolic left ventricular volume ($\geq 30\,ml\,m^{-2}$ body surface area) persists despite medical therapy (ACE inhibitors and diuretics). Repair and reconstruction of the valve (valvuloplasty) and its ring (annuloplasty), if feasible (particularly in young adult women), is preferable because of its low perioperative mortality and the lack of requirement for long-term anticoagulation. As for other volume-loading pathology, signs of progressive left ventricular dilatation (demonstrated by serial echocardiography) are the key to decisions relating to timing of surgery. Acute severe mitral incompetence (e.g. infective endocarditis, ruptured chordae tendinae) may require emergency valve replacement.

---

* If the posterior leaflet is predominantly involved the systolic murmur is best heard at the left sternal edge whereas if the anterior leaflet is involved the murmur is best heard over the spine.

Case 3 | Mixed aortic valve disease

Frequency in survey: main focus of a short case in 9% of attempts at PACES station 3, cardiovascular.

Record 1

The pulse is regular (give rate) and *slow rising* (may have a *bisferiens* character). The venous pressure is not raised. The apex beat is palpable 1 cm to the left of the mid-clavicular line as a *forceful, sustained heave* (*pressure loaded*). There is a *systolic thrill* palpable at the apex, in the aortic area and also in the carotid. There is a *harsh ejection systolic murmur* in the aortic area radiating into the neck, the *aortic component* of the second sound is *soft,* and there is an *early diastolic murmur* down the *left sternal edge* audible when the patient is sitting forward in expiration.

The diagnosis is mixed aortic valve disease. Since the pulse is slow rising rather than collapsing, there is a systolic thrill, the second sound is soft and the apex has a forceful heaving quality, I think there is predominant aortic stenosis. (Systolic blood pressure will be low with a low pulse pressure.)

Record 2

The pulse is regular (give rate), of *large volume* and *collapsing* (may have a *bisferiens* character). The venous pressure is not raised. The apex beat is *thrusting* (*volume loaded*) in the *anterior axillary line* in the sixth intercostal space. There is a harsh *ejection systolic murmur* in the aortic area radiating into the neck and an *early diastolic murmur* down the *left sternal edge* (loudest with the patient sitting forward in expiration).

The diagnosis is mixed aortic valve disease. Since the pulse is collapsing rather than plateau in character and the apex is displaced and thrusting, I think the predominant lesion is aortic incompetence. (Blood pressure will show a wide pulse pressure.)

Often mixed aortic murmurs will be due to either aortic stenosis with incidental aortic incompetence or severe aortic incompetence with a systolic flow murmur.* In such cases commenting on dominance is easy. If it is not clear clinically which lesion is predominant and the examiners wish your opinion, point out the factors in favour of each (Table C3.1), stress that you would like to measure the blood pressure and how this would help and lean towards or, if possible, come down in favour of the one you think most likely, giving the reasons; but point out that in this case cardiac catheter studies with left ventricular angiography and an aortogram to show the aortic regurgitation would be required to be certain (see p. 143) for an example of how this might be done in the case of mixed mitral valve disease). Echocardiography may help but Doppler valve gradient is inaccurate in the presence of significant aortic incompetence; TOE may be helpful in more precisely delineating the anatomy of the aortic valve.

Treatment

There is a trend towards aortic valve *repair* if at all possible, particularly in younger patients with congenital aortic valve disease.

As for any valve lesion, surgery is generally indicated for *symptoms* in stenotic lesions (pressure overload), and

* NB The causes of aortic incompetence in this latter case — see p. 150)

for signs of *left ventricular compromise* in regurgitant lesions (volume overload) Exercise testing is advocated in all but severe aortic stenosis to objectively assess exercise tolerance. Echocardiography is vital for follow-up for subtle signs of deteriorating function of the volume-loaded ventricle.

Table C3.1 Factors pointing to a predominant lesion in mixed aortic valve disease

	Aortic incompetence	Aortic stenosis
Pulse	Mainly collapsing	Mainly slow rising
Apex	Thrusting, displaced	Heaving, not displaced much
Systolic thrill	Absent	Present
Systolic murmur	Not loud, not harsh	Loud, harsh
Blood pressure		
systolic	High	Low
pulse pressure	Wide	Narrow

Case 4 | **Mixed mitral valve disease**

Frequency in survey: main focus of a short case in 9% of attempts at PACES station 3, cardiovascular.

Record 1

There is a *malar flush* and a *left thoracotomy scar*. The pulse is irregularly irregular (give rate) in rate and volume and the venous pressure is not raised. The cardiac impulse is *tapping* and the apex beat is *not displaced*. There is a *left parasternal heave*. On auscultation there is a *loud* first heart sound, a *pansystolic murmur** radiating to the axilla, a loud pulmonary second sound, and an *opening snap* followed by a *mid-diastolic rumbling murmur* localized to the apex.

The patient has mixed mitral valve disease. In view of the tapping cardiac impulse, the loud first heart sound and the undisplaced apex, I think this is predominant mitral stenosis. There are signs of pulmonary hypertension.

Record 2

There is a left thoracotomy scar. The pulse is irregularly irregular (give rate) in rate and volume and the venous pressure is not raised. The apex beat is *thrusting* (volume loaded) and *displaced* to the sixth intercostal space in the anterior axillary line and there is a *left parasternal heave*. On auscultation the first heart sound is *soft* and there is a loud *pansystolic murmur* at the left sternal edge and/or apex radiating to the axilla. There is a loud pulmonary second sound and with the patient in the left lateral position I could hear a *mid-diastolic rumbling murmur* following an opening snap.†

The patient has mixed mitral valve disease with pulmonary hypertension. In view of the soft first heart sound and displaced and vigorous apex beat, I think this is predominant mitral incompetence.

If it is not clear clinically which lesion is predominant (e.g. loud first heart sound but enlarged left ventricle) and the examiners want your opinion, point out the factors in favour of each (Table C3.2) then come down in favour of the one you think most likely, but point out that in this case cardiac catheter studies would be required to be certain, e.g. 'It is difficult in this case. The loud first heart sound would suggest predominant mitral stenosis; however, the enlarged left ventricle suggests mitral incompetence as the more important lesion. I think cardiac catheter studies would be required to resolve the issue.'

---

* In the patient with severe pulmonary hypertension when a very large right ventricle displaces the left ventricle posteriorly, the murmur of tricuspid incompetence (p. 162) can mimic that of mitral incompetence. The murmur of tricuspid incompetence is ordinarily heard best at the lower left sternal border, increases with inspiration and is not heard in the axilla or over the spine posteriorly. In tricuspid incompetence giant *v* waves will be present.

† In severe mitral incompetence without mitral stenosis a mid-diastolic flow murmur may be heard without an opening snap. The presence of a third heart sound (due to rapid ventricular filling in severe mitral incompetence) is incompatible with any significant degree of mitral stenosis.

Table C3.2 Factors pointing to a predominant lesion in mixed mitral valve disease

	Mitral stenosis	Mitral incompetence
Pulse	Small volume	Sharp and abbreviated
Apex	Not displaced; tapping impulse present	Displaced, thrusting
First heart sound	Loud	Soft
Third heart sound	Absent	Present

Case 5 | Other combinations of mitral and aortic valve disease

Frequency in survey: main focus of a short case in 8% of attempts at PACES station 3, cardiovascular.

Survey note: patients with any combination of aortic and mitral valve disease may be found in the examination (including, very rarely, lesions of one valve in combination with a prosthetic valve—see p. 138). Whenever you are examining the heart it is essential that, having found some obvious murmurs, you go in search of the others which may be present and less obvious, before presenting your findings (see experience 75, vol. 2, p. 334 and anecdote 29, vol. 2, p. 364).

If the examiner seeks an opinion as to which are the main lesions, or if you feel confident to offer one, the criteria used are the same as those described under mixed mitral valve disease (p. 143) and mixed aortic valve disease (p. 141). The example here is of a *record* of mixed mitral and aortic valve disease.

Record

There is a left thoracotomy scar, and the patient has a malar flush. The pulse is irregularly irregular (give rate) and *slow rising* (can be difficult to assess if the patient is in atrial fibrillation) in character. The venous pressure is not elevated. The apex is . . . (give appropriate word on the basis of what you find; e.g. thrusting, heaving, lifting, etc.) in the anterior axillary line and there is a *left parasternal heave*. There is a *systolic thrill* at the apex, in the aortic area and in the neck. The first heart sound is *loud*, there is a harsh *ejection systolic murmur* in the aortic area radiating into the neck, a *pansystolic murmur* at the lower left sternal edge radiating to the *apex* and to the *axilla*, an *early diastolic murmur* just audible in the aortic area and down the *left sternal edge* with the patient *sitting forward in expiration*, and an *opening snap* followed by a *mid-diastolic rumbling murmur* localized to the apex.

The findings suggest mixed aortic and mitral valve disease. The slow rising pulse suggests aortic stenosis is the dominant aortic valve lesion. It is not possible to ascertain clinically which is the major mitral valve lesion.* Further investigation involving transthoracic echocardiography, probably leading on to transoesophageal echo and/or cardiac catheterization with left ventricular angiography, would be required to assess the haemodynamic significance of each lesion.

---

* In the case of severe mitral stenosis the signs of significant aortic stenosis may be underestimated. A displaced apex in the above setting would tend to suggest that mitral incompetence is haemodynamically dominant.

Case 6 | Mitral stenosis (lone)

Frequency in survey: main focus of a short case in 7% of attempts at PACES station 3, cardiovascular.

Record

There is a *malar flush* and a *left thoracotomy scar.* The pulse is *irregularly irregular* (give rate) in rate and volume (if sinus rhythm the volume is usually small). The venous pressure is not raised, and there is no ankle or sacral oedema (unless in cardiac failure). The cardiac impulse is *tapping* (palpable first heart sound) and the apex is not displaced. There is a *left parasternal heave.* The *first heart sound* is *loud,* there is a loud pulmonary second sound and an *opening snap* followed by a *mid-diastolic rumbling murmur* (with *presystolic accentuation* if the patient is in sinus rhythm) *localized* to the apex and heard most loudly with the patient in the *left lateral* position.*

The diagnosis is mitral stenosis. The patient has had a valvotomy in the past. There are signs of pulmonary hypertension.

Other signs which may be present

Giant *v* waves (tricuspid incompetence—usually secondary; may be primary—see p. 162)

Graham Steell† murmur—rare (secondary pulmonary incompetence; a high-pitched, brief, early diastolic whiff in the presence of marked signs of pulmonary hypertension and a pulse which is not collapsing).

The opening snap soon after the second sound‡ in tight mitral stenosis (<0.09 seconds—mean left atrial pressure above 20 mmHg); longer after the second sound in mild mitral stenosis (>0.1 seconds—mean left atrial pressure below 15 mmHg); absent if the mitral valve is calcified (first heart sound soft).

Indications for intervention (surgery or percutaneous transcatheter valvuloplasty)

Significant symptoms which limit normal activity

An episode of pulmonary oedema without a precipitating cause

Recurrent emboli§

Pulmonary oedema in pregnancy (emergency valvotomy)

Deterioration due to atrial fibrillation which does not respond to medical treatment

Haemoptysis.

Criteria for valvotomy (open or transcatheter)¶

Mobile valve (loud first heart sound, opening snap, absence of calcium in submitral apparatus on TOE)**

Absence of mitral incompetence.

---

* If unsure about the presence of the murmur, it can be accentuated by excrcise—get the patient to touch her toes and then recline 10 times.

† Though associated eponymously with Graham Steell, the original source of the observation was probably George Balfour of Edinburgh, for whom Steell worked as house physician (*Journal of the Royal College of Physicians* 1991, **25**: 66–70).

‡ The interval from the second sound to the opening snap varies with heart rate. If the interval is ≤0.07 seconds with the heart rate <100, the mitral stenosis is usually of haemodynamic significance.

§ Anticoagulation is recommended in all but very mild mitral stenosis, even if in sinus rhythm (particularly if the left atrium is enlarged on transthoracic echo).

¶ Should be considered, particularly in the young female who has a desire for pregnancy. Sometimes it can be performed before the development of significant symptoms.

** Transoesophageal echo (TOE) is by far the best way to image the mitral valve. It is possible to perform transcatheter mitral valvuloplasty using TOE alone, obviating the need for ionizing radiation—particularly useful in pregnancy.

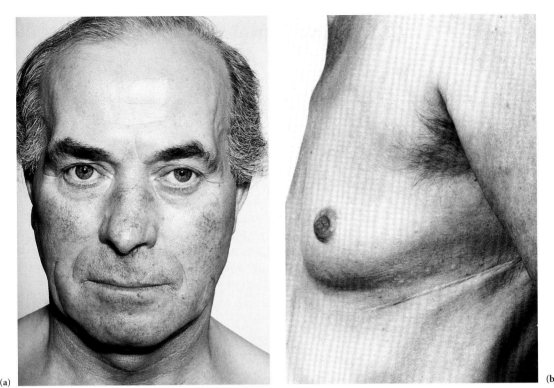

(a)

(b)

Figure C3.1 (a) Mitral facies. (b) Thoracotomy scar for mitral valvotomy.

Case 7 | Aortic stenosis (lone)

Frequency in survey: main focus of a short case in 7% of attempts at PACES station 3, cardiovascular.

Record 1

The *pulse* is regular (give rate), of *small volume* and *slow rising*. The venous pressure is not raised (unless there is cardiac failure). The apex beat is palpable 1 cm to the left of the mid-clavicular line in the fifth intercostal space (the apex position is normal or only slightly displaced in pure aortic stenosis unless the left ventricle is starting to fail) as a forceful *sustained heave* (pressure overload).* There is a *systolic thrill* palpable over the aortic area and the carotids (may be felt over the apex). Auscultation reveals a *harsh ejection systolic murmur* in the aortic area *radiating* into the *neck*, and the *aortic second sound* is *soft* (or absent). (An associated ejection click is usually present if the valve is bicuspid.) (The blood pressure is usually low normal with a decreased difference between systole and diastole — pulse pressure.)

The diagnosis is aortic stenosis.

Possible causes

1 Rheumatic heart disease (mitral valve is usually involved as well and aortic incompetence is often present)
2 Bicuspid aortic valve (commoner in males; typically presents in the sixth decade)
3 Degenerative calcification (in the elderly; the stenosis is usually relatively mild)
4 Congenital (may worsen during childhood and adolescence due to calcification).

In the late stages of aortic stenosis when cardiac failure with low cardiac output supervenes, the murmur may become markedly diminished in intensity. The murmur of associated mitral stenosis should be carefully sought, particularly in the female patient, because the association of these two obstructive lesions tends to diminish the physical findings of each. Mitral stenosis is easily missed and the severity of aortic stenosis underestimated. As with all valvular heart diseases, echocardiography is of great value in a situation like this.

Indications for surgery

In the adult patient valve replacement is indicated for symptoms or a systolic pressure gradient greater than 50–60 mmHg (lower when the left ventricle has failed), as without operation the outlook for these patients is poor. Critical coronary lesions which can exacerbate the symptoms of aortic stenosis (and vice versa) should be bypassed at the same time. Asymptomatic children and young adults can be treated with valvotomy if the obstruction is severe, as the operative risk appears to be less than the risk of sudden death. This is only temporary but may postpone the need for valve replacement for many years. Valve repair is increasingly advocated, particularly in younger patients.

Beta-blockers — to slow the heart rate and hence increase ejection time — can be used in symptomatic patients pending surgery or in those unfit for surgery. Beta-blockers also reduce cardiac work by reducing the

---

* There may also be a presystolic impulse due to left atrial overactivity (this is also felt in moderately severe cases of hypertrophic obstructive cardiomyopathy). The result is a double apical impulse best felt in the left lateral recumbent position. Other signs which may be present include: a fourth heart sound; a single second sound or even paradoxical splitting of the second sound, which are both due to prolonged left ventricular ejection.

rate of rise of systolic pressure and thus the effective valve gradient.

Calcific aortic stenosis is increasingly common and, due to the proximity of the atrioventricular node (and its subsequent involvement in the calcific process), may be associated with atrioventricular nodal block, particularly in the postsurgical population. Look for the small scar(s) of pacemaker implantation inferior to either clavicle.

Record 2

The *carotid pulses* are *normal*, the apical impulse is just palpable and not displaced. There are *no thrills*. There is an *ejection systolic murmur* which is not (usually) harsh or loud and is audible in the aortic area but only faintly in the neck. The aortic component of the second sound is well heard. The blood pressure is normal (or may be hypertensive—there may be a resultant ejection click).

These findings suggest aortic sclerosis* (or minimal aortic stenosis) rather than significant aortic stenosis. (NB The differentiation of this from the other causes of a short systolic murmur are: prolapsing mitral valve, p. 159; trivial mitral incompetence and hypertrophic cardiomyopathy, p. 155.)

---

* Aortic sclerosis on echocardiography, even without haemodynamically significant obstruction to left ventricular outflow, is associated with a 50% increased risk of death from cardiovascular causes and risk of myocardial infarction.

Case 8 | Aortic incompetence (lone)

Frequency in survey: main focus of a short case in 5% of attempts at PACES station 3, cardiovascular. Additional feature in a further 1% (not counting where additional to other valve lesions).

Record

The pulse is regular* (give rate), of large volume and *collapsing* in character. The venous pressure is not raised but *vigorous arterial pulsations* can be seen in the neck (Corrigan's sign†). The apex beat is *thrusting* (volume overload) in the anterior axillary line, in the sixth intercostal space. There is a high-pitched *early diastolic murmur* audible down the left sternal edge and in the aortic area; it is *louder* in *expiration* with the patient *sitting forward.* (The blood pressure may be wide with a high systolic and low diastolic. In severe cases it may be 250–300/30–50.)

The diagnosis is aortic incompetence (now consider looking for *Argyll Robertson pupils, high-arched palate* or *marfanoid* appearance, or obvious features of an arthropathy especially *ankylosing spondylitis.* If these are not present the aortic incompetence is likely to be rheumatic in origin — rheumatic fever and infective endocarditis are the commonest identifiable causes, although hypertension-induced aortic root dilatation with secondary aortic incompetence is being increasingly recognized).

The early diastolic murmur can be difficult to hear and is easily overlooked (see anecdote 29, vol. 2, p. 364). It should be specifically sought with the patient sitting forward in expiration. Listen for the 'absence of silence' in the early part of diastole. The murmur is usually best heard over the mid-sternal region or at the lower left sternal edge. In some cases, particularly syphilitic aortitis, it is loudest in the aortic area. There is often an accompanying systolic murmur due to increased flow which does not necessarily indicate coexistent aortic stenosis (see p. 141).

If there is a mid-diastolic murmur at the apex it may be an Austin Flint murmur‡ or it may represent some associated mitral valve disease. These two may be clinically indistinguishable, though the presence of a loud first heart sound and an opening snap suggest the latter. Though the first heart sound in the Austin Flint may be loud, it is never palpable (i.e. no tapping impulse).

Causes of aortic incompetence

Rheumatic fever

Infective endocarditis (usually occurs on a deformed valve)

Long-standing hypertension (by causing aortic dilatation; complications of hypertension such as ascending aortic aneurysm or dissecting aneurysm may also cause aortic incompetence)

Marfan's syndrome (?tall with long extremities, arachnodactyly and high-arched palate, etc. — p. 156)

Ankylosing spondylitis (?male with fixed kyphosis and stooped 'question mark' posture — p. 401; aortic incompetence may also occur in the other seronegative arthropathies — psoriatic, ulcerative colitis and Reiter's sydrome)

Rheumatoid arthritis (?hands, nodules)

---

* The pulse is usually regular unless there is associated mitral valve disease.

† Other physical signs which result from a large pulse volume and peripheral vasodilatation include de Musset's sign (the head nods with each pulsation) and Quincke's sign (capillary pulsation visible in the nail beds). Of greater clinical value is Duroziez's sign — the femoral artery is compressed and auscultated proximally with a stethoscope; a diastolic murmur implies retrograde flow and aortic incompetence of at least moderate severity.

‡ The Austin Flint murmur occurs in severe aortic incompetence. It is probably attributable to: (i) the regurgitant jet interfering with the opening of the anterior mitral valve leaflet; and (ii) the left ventricular diastolic pressure rising more rapidly than the left atrial diastolic pressure.

Coarctation of the aorta (in association with a bicuspid aortic valve)

Associated perimembranous ventricular septal defect (loss of support of valve—not a feature of muscular VSDs)

Syphilitic aortitis (?Argyll Robertson pupils; there may be an aneurysm of the ascending aorta)

Hurler's syndrome.

Indications for surgery

Although patients tolerate aortic incompetence longer than aortic stenosis (p. 148), the clinician's aim is to replace the valve *before* serious left ventricular dysfunction occurs. Every effort should be made to recognize any reduction in left ventricular function or reserve as early as possible (i.e. before symptoms appear). Serial echocardiograms will show a gradual increase in left ventricular dimensions. Radionuclear angiography can be particularly useful in showing evidence of early left ventricular dysfunction in asymptomatic patients. Vasodilators, particularly ACE inhibitors and calcium antagonists, are thought to reduce the rate of deterioration in mild to moderate aortic incompetence, and should be considered even in asymptomatic patients. The left ventricular ejection fraction, though normal at rest, may show a subnormal rise during exercise. Aortic valve replacement may have to be undertaken as a matter of urgency in patients with infective endocarditis in whom the leaking valve causes rapidly progressive left ventricular dilatation.

Case 9 | Ventricular septal defect

Frequency in survey: main focus of a short case in 3% of attempts at PACES station 3, cardiovascular. Additional feature in a further 1%.

Survey note: youthfulness of patient is sometimes a clue to the diagnosis.

Record

The pulse is regular (give rate) and the venous pressure is not raised. The apex beat is (may be) palpable half-way between the mid-clavicular line and the anterior axillary line, and there is a *left parasternal heave* (there may be a systolic thrill). There is a *pansystolic murmur* at the lower left sternal edge which is also audible at the apex. (The pulmonary second sound may be loud due to pulmonary hypertension and there may be an early diastolic murmur of secondary pulmonary incompetence.)*

The diagnosis is ventricular septal defect.

Other features of ventricular septal defect

Maladie de Roger (small haemodynamically insignificant hole, loud murmur, normal heart size, etc.; tends to close spontaneously)

Development of Eisenmenger's complex (p. 157) if a significant defect is left untreated

Susceptibility to subacute bacterial endocarditis (defects of all sized — NB chemoprophylaxis)

Association with aortic incompetence in 5% of cases (10% in Japan)†

Possibility of a mitral mid-diastolic flow murmur if shunt is large

May occur following acute myocardial infarction with septal rupture

Sometimes associated with Down's syndrome and Turner's syndrome

Newer technology allows percutaneous transcatheter closure of suitable VSDs, including those secondary to acute myocardial infarction.

---

* Although cases like the one presented here are occasionally seen in the exam, it is very unlikely that there would be a haemodynamically significant VSD, as this would have been operated upon in childhood. There may be no evidence of right ventricular overload and the P2 may be normal. Candidates are advised to present the signs as they find them, and conclude whether there is/is not haemodynamically significant VSD. Generally, the defects that have been 'allowed' to persist into adult life are likely to be small.

The smaller the hole, the greater the pressure difference between the two ventricles, and the louder the murmur.

† Defects in the membranous region (just under the aortic valve) persist and are associated with late aortic incompetence which may require surgery-echocardiography is mandatory during follow-up. Defects in the muscular part of the septum close spontaneously during childhood.

Case 10 | Irregular pulse

Frequency in survey: main focus of a short case in 2% of attempts at PACES station 3, cardiovascular. Additional feature in a further 13%.

Survey note: though an irregular pulse was usually encountered in the examination as a feature in the common valvular short cases, occasionally it was itself the main focus of a short case. This was often because the patient had a goitre.

Record

The pulse is . . . /min and *irregularly irregular* in rate and volume suggesting atrial fibrillation with a controlled* ventricular response (uncontrolled if the rate is >90/min). Now look at the *neck* (goitre), *eyes* (exophthalmos), *face* (mitral facies, hypothyroidism,† or hemiplegia due to an embolus) and *chest* (thoracotomy scar).‡

Differential diagnosis

The differentiation of an irregular pulse due to controlled atrial fibrillation from that of multiple extrasystoles, will depend upon the observation that only in atrial fibrillation do long pauses occur in groups of two or more (with ectopic beats the compensatory pause follows a short pause because the ectopic is premature). Furthermore, exercise may abolish extrasystoles but worsen the irregularity of atrial fibrillation. Without recourse to an electrocardiogram, atrial fibrillation can be difficult to distinguish from atrial flutter with variable block, from multiple atrial ectopics due to a shifting pacemaker, and sometimes from paroxysmal atrial tachycardia with block. Only in atrial fibrillation is the ventricular rhythm truly *chaotic*.

Causes of atrial fibrillation

Ischaemic heart disease (especially myocardial infarction)

Sinoatrial (sick sinus syndrome) disease with primary involvement of the conduction tissue

Rheumatic heart disease

Hypertensive heart disease

Thyrotoxicosis

Cardiomyopathy§

Acute infections (especially lung)

Constrictive pericarditis

Local neoplastic infiltration (particularly lymphoma).

---

* Though controlled atrial fibrillation may sometimes feel regular initially, if you concentrate there is a definite irregular variation in the beat to beat time interval (NB experience 79, vol. 2, p. 334).

† Previously treated Graves' disease now on inadequate thyroxine replacement — pulse rate slow, ankle jerk relaxation slow, etc.

‡ If allowed, follow up any positive findings from this *visual survey* by appropriate examination of the relevant system. If there is no visible abnormality proceed, if allowed, to examine the heart, the neck for a goitre, and thyroid status.

§ In many patients with cardiomyopathy no cause can be found ('idiopathic'). It is thought that most of these are a result of viral myocarditis. Often the index event cannot be recalled by the patient, and may have occurred some decades earlier. Occult ischaemic heart disease is the commonest form of 'dilated cardiomyopathy' and the label 'idiopathic' should only be used after coronary artery disease has been excluded by angiography. Sometimes the causal disorder can be identified. Some of the usual causes can be grouped as follows:

1 Toxic (alcohol, adriamycin, cyclophosphamide, emetine, corticosteroids, lithium, phenothiazines, etc.)

2 Metabolic (thiamine deficiency, kwashiorkor, pellagra, obesity, porphyria, uraemia, electrolyte imbalance)

3 Endocrine (thyrotoxicosis, acromegaly, myxoedema, Cushing's, diabetes mellitus)

4 Collagen diseases (SLE, polyarteritis nodosa, etc.)

5 Infiltrative (amyloidosis, haemochromatosis, neoplastic, glycogen storage disease, sarcoidosis, mucopolysaccharidosis, Gaucher's disease, Whipple's disease)

6 Infective (viral, rickettsial, mycobacterial)

7 Genetic (hypertrophic cardiomyopathy, muscular dystrophies)

8 Fibroplastic (endomyocardial fibrosis, Löffler's endocarditis, carcinoid)

9 Miscellaneous (postpartum, incessant atrial tachycardia).

Treatment

Oral anticoagulants and atrial fibrillation: the advice relating to this topic is changing rapidly. It is, however, a *perfect* subject for PACES—so make sure you are up to date! Likewise, the best management of atrial fibrillation. If asked, chose a scenario to discuss—e.g. acute onset atrial fibrillation in an elderly person associated with a chest infection or paroxysmal atrial fibrillation in an otherwise fit 40-year old, etc. Do not forget the role of cardioversion, and remember that management depends on the treatment aim, i.e. restoration and maintenance of sinus rhythm *or* control of the resulting irregular ventricular rate.

Case 11 | Hypertrophic cardiomyopathy

Frequency in survey: main focus of a short case in 2% of attempts at PACES station 3, cardiovascular.*

Record

The pulse is regular (may be irregular if patient is in atrial fibrillation) and of normal volume (in severe cases the carotid pulse has a '*jerky*' character) and the JVP is not elevated (may show a prominent *a* wave). The cardiac apex is forceful in the left fifth intercostal space just outside the mid-clavicular line, there is (may be) a strong *presystolic impulse* (*double apical impulse* caused by atrial systole), and a *systolic thrill* is palpable over the left sternal border. There is a *fourth heart sound*, and an *ejection systolic murmur* (may be harsh) over the left third interspace, which radiates widely to the base and to the axilla (perhaps because it merges with the pansystolic murmur of mitral incompetence which frequently accompanies hypertrophic cardiomyopathy). The intensity of the ejection murmur is enhanced by minimal exercise.

The findings suggest hypertrophic cardiomyopathy (HCM).

Other features of hypertrophic cardiomyopathy

Patients may be asymptomatic. Severe cases are marked by symptoms such as dyspnoea, palpitations, angina, dizziness and syncope (often after cessation of exercise due to temporary reduction in cardiac output or secondary to paroxysmal ventricular arrhythmia; cf. aortic stenosis where syncope usually occurs during exercise)

ECG: normal in 25%. ST–T and T wave changes, tall QRS in mid-precordial leads. Q wave in inferior and lateral precordial leads (due to septal hypertrophy). Sometimes left-axis deviation

Chest X-ray may be normal, or it may show left atrial enlargement

Echocardiography is diagnostic and characteristically shows asymmetrical septal hypertrophy, and may show systolic anterior motion of the anterior mitral valve leaflet

HCM is an autosomal dominant condition associated with several genes coding for myosin (with hundreds of different mutations described). Many cases arise *de novo* and the condition may have variable penetrance making genetic studies difficult. All first-degree relatives of an affected individual should be offered clinical screening for the condition

The risk of a poor outcome for any given individual can be assessed using the following criteria: history of syncope, family history of sudden cardiac death, poor blood pressure response to exercise, the presence of ventricular arrhythmias on Holter monitoring, outflow tract gradient of >40 mmHg at rest, and a septal thickness of >18 mm on echocardiography

Treatment options include beta blockers, rate-limiting calcium antagonists, septal ablation or myomectomy and pacing technologies, including implantable defibrillators for high risk individuals.

---

* Hypertrophic cardiomyopathy did not occur in our extensive pre PACES surveys. A case of hypertrophic obstructive cardiomyopathy (HOCM), as it was referred to, was included in one mock Membership examination. One of the examiners commented to us that none of his prospective candidates got the correct diagnosis. It is of course possible that conditions such as HCM did occur in the examination sittings covered by our survey, but the candidates concerned did not get, or even suspect, the diagnoses and were not enlightened by their examiners. These days, the word 'obstructive' has been removed as it is not essential for the diagnosis, and the risk profile is the same for both the obstructive and non-obstructive forms of HCM.

Case 12 | **Marfan's syndrome**

Frequency in survey: main focus of a short case in 2% of attempts at PACES station 3, cardiovascular.

Survey note: see CVS PACES experience 9, vol. 2, p. 297

Marfan's syndrome is dealt with on p. 407

Case 13 | Eisenmenger's syndrome

Frequency in survey: did not occur in the small initial survey of PACES station 3, cardiovascular.

Predicted frequency from older, more extensive MRCP short case surveys: main focus of a short case in 2% of attempts at PACES station 3, cardiovascular. Additional feature in a further 1%.

Record

There is *central cyanosis* and *clubbing* of the fingers (may be only in the toes in patent ductus arteriosus). The pulse (give rate) is regular (and small in volume). A large *a* wave is (may be) seen in the venous pulse (due to forceful atrial contraction in the face of the right ventricular hypertrophy). There is a marked *left parasternal heave* and (often) a palpable (pulmonary) second heart sound. On auscultation (the signs of pulmonary hypertension are heard) the *second heart sound* is *loud* and single, there is (may be) a right ventricular fourth heart sound, (may be) a pulmonary early systolic ejection click, (may be) an early diastolic murmur (dilated pulmonary artery leads to secondary pulmonary incompetence), and (may be) a pansystolic murmur (secondary tricuspid incompetence — *v* wave in JVP).

These findings suggest Eisenmenger's syndrome with pulmonary hypertension.

Causes

1 Large, non-restrictive ventricular septal defect (VSD)* (cyanosis due to bidirectional shunt at the ventricular level)
2 Primary pulmonary hypertension (cyanosis due to intrapulmonary shunting)
3 Atrial septal defect (fixed and wide splitting of the second sound)
4 Patent ductus arteriosus† (normal splitting of the second sound — *P2* follows *A2* and the split widens with inspiration; only the lower limbs are cyanosed — differential cyanosis)
5 Other complex congenital heart disease (cyanosis usually due to bidirectional shunt at the ventricular level)
6 Fallot's tetralogy — palliated or untreated (see p. 163)

Once Eisenmenger's syndrome has developed it is too late (high mortality) for correction of the cardiac anomaly. A palliative procedure involving redirection of the venous return has been successful in the presence of transposition of the great arteries, VSD and severe pulmonary vascular disease. Heart/lung transplantation is an option but has a much poorer prognosis than heart transplantation alone. Death commonly occurs between

* When due to a VSD it is termed Eisenmenger's complex. The classic pansystolic murmur of the VSD tends to disappear as the right and left ventricular pressures equalize. A pansystolic murmur in Eisenmenger's complex is more likely to be from tricuspid incompetence.

† Again the classic patent ductus arteriosus murmur tends to shorten to a soft systolic murmur, and then disappear as the pressures in the pulmonary artery and descending aorta equalize. Untreated patent ductus arteriosus is very rare these days as it can be repaired surgically without the need for cardiopulmonary bypass.

Table C3.3 The features which may be helpful in differentiating Eisenmenger's syndrome from tetralogy of Fallot

	Eisenmenger's syndrome	Fallot's tetralogy
Pulmonary systolic thrill	Absent	Present
Pulmonary systolic murmur	Absent	Intense (unless such severe stenosis that there is no flow)
Right ventricle	Very hypertrophied	Hypertrophied
Chest X-ray	Large pulmonary arteries	Small pulmonary arteries

the ages of 20 and 40 years and is usually due to pulmonary infarction, right heart failure, dysrhythmias and, less often, infective endocarditis or cerebral abscess.

With the advent of cardiopulmonary bypass in the 1960s, VSD repair was possible, and the prevalence of Eisenmenger's syndrome due to congenital heart disease in the adult population is falling all the time.

It is generally now agreed that untreated isolated atrial septal defect does *not* lead to Eisenmenger's sydrome. The absence of chest signs help to differentiate Eisenmenger's syndrome from the cyanosis and pulmonary hypertension of cor pulmonale. The features which may be helpful in differentiating Eisenmenger's syndrome from Fallot's tetralogy (the commonest cause of central cyanosis in the adolescent or young adult) are shown in Table C3.3. Furthermore, the patient with Fallot's tetralogy in the examination may well have thoracotomy scars and a pulse which is weaker on the left than on the right, from a previous Blalock shunt operation (see p. 163).

Case 14 | **Mitral valve prolapse**

Frequence in survey: did not occur in the small initial survey of PACES station 3, cardiovascular.

Predicted frequency from older, more extensive MRCP short case surveys: main focus of a short case in 2% of attempts at PACES station 3, cardiovascular.

Record

The pulse (in this well-looking patient) is regular (give rate) and the venous pressure is not raised. The apex beat is palpable in the fifth intercostal space in the mid-clavicular line. There are no heaves or thrills. On auscultation the heart sounds are normal but there is a *midsystolic click** (which is usually but not always) followed by a late *systolic crescendo-decrescendo murmur* loudest at the left sternal edge (as the condition progresses the murmur develops the characteristics of mitral incompetence — p. 139).

These findings suggest mitral valve prolapse (floppy posterior mitral valve leaflet — echocardiography is useful for confirmation).

The prolapse is increased by anything which decreases cardiac volume (standing position; Valsalva manoeuvre) and as a result the click and murmur occur earlier during systole and the murmur is prolonged. Increasing cardiac volume (squatting position, propranolol) has the reverse effect. Phonocardiography documents these effects well. Mitral valve prolapse (said to occur in 5–10% of the population,† more commonly in females) is usually asymptomatic but may be associated with atypical chest pain, palpitation, fatigue and dyspnoea. The symptoms may become worse once the patient knows there is a murmur. The prognosis is good† but complications can include infective endocarditis, atrial and ventricular dysrhythmias, worsening mitral incompetence, embolic phenomena (transient ischaemic attacks, amaurosis fugax, acute hemiplegia), rupture of the mitral valve (age-related degenerative changes) and sudden death. The condition may be familial and there may be a family history of sudden death. There is a serious risk of precip-

itating cardiac neurosis which may, at least in part, contribute to the association with atypical chest pain. There is often myxomatous degeneration of the mitral valve, deposition of acid mucopolysaccharide material and redundant valve tissue.

Causes and associations
Marfan's syndrome
Polycystic kidney disease
Congenital heart disease
Congestive cardiomyopathy
Hypertrophic cardiomyopathy
Myocarditis
Mitral valve surgery
Fabry's disease
Ehlers–Danlos syndrome
Osteogenesis imperfecta
Systemic lupus erythematosus (after Libman–Sachs endocarditis)

---

* The click is characteristic but easily missed if you have not heard one before. This may be because of the distraction of the murmur. Concentrate on listening for other sounds at different frequencies from the murmur and you will hear it.

† It may be that the clinically silent, echocardiographic mitral valve prolapse which is common in thin, young women is a variant of normal, distinct from the floppy valve or complication of chordal lengthening or rupture needing mitral valve replacement, which is

commonest in elderly men. It seems likely that 'echo only' mitral valve prolapse carries a good prognosis whereas complications are associated with the clinical variety. Since patients with auscultatory and echocardiographic evidence of mitral valve prolapse may be candidates for endocarditis, they should be recommended for antimicrobial prophylaxis before dental procedures, etc. This prophylaxis is only required if a murmur is audible. 'Click only' patients have a very low incidence of subacute bacterial endocarditis.

Muscular dystrophy
Turner's syndrome
Primary mitral valve prolapse.

Other points of note

Mitral valve prolapse (MVP) can be an incidental finding during echocardiography (a technical MVP). Endocarditis prophylaxis is generally recommended only in cases where MVP is associated with an audible click or murmur.

Indications for surgery are as for mitral regurgitation (see p. 139); surgical repair rather than valve replacement is favoured.

Palpitations are usually due to benign ventricular ectopy and generally respond well to beta blockade if symptoms are troublesome.

Other causes of a short systolic murmur

audible at the apex should always be thought of and excluded. These are:

Trivial mitral incompetence (the usual cause—the murmur may not be pansystolic but there is no click)

Aortic stenosis/sclerosis (see p. 148)

Hypertrophic cardiomyopathy (see p. 155).

Case 15 | **Patent ductus arteriosus**

Frequence in survey: did not occur in the small initial survey of PACES station 3, cardiovascular.

Predicted frequency from older, more extensive MRCP short case surveys: main focus of a short case in 2% of attempts at PACES station 3, cardiovascular.

Record

The *pulse* is *collapsing* (may be normal if the duct is narrow and the 'run-off' from the aorta to the left pulmonary artery is small) in character, regular (give rate) and the venous pressure is not raised. The apex is *thrusting* (volume overload) in the anterior axillary line (may be normal if the ductus is small), and there is (sometimes) a *left parasternal heave* (if there is associated pulmonary hypertension). On auscultation there is a continuous '*machinery' murmur** with systolic *accentuation* heard in the second left intercostal space near the sternal edge (but maximal 5–7.5 cm above or to the left of this, *beneath the clavicle*, and also *heard posteriorly*).

The diagnosis is patent ductus arteriosus.

Male to female ratio is 1 : 3.

The incidence is higher in patients born at a high altitude. Spontaneous closure is rare except in premature infants. The diagnosis is made by echocardiography or MRI. Closure can usually be effected using percutaneous transcatheter technology although surgical repair is still advocated for large calcified ducts.

Other causes of a continuous murmur†
With collapsing pulse

Mitral incompetence and aortic incompetence
Ventricular septal defect and aortic incompetence.

Without collapsing pulse

Venous hum (common in normal children—maximal to the right of the sternum—diminishes or disappears when the child lies flat or when the right JVP is compressed)
Pulmonary arteriovenous fistula or shunt (e.g. Blalock).

Complications of patent ductus arteriosus

Infective endocarditis (infection of the ductus—even small ones; therefore closure is always recommended unless Eisenmenger's is already present)
Heart failure
Eisenmenger's syndrome (p. 157).

---

* The murmur seldom lasts for the whole of systole and diastole. It may occupy only the latter part of systole and the early part of diastole. Occasionally, particularly in young children, it may occur as a crescendo in late systole only. The unwary may mistake the systolic component of this murmur for pulmonary stenosis—listen posteriorly: the murmur of a patent ductus will still be as loud as that anteriorly, whereas that of pulmonary stenosis will be much softer.
† NB the murmur of patent ductus distinguishes itself by being loudest below the left clavicle. There should not usually be any diagnostic difficulty.

Case 16 | Tricuspid incompetence

Frequency in survey: did not occur in the small initial survey of PACES station 3, cardiovascular.

Predicted frequency from older, more extensive MRCP short case surveys: main focus of a short case in 2% of attempts at PACES station 3, cardiovascular. Additional feature in some others.

Record

The JVP is elevated (say height*) and shows *giant v waves*† which oscillate the earlobe (if the venous pressure is high enough) and which are diagnostic of tricuspid incompetence. (Now, if allowed, examine the heart, respiratory system and abdomen.‡)

The commonest cause of tricuspid incompetence is *not* organic, but dilatation of the right ventricle and of the tricuspid valve ring due to right ventricular failure§ in conditions such as:
Mitral valve disease
Cor pulmonale
Eisenmenger's syndrome
Right ventricular infarction (rare)
Primary pulmonary hypertension.

Causes of primary tricuspid incompetence
Infective endocarditis (especially intravenous drug addicts—recurrent septicaemia with pulmonary infiltrates should raise suspicion)

Congenital heart disease (e.g. Ebstein's anomaly)
Carcinoid syndrome (flushing, diarrhoea, hepatomegaly, sometimes asthma; fibrous plaques on the endothelial surface of the heart are associated with tricuspid incompetence and pulmonary stenosis)
Myxomatous change (may be associated with mitral valve prolapse or atrial septal defect)
Rheumatic heart disease (extremely rare and usually associated with tricuspid stenosis; almost invariably associated with other valvular disease—if there is pulmonary hypertension it may not be possible to differentiate organic from functional tricuspid incompetence on clinical grounds alone)
Trauma.

---

*In centimetres vertically above the sternal angle, not the suprasternal notch or supraclavicular fossa. In tricuspid incompetence which is secondary to right ventricular dilatation, the venous pressure is usually of the order of 8–10 cm or more.
† These *v* waves are in fact *cv* waves because systole spans the time between *c* and *v* waves of the normal jugular pulse.
‡ In the *heart* you would expect to find the pansystolic murmur of tricuspid incompetence which may be louder on inspiration (Carvallo's sign) and augmented by the Müller manoeuvre (attempted inspiration against a closed glottis). The murmur may be audible at the lower right sternal edge if the right-sided pressures are high. There may be murmurs of associated or underlying disease of the heart valves, especially mitral. There may be a tricuspid

diastolic murmur louder on inspiration and augmented by the Müller manoeuvre. This could be due to increased flow across the tricuspid valve or to concomitant tricuspid stenosis. In the *respiratory system* you would be looking for signs of the condition leading to underlying cor pulmonale. In the *abdomen* you may find forceful epigastric pulsations and hepatomegaly which is tender and pulsatile. In severe, long-standing tricuspid incompetence, ascites and signs of chronic liver disease (p. 106) can occur.
§ The importance of a functional tricuspid valve in maintaining normal right ventricular function is increasingly recognized and a surgeon will often place an annuloplasty ring for secondary tricuspid regurgitation when operating for the primary condition. Tricuspid valve replacement is rarely indicated or performed.

Case 17 | Fallot's tetralogy with a Blalock shunt

Frequency in survey: main focus of a short case in 0.9% of attempts at PACES station 3, cardiovascular.

Survey note: the cases of Fallot's tetralogy in our survey all had a Blalock shunt.

Record

There is a thoracotomy scar. There is *central cyanosis* and *clubbing* of the fingers. The pulse is regular (give rate) and the *left pulse is weaker than the right* (or vice versa). The venous pressure is normal. The apex beat is (may be) palpable (say where), there is a *left parasternal heave* and a *systolic thrill* is palpable in the pulmonary area. There is a loud *ejection systolic murmur** (unless the stenosis is so severe that virtually no blood traverses it) in the *pulmonary area*. There is (may be) a soft early diastolic murmur of aortic regurgitation (common in adult survivors).

It is likely that this patient has had a Blalock shunt† for Fallot's tetralogy (pulmonary stenosis, ventricular septal defect,‡ right ventricular hypertrophy and overriding aorta).

The features that may be helpful in differentiating Fallot's tetralogy from Eisenmenger's are shown in Table C3.3 (p. 158).

---

*There may be a continuous murmur over the shunt (front or back of chest).

† Anastomosis of the subclavian artery to the pulmonary artery. This operation is not often performed nowadays as total correction on cardiopulmonary bypass is usually the treatment of choice.

‡ There is no murmur from the VSD as it is large and non-restrictive, i.e. both ventricles are at the same pressure.

Case 18 | Raised jugular venous pressure

Frequency in survey: did not occur in the small initial survey of PACES station 3, cardiovascular.

Predicted frequency from older, more extensive MRCP short case surveys: main focus of a short case in 0.9% of attempts at PACES station 3, cardiovascular. Additional feature in many others.

Record

The JVP is elevated (measure) at . . . cm above the sternal angle (look for individual waves and time against the opposite carotid artery). The predominant wave is the systolic *v* wave which reaches the ear lobes. (If there is no oscillation of the blood column, sit the patient up to find the upper level. Make sure that there is no superior vena caval obstruction with congestion of the face and neck, and prominent veins on the upper chest — p. 90). The carotid pulsation is irregularly irregular and the rhythm is atrial fibrillation (look for the evidence of congestive cardiac failure: ankle and sacral oedema, hepatomegaly, which may be pulsatile in tricuspid incompetence).

The large *v* wave suggests tricuspid incompetence either organic or due to congestive cardiac failure (see p. 162)

Causes of a raised JVP (if venous obstruction is excluded)

Congestive cardiac failure (ischaemic heart disease, valvular heart disease, hypertensive heart disease, cardiomyopathy)

Cor pulmonale (?signs of chronic small airways obstruction, cyanosis, etc. — p. 92)

Pulmonary hypertension (large *a* wave in the JVP when in sinus rhythm — primary (young females) and secondary to mitral valve disease or thrombo-obliterative disease)

Constrictive pericarditis (abrupt *x* and *y* descent, loud early *S3* ('pericardial knock') though heart sounds often normal, slight 'paradoxical' pulse, *no signs in the lungs*; chest X-ray may show calcified pericardium)

Large pericardial effusion (*x* descent, pulsus paradoxus, breathlessness, chest X-ray shows cardiomegaly, echocardiogram shows effusion).

Case 19 | **Coarctation of the aorta**

Frequency in survey: did not occur in the small initial survey of PACES station 3, cardiovascular.

Predicted frequency from older, more extensive MRCP short case surveys: main focus of a short case in 0.9% of attempts at PACES station 3, cardiovascular. Additional feature in a further 1%.

Record 1

The radial pulses (in this young adult with a well-developed upper torso) are regular, equal* and of large volume (give rate). The *carotid pulsations* are *vigorous*,† and the JVP is not elevated (unless there is heart failure). The *femorals* are *delayed* and of *poor volume* (palpate the radial and femoral simultaneously). The *blood pressure* in the right arm is elevated at 190/110 mmHg (it will be *low in the legs*). There are *visible arterial pulsations*‡ and *bruits* can be heard over and around the *scapula*, *anterior axilla* and over the *left sternal border* (internal mammary artery). The cardiac impulse is heaving but not displaced (unless in failure). Systolic *thrills* are palpable over the collaterals and suprasternally. There is a *systolic murmur* which is loudest at the level of the *fourth intercostal space posteriorly* (the level of the coarctation), but is also audible in the *second intercostal spaces* close to the sternum (the murmur — if present — of the associated bicuspid aortic valve is often obscured by that from the coarctation).§

These findings suggest a diagnosis of coarctation of the aorta.

Record 2

There is a left-sided thoracotomy scar. The right radial pulse is normal, whilst the left is diminished (or absent). The carotid pulses are normal and the JVP is not elevated. The femorals are palpable and there is no radiofemoral delay. The apex beat is normal, and there is an ejection click associated with a soft systolic murmur in the aortic area.

The left thoracotomy scar and absent/reduced left radial pulse suggest repaired coarctation of the aorta whilst the aortic signs are compatible with associated bicuspid aortic valve. (The left radial pulse is commonly reduced or absent as a result of the surgical repair — the origin of the left subclavian artery is in close proximity to the coarctation and the left subclavian can actually form part of the repair in some cases.)

---

* Rarely (2%) the coarctation is proximal to the origin of the left subclavian artery and the left arm pulses will be weaker than the right; rib notching will be unilateral and right sided.

† If you see vigorous carotid pulsations the likeliest cause is aortic incompetence (?collapsing pulse). The occasional patient, however, will have coarctation.

‡ Collaterals are best observed with the patient sitting up and leaning forward with the arms hanging by the side.

§ A continuous murmur in systole and diastole, arising from the dilated collaterals, may be heard over the back. An early diastolic murmur arising because of the dilated ascending aorta may be heard especially in older patients.

Following repair

It can be useful to assess the brachial/ankle index with a Doppler probe to assess the functional state of the repair.

Echocardiography is a poor imaging modality after coarctation repair; MRI is much preferred and is recommended for follow-up.

Balloon dilatation of the coarctation and/or recoarctation is useful in selected cases. Stent implantation is under assessment.

Complications following repair

1 Aortic valve degeneration
2 Aneurysm formation at site of repair (can become infected — mycotic aneurysm)
3 Aneurysm rupture
4 Recoarctation
5 Aortic dissection in later life (anywhere from top to bottom).

Male to female ratio is 2 : 1.

Other features and associations of coarctation of the aorta

Rib notching* and poststenotic dilatation on chest X-ray

Bicuspid aortic valve in 25% (site of infective endocarditis and may lead to coexisting aortic incompetence; diagnosis can be made by echocardiography)

Berry aneurysms of the circle of Willis (may cause death even in corrected cases)

Patent ductus arteriosus (?machinery murmur, etc. — p. 161)

Turner's syndrome (check for features of Turner's if your patient is female — webbed neck, increased carrying angle, short stature, etc. — p. 456)

Marfan's syndrome (?tall, arachnodactyly, high arched palate, lens dislocation, etc. — p. 407)

High mortality after the age of 40. Hypertension* may not be cured even in corrected cases (low perfusion of kidneys may involve the renin — angiotensin system).

Other causes of rib notching

Neurofibromatosis (multiple neuromata on the intercostal nerves)

Enlargement of nerves (amyloidosis, congenital hypertrophic polyneuropathy)

Inferior vena cava obstruction

Blalock shunt operation (left-sided unilateral rib notching)

Congenital.

---

* Coarctation in adults usually presents clinically with hypertension.

Case 20 | **Slow pulse**

Frequency in survey: did not occur in the small initial survey of PACES station 3, cardiovascular.

Predicted frequency from older, more extensive MRCP short case surveys: main focus of a short case in 0.9% of attempts at PACES station 3, cardiovascular.

Record

The pulse rate is regular at 40/min (irregularly irregular pulse with beat-to-beat variation may be atrial fibrillation with a slow ventricular response) and there is *no increase* in the rate on *standing* (complete heart block; mostly in older patients). The JVP is not elevated (unless there is heart failure) but just visible, and there is a complete dissociation of *a* and *v* waves with frequent *cannon waves* (flicking *a* waves occurring during ventricular systole). (The pulse pressure is large and this may be evident clinically.)

This patient has complete heart block.

Other causes of bradycardia

Beta-blocker therapy: about 2% of patients receiving β-blockers have excessive bradycardia (heart rate increases by a few beats on standing and during exercise)

Atrial fibrillation with a slow ventricular response (may be regular if there is associated complete heart block): the patient may be on β-blockers and/or digoxin

Hypothyroidism (?facies, ankle jerks, etc. — p. 438)

Sinoatrial disease: bradycardia–tachycardia syndrome

Digoxin toxicity.

Cardiac pacing

Most patients with complete heart block will benefit from a demand pacemaker (even asymptomatic patients with a heart rate <40). Cardiac pacing is recommended for all symptomatic patients with bradycardia, and for those with brady–tachy syndrome who will need anti-arrhythmic therapy to control episodes of tachycardia.

Most authorities would agree that all patients with complete heart block, and those with Mobitz type 2 block, should be offered cardiac pacing, even if the arrhythmia is intermittent (unless associated with acute ischaemia or other reversible events) and/or the patient is asymptomatic.

Case 21 | **Dextrocardia**

Frequency in survey: did not occur in the small initial survey of PACES station 3, cardiovascular.

Predicted frequency from older, more extensive MRCP short case surveys: main focus of a short case in 0.5% of attempts at PACES station 3, cardiovascular.

Record

The pulse is regular (give rate) and of good volume. The JVP is not raised. The apex beat is *not palpable on the left side*, but can be felt in the fifth *right* intercostal space in the mid-clavicular line.

This patient has dextrocardia.* (If allowed, listen to the lung fields — Kartagener's syndrome — and feel the abdomen to see which side the liver is on — situs inversus.)

If situs inversus is present the patient is usually otherwise normal. Dextrocardia without situs inversus is usually associated with cardiac malformation. Dextrocardia may occur in Turner's syndrome.

Kartagener' syndrome: dextrocardia, bronchiectasis, situs inversus, infertility, dysplasia of frontal sinuses, sinusitis and otitis media. Patients have ciliary immotility.

---

* Consider the possibility of this diagnosis if you cannot feel the apex beat and than have difficulty hearing the heart sounds. As you gradually move the stethoscope towards the right side of the chest, they get louder.

Case 22 | **Pulmonary stenosis**

Frequency in survey: did not occur in the small initial survey of PACES station 3, cardiovascular.

Predicted frequency from older, more extensive MRCP short case surveys: main focus of a short case in 0.5% of attempts at PACES station 3, cardiovascular.

Record

The pulse is regular and the JVP is not elevated (prominent *a* wave in severe cases).* The cardiac apex is not palpable but there is (may be) a *left parasternal heave*. A *systolic thrill* is palpable over the left second and third interspaces. An *ejection click* and a *systolic murmur* (and maybe also a fourth heart sound) are heard over the *pulmonary area*. The murmur is louder during inspiration and radiates to the suprasternal notch. The second sound is (may be) split (the pulmonary component is soft).†

The diagnosis is pulmonary stenosis.

Poststenotic dilatation of the pulmonary arteries may be seen on the chest X-ray and, in the severe case, right ventricular hypertrophy and diminution of pulmonary vascular markings. A minor degree of pulmonary stenosis is compatible with a normal life span. Surgical relief is required in symptomatic cases or if there is a gradient of more than 50 mmHg across the pulmonary valve. Balloon valvotomy is becoming the technique of choice in children and young adults, especially if the valve is not dysplastic. If treatment is delayed too long in severe pulmonary stenosis an irreversible fibrotic change can take place in the hypertrophied right ventricle.

Pulmonary stenosis may occur in the setting of surgically corrected tetralogy of Fallot. In this case there will usually be a left or right thoracotomy scar associated with a previous Blalock shunt (see p. 163) *and* a midline scar from the later complete Fallot repair. The dysplastic pulmonary valve was often replaced with a valved conduit which can calcify and obstruct in later life. If there is a single midline scar, the patient may have had an open pulmonary valvotomy in childhood, which often leaves a loudish murmur without any objective evidence of obstruction. Echocardiography is the key investigation.

---

* A patient with severe pulmonary stenosis may have cyanosis (check buccal mucosa) if the foramen ovale is unsealed and this may be intermittent.

† Pulmonary incompetence is commonly associated with many causes of pulmonary stenosis (particularly after repair of tetralogy of Fallot and after pulmonary valvuloplasty). One should specifically listen for the tell-tale early diastolic murmur radiating from the pulmonary area down the left sternal edge. Like the murmur of aortic incompetence, it is easily missed unless specifically sought.

Case 23 | **Cannon waves**

Frequency in survey: did not occur in the small initial survey of PACES station 3, cardiovascular.

Predicted frequency from older, more extensive MRCP short case surveys: main focus of a short case in 0.5% of attempts at PACES station 3, cardiovascular.

Survey note: one candidate was asked to examine the heart only, another was asked to look at the patient's neck and then examine the heart, and a third was asked to take the patient's pulse.

Record

There are sharp *a* waves* (cannon waves*) visible in this patient's jugular veins. (Feel the carotid pulse on the opposite side.) These waves occur irregularly even though the pulse is regular but slow at 48/min.

As the waves are irregular and the pulse is slow the explanation is that this patient has complete heart block. (The patient may have a demand pacemaker and it will be felt as a solid, mobile mass below the right or left clavicle with an associated scar(s). He/she may have been admitted for changing the defunct generator.)

If allowed to auscultate you will hear an S1 of variable intensity; the sound coinciding with the cannon wave will be soft.

Causes of cannon waves

Regular cannon waves—nodal rhythm, paroxysmal nodal tachycardia, partial heart block with very long PR interval

Irregular cannon waves—complete heart block, multiple ectopic beats.

---

* Candidates who have never seen cannon waves have been known to confuse them with giant *v* waves (see p. 162). Cannon waves are seen like sharp flicks and are quite characteristic in appearance. You should attempt to see some in the pacemaker clinic of a cardiology unit. Cannon waves are giant *a* waves and these occur whenever the right atrium contracts against a closed tricuspid valve, and the whole of the energy released by the right atrial contraction is transmitted to the JVP, as forward flow is impossible (the ECG complex associated with a cannon wave shows that the P wave falls between the end of the QRS and the T wave or at the end of the T wave).

Case 24 | Pulmonary incompetence

Frequency in survey: did not occur in the small initial survey of PACES station 3, cardiovascular.

Predicted frequency from older, more extensive MRCP short case surveys: main focus of a short case in 0.3% of attempts at PACES station 3, cardiovascular.

Record 1*

This patient has features of *mitral stenosis* (state them—p. 146) combined with evidence of *pulmonary hypertension* and *pulmonary incompetence* suggested by a *palpable second sound* in the pulmonary area, followed by an *early diastolic murmur*, which has a sharp whiffing quality, most loudly heard in the pulmonary area but radiating only for a few centimetres down the left sternal edge. There is also an early ejection systolic murmur audible over the pulmonary area.

The patient has a Graham Steell murmur complicating mitral stenosis with pulmonary hypertension.

Record 2*

This patient has *cyanosis* and a weak peripheral pulse. The JVP is *elevated* with both *a* and *v* waves being prominent. The apex beat is not palpable, but there is a strong right ventricular heave. The auscultatory signs are a *gallop of the fourth heart sound*, a *pansystolic murmur* over the tricuspid area (sometimes associated with a *thrill*), a *pulmonary ejection click*, grade 2/6 midsystolic murmur over the pulmonary area and an *early diastolic murmur* heard over the same region. In addition she† also has ankle oedema.

These features suggest that she has *primary pulmonary hypertension* associated with pulmonary incompetence.

Record 3‡

The JVP is elevated with a large *v* wave reaching the right earlobe (there may be secondary *tricuspid incompetence*). There is a right ventricular lift but the apex beat is not palpable. There is a pansystolic murmur heard over the left third interspace and a high-pitched mid-diastolic murmur.§

The patient has pulmonary incompetence and tricuspid incompetence.

---

*The most likely scenario of a case where there is a focus on pulmonary incompetence is that of a patient who has established pulmonary hypertension and its associated features. Pulmonary hypertension results in dilatation of both the main pulmonary artery and the valve ring; the valve cusps do not close completely and a regurgitant murmur, known as the Graham Steell murmur, is produced. In some cases this becomes the focus of the examiners' attention and your record should take account of it.

†In primary pulmonary hypertension the ratio of males to females is 1:4.

‡Rarely there may be a patient with a valvular pulmonary incompetence caused either by carcinoid (see p. 125) involvement of the pulmonary valve or due to endocarditis (the patient may have been a drug addict). In patients with a valvular pulmonary incompetence there is unlikely to be any evidence of pulmonary hypertension. Other possible causes of valvular incompetence are congenital malformation or a previous surgical procedure.

§The diastolic murmur of valvular pulmonary incompetence occurs after the delayed P₂ which is more like mid-diastolic than early diastolic in timing.

Causes of pulmonary hypertension

Primary: primary pulmonary hypertension—rare, favours women with a female to male ratio of 4 : 1.

Secondary:

Acquired heart disease: mitral valve disease, congestive cardiomyopathy

Congenital heart disease: atrial/ventricular septal defect, patent ductus arteriosus

Pulmonary vascular disease:

(a) vasoactive: autoimmune disease, high altitude

(b) obliterative: thromboembolic disease, schistosomiasis

Structural lung disease: emphysema, cystic fibrosis, etc.

Case 25 | Infective endocarditis

Frequency in survey: did not occur in the small initial survey of PACES station 3, cardiovascular.

Predicted frequency from older, more extensive MRCP short case surveys: main focus of a short case in 0.3% of attempts at PACES station 3, cardiovascular.

Record

This patient has mitral incompetence* suggested by a pansystolic murmur over the precordium, radiating to the left axilla, a third heart sound, a dilated left ventricle with the point of maximum impulse in the left sixth intercostal space in the anterior axillary line, and a right ventricular lift. There are (may be) *splinter haemorrhages*, the conjunctivae are pale† and there is a *petechial haemorrhage* inside the right lower eyelid (look for *cutaneous manifestations* elsewhere on the body). There is no clubbing‡ (ask to look for *splenomegaly* and for *Roth's spots*§).

There is an infusion line and I strongly suspect that this patient has infective endocarditis.

Cutaneous manifestations of infective endocarditis

Four lesions involving the *skin* and *its appendages* have traditionally been considered as the peripheral manifestations of infective endocarditis: *petechiae, subungual ('splinter') haemorrhages, Osler nodes* and *Janeway lesions*. Since the advent of effective antibiotic therapy and early diagnosis in most cases, these signs have become less frequent in real life but, whenever available, would be presented in the MRCP clinical examination.

Petechiae are often present in the *conjunctivae*, on the skin of the *dorsum* of the *hands* and *feet*, the anterior chest and abdominal wall and on the oropharynx. Petechiae are common in both acute and subacute endocarditis but are not specific and may occur in *thrombocytopenia, scurvy, renal failure, bacteraemia* without endocarditis (e.g. *meningococcaemia*) and after

cardiopulmonary bypass in the absence of infection (presumably due to fat microemboli).

Subungual (splinter) haemorrhages are more commonly seen after trauma and in *psoriasis* but they are also seen in all forms of endocarditis.* A true splinter almost always occurs about 3–5 mm proximal to the free edge of the nail.

Osler nodes are small, raised, red to purple, *tender* lesions that are most often seen on the pulps of the fingers and toes. They may also be seen on the soles and palms. Osler nodes are not common, and they are almost always associated with a more protracted course of the disease.

Janeway lesions are small (1–4 mm in diameter), irregular, flat, erythematous, *non-tender macules* present most often on the palms, soles and around the ankles. They may appear on the tips of the fingers and toes and

---

* In the examination setting one usually expects a valvular lesion when asked to examine the heart of a patient with infective endocarditis. However, murmurs are not essential for this diagnosis.

† *Pallor* in a patient with a *valvular lesion* (though uncommon these days when patients are diagnosed and treated early) should alert the candidate to look for other circumstantial evidence (e.g. temperature chart, intravenous line) and cutaneous manifestations of SBE.

‡ Clubbing is rare in endocarditis and only occurs in the subacute variety.

§ *Roth's spots* (infrequent; usually subacute variety) are seen on the retina as cotton-wool exudates, often surrounded by a haemorrhage. Histologically, these lesions are collections of lymphocytes in the nerve layer of the retina surrounded by oedema and/or haemorrhage. Roth's spots may occur in association with other infections

occasionally on the extremities and the trunk. These lesions *blanch on pressure*. They are not common and usually occur in acute fulminant endocarditis but seldom occur in bacteraemia without endocarditis.

Acute versus subacute bacterial endocarditis

Many authorities now recommend abandoning the terms acute (ABE) and subacute (SBE) bacterial endocarditis and recommend the use of 'infective endocarditis' instead. Nevertheless, a comparison between the two extremes of the spectrum does provide a useful reminder that very different presentations of infective endocarditis can occur. The clinical course in classic *acute bacterial endocarditis* (commonest organism *Staphylococcus aureus*—50–70% of cases) is usually measured in *days*, the associated systemic illness is more severe and *early mortality higher*, the patient is more likely to suffer rapid destruction of the valve and more likely to have one or more focal collections outside the heart. Treatment in the acute variety should not be delayed until blood culture results are available. Classic *subacute bacterial endocarditis* (commonest organism *Streptococcus viridans*) may have a course measured in *weeks or months* with vague non-specific complaints of general malaise, anorexia, aches and pains, weakness and fatigue, low grade fevers and night sweats.

Intravenous drug abuse is a common cause of either left- or right-sided endocarditis and commonly presents late and with staphylococcal infection. Paradoxically, the florid signs of acute endocarditis are thus becoming commonplace, as are the myriad infective complications of the condition (cerebral abscess, spinal abscess, mycotic pulmonary emboli, etc.).

Infective endocarditis can be a fatal complication of central line incision, particularly in the immunocompromised where endocarditic infection with fungal agents is a real risk.

Aortic root abscess may develop in association with aortic valve endocarditis. This can cause heart block (ask to see the ECG and examine the PR interval; the ward review should include serial ECGs).

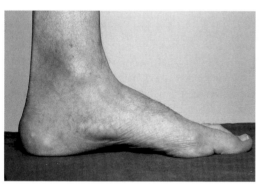
(a)

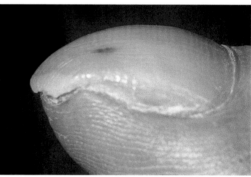
(b)

Figure C3.2 (a) Janeway lesions above the ankle. (b) Splinter haemorrhage.

Case 26 | **Atrial septal defect**

Frequency in survey: did not occur in the small initial survey of PACES station 3, cardiovascular.

Predicted frequency from older, more extensive MRCP short case surveys: main focus of a short case in 0.1% of attempts at PACES station 3, cardiovascular.

Record 1

The pulse in this middle-aged female is irregularly irregular (onset of atrial fibrillation is usually the cause of symptoms after the third or fourth decade, otherwise asymptomatic). The JVP is not elevated (unless in right heart failure). The apex beat is just palpable and not displaced. The second heart sound is widely split and the two-component split is not influenced by respiration (*fixed splitting*). There is an *ejection systolic murmur* (due to increased flow across the pulmonary valve) over the pulmonary area. (Occasionally there may be an ejection click due to pulmonary artery dilatation.)

The diagnosis is atrial septal defect of little haemodynamic significance.

Record 2

The pulse is irregularly irregular (atrial fibrillation) in this middle-aged woman. There is no oedema and the JVP is not elevated. The apex beat is just palpable in the left fifth intercostal space just outside the mid-clavicular line, there is a *left parasternal heave* (right ventricular volume overload), and there is (may be) a systolic thrill over the pulmonary area (large left-to-right shunt). The second sound is *widely split*. There is an *ejection systolic murmur*, and an *ejection click* (may be palpable) over the pulmonary area, and a *mid-diastolic rumble* over the tricuspid area (a large left-to-right shunt causes increased flow through the tricuspid valve).

The diagnosis is a haemodynamically significant atrial septal defect.

Male to female ratio is 1 : 3

Other features of atrial septal defect

Ostium secundum defect is the commonest type and may be multiple (fenestrated ASD) — small defects can easily pass unnoticed clinically

Ostium primum defect is common in Down's syndrome (see p. 517) and is associated with mitral regurgitation (due to the cleft in the anterior leaflet of the mitral valve)

rSR in the right precordial leads on ECG. Right-axis deviation is associated with an ostium secundum defect, left-axis deviation suggests an ostium primum defect

Dilated proximal pulmonary arteries and an enlarged right heart with pulmonary plethora* on chest X-ray. The aortic knuckle is small and left heart border is straight. The peripheral pulmonary vascularity is replaced by clear lung fields with the advent of pulmonary hypertension. The superior vena cava is enlarged in the sinus venosus type

* The main differential diagnosis of *pulmonary plethora* due to a left-to-right shunt is atrial septal defect, ventricular septal defect (p. 152), patent ductus arteriosus (p. 161). It may be possible to differentiate these on chest X-ray by looking at the left atrium and aorta. Small left atrium and normal aorta suggests atrial septal defect, large left atrium and normal aorta suggests ventricular septal defect, large left atrium and large or abnormal aorta suggests patent ductus arteriosus.

Diagnosis is confirmed by TOE. If performed, cardiac catheterization will show a step up in oxygen saturation in the mid right atrium, suggestive of a left-to-right shunt

Surgical closure for ostium secundum defect is recommended if the pulmonary to systemic flow ratio is 2 : 1 or more, or if the patient is symptomatic. Anatomically suitable defects can be closed using percutaneous transcatheter technology. At present, surgical closure is required for ostium primum and sinus venosus ASDs. Closure does not seem to prevent the early development of atrial fibrillation

There is a risk of paradoxical emboli in patients, even with small ASDs. Anticoagulation should be considered—particularly if there is echocardiographic evidence of bidirectional shunting

Patients with pulmonary hypertension are cyanosed and may have clubbing of the fingers (Eisenmenger's syndrome—p. 157). The systolic murmur becomes faint and an early diastolic murmur with a loud P_2 appears. Operative repair is contraindicated

Usual causes of death: right heart failure, arrhythmias, pulmonary embolism, brain abscess, rupture of the pulmonary artery.

Case 27 | **Normal heart**

Frequency in survey: did not occur in the initial small survey of PACES station 3.

The College have made it clear that 'normal' is an option in stations 1, 3 and 5 of PACES. Because of the change in the structure of the exam compared to the old short cases format, it is likely to occur more frequently than it did before. This is because in order for PACES to proceed there must be a cardiovascular case in station 1, cardiovascular. If, at the last minute, neither of the scheduled heart cases turn up on the day; or if in the middle of a carousel the only one who did turn up decides not to continue or is too ill to continue, a substitute case has to be found at short notice. In the old, pre PACES, days the exam would have proceeded without a heart case whilst the wards were searched and one was found. In the case of PACES, if there is not time for this, one option is to proceed with a patient with a heart that is normal and make up an appropriate scenario. One simply has to imagine oneself as the invigilating registrar to think what that might be. One would first look amongst any surplus cases in the other stations for a volunteer or one might ask a member of the nursing, portering or other support staff, and come up with a scenario such as:

'This . . . -year-old patient complains of palpitations. Please examine the heart . . .'

There may thus be a clue in the case scenario and the fact that the scenario has been hurriedly hand-scribbled.

From the pre PACES surveys it was clear that the commonest reason for finding no abnormality is missing the physical signs that are present (probably anecdote below; possibly anecdote 2 on p. 135; see also experience 49, vol. 2, p. 331). Other reasons for cases of 'normal' will be either because the physical signs are no longer present by the time the patient comes to the examination (see the anecdote on p. 277), or that the examiners and candidate disagree with the selectors of the cases about the presence of physical signs (this may have happened in the anecdote on p. 508; see also experience 87b and anecdote 55, vol. 2, pp. 335 and 367). The following anecdote is from our original, pre PACES, surveys.

Anecdote

A candidate was asked to examine the heart. He could find no abnormality and said so because he thought he had to be honest. He has no idea what the diagnosis was. He failed.

Station 3
Central nervous system

1 Peripheral neuropathy
2 Myotonic dystrophy (dystrophia myotonica)
3 Hemiplegia
4 Cerebellar syndrome
5 Charcot–Marie–Tooth disease (hereditary motor and sensory neuropathy)
6 Motor neurone disease
7 Ulnar nerve palsy
8 Visual field defect
9 Spinal cord compression
10 Spastic paraparesis
11 Abnormal gait
12 Ocular palsy
13 Parkinson's disease
14 Multiple sclerosis
15 Lower motor neurone VIIth nerve palsy
16 Drug-induced extrapyramidal syndrome
17 Choreoathetosis
18 Carpal tunnel syndrome
19 Diabetic foot
20 Friedreich's ataxia
21 Proximal myopathy
22 Subacute combined degeneration of the cord
23 Muscular dystrophy
24 Wasting of the small muscles of the hand
25 Nystagmus
26 Horner's syndrome
27 Old polio

28 Cervical myelopathy
29 Bulbar palsy
30 Dysarthria
31 Dysphasia
32 Myasthenia gravis
33 Guillain–Barré syndrome (acute inflammatory demyelinating polyradiculopathy)
34 Pseudobulbar palsy
35 Syringomyelia
36 Holmes–Adie–Moore syndrome
37 Jugular foramen syndrome
38 Polymyositis
39 Argyll Robertson pupils
40 Congenital syphilis
41 Cerebellopontine angle lesion
42 Absent ankle jerks and extensor plantars
43 Lateral popliteal (common peroneal) nerve palsy
44 Ptosis
45 Tabes
46 Subclavian-steal syndrome
47 Infantile hemiplegia
48 Thalamic syndrome
49 Radial nerve palsy
50 Lateral medullary syndrome (Wallenberg's syndrome)
51 Psychogenic/factitious
52 Normal central nervous system

Case 1 | Peripheral neuropathy

Frequency in survey: main focus of a short case in 9% of attempts at PACES station 3, CNS. Additional feature in a further 8%.

Record

There is *impairment* of *sensation* to light touch, vibration sense, joint position sense and pinprick over a *stocking* and, to a lesser extent, a *glove distribution* (much less common).

The patient has a peripheral neuropathy.

Most likely causes

1 Diabetes mellitus (?fundi, amyotrophy)

2 Carcinomatous neuropathy (?evidence of primary, cachexia, clubbing)

3 Vitamin B$_{12}$ deficiency (subacute combined degeneration not always present; ?plantars)

4 Vitamin B deficiency (alcoholics*)

5 Drugs (e.g. isoniazid, vincristine, nitrofurantoin, gold, ethambutol, phenytoin, hydrallazine, metronidazole, amiodarone, chloramphenicol, cyclosporin)

6 Idiopathic (in 10–20% of patients with chronic peripheral neuropathy for >1 year, no cause can be found).

There are many rare causes (see below).

Leprosy is a cause of major importance worldwide.

Important rare causes

Guillain–Barré syndrome (also motor involvement, absent reflexes, ?bilateral lower motor neurone VIIth nerve palsy; ?peak flow rate — p. 246)

Polyarteritis nodosa (?arteritic lesions)

Rheumatoid arthritis and other collagen disease (hands, facies)

Amyloidosis (?thick nerves, autonomic involvement)†

AIDS‡

Causes of predominantly motor neuropathy

Carcinomatous neuropathy (?evidence of primary, cachexia)

Lead (wrists mainly)

Porphyria

Diphtheria

Charcot–Marie–Tooth disease (?atrophy of peronei, pes cavus, etc. — p. 188).

---

* Can also occur with nutritional deficiencies from other causes, e.g. dialysis for chronic renal failure, prison camp victims.

† Neuropathy is a feature of primary and myeloma-associated amyloidosis (it is exceptional in secondary amyloidosis). Carpal tunnel syndrome is not uncommon. Sensory or mixed sensory and motor neuropathy are commonest. Signs of autonomic involvement would be orthostatic hypotension, impotence, impairment of sweating and diarrhoea. The other organs mainly involved in primary and myeloma-associated amyloidosis include heart (car-

diomyopathy), tongue (dysarthria), skeletal and visceral muscle and alimentary tract (rectal biopsy). See also footnote on p. 108).

‡ Acute (Guillain–Barré type) or chronic inflammatory neuropathy may be the presenting feature of HIV infection but with a cerebrospinal fluid pleocytosis which is not usually seen in these conditions. A distal sensory neuropathy may also occur in AIDS, sometimes but not always caused by cytomegalovirus infection.

Other rare causes of peripheral neuropathy

Myxoedema (?facies, pulse, reflexes, etc. — p. 438)

Acromegaly (?facies, hands, etc. — p. 429)

Sarcoidosis (?lupus pernio, chest signs)

Uraemia (?pale brownish yellow complexion)

Lyme disease

Tetanus

Botulism (can be mistaken for Guillain–Barré, encephalitis, stroke or myasthenia gravis; EMG resembles Eaton–Lambert)

Paraproteinaemia*

Hereditary ataxias

Refsum's disease (cerebellar ataxia, pupillary abnormalities, optic atrophy, deafness, retinitis pigmentosa, cardiomyopathy, ichthyosis)

Arsenic poisoning (e.g. pesticides; Mee's transverse white lines may occur on the fingernails and rain-drop pigmentation may occur on the skin)

Other chemical poisoning (e.g. tri-ortho-cresyl phosphate).

---

*NB The rare POEMS syndrome: Polyneuropathy, Organomegaly, Endocrinopathy, Monoclonal gammopathy, Skin changes. These are associated with osteosclerotic myeloma.

Case 2 | Myotonic dystrophy (dystrophia myotonica)

Frequency in survey: main focus of a short case in 8% of attempts at PACES station 3, CNS.

Record

The patient has *myopathic facies* (drooping mouth and long, lean, sad, lifeless, somewhat sleepy expression) frontal *balding* (in the male), *ptosis* (may be unilateral) and *wasting of the facial muscles*, temporalis, masseter, *sternomastoids*, shoulder girdle and quadriceps. The forearms and legs are involved and the *reflexes* are *lost*. The patient has *cataracts*. After he made a fist he was unable to quickly open it, especially when asked to do this repetitively (this gets worse in the cold and with excitement). He has difficulty opening his eyes after firm closure. When he shook hands there was a delay before he released his grip* (these are all features of *myotonia*). When dimples and depressions are induced in his muscles by percussion, they fill only slowly (*percussion myotonia*—e.g. tongue and thenar eminence).

The diagnosis is myotonic dystrophy.

Males > females.
Autosomal dominant.

Other features

Cardiomyopathy (?small volume pulse, low blood pressure, splitting of first heart sound in mitral area; low voltage P wave, prolonged PR interval, notched QRS and prolonged QT_c on the ECG; dysrythmias; sudden death may occur)

Intellect and personality deterioration

Slurred speech due to combined tongue and pharyngeal myotonia

Testicular atrophy (small soft testicles but secondary sexual characteristics preserved; usually develops after the patient has had children and thus the disease is perpetuated; evidence regarding ovarian atrophy is indefinite)

Diabetes mellitus (end-organ unresponsiveness to insulin)

Nodular thyroid enlargement, small pituitary fossa but normal pituitary function, dysphagia, abdominal pain, hypoventilation, and postanaesthetic respiratory failure may also occur.

The condition may show 'anticipation'—progressively worsening signs and symptoms in succeeding generations; e.g. presenile cataracts may be the sole indication of the disorder in preceding generations. Genetic testing can be confirmatory, demonstrating expanded trinucleotide repeats in a region on chromosome 19 in the myotonin protein kinase gene.

Myotonia congenita (Thomsen's disease)

There is difficulty in relaxation of a muscle after forceful contraction (myotonia) but none of the other features of myotonic dystrophy (e.g. weakness, cataracts, baldness, gonadal atrophy, etc.). The *reflexes are normal*. Some patients have a 'Herculean' appearance from very developed musculature (?related to repeated involuntary isometric exercise). Myotonia congenita is usually autosomal dominant, but autosomal recessive forms are also recognized. It is now understood that these conditions are due to disorders of ion channels (channelopathies). The finding of paramyotonia—myotonia worsening with exercise and cold—may be useful clinically in differentiating various subtypes of channelopathy.

---

* There may be absence of grip myotonia in advanced disease because of progressive muscle wasting. Though myotonia can be relieved by phenytoin, quinine or procainamide, it is weakness (for which there is no treatment) rather than the myotonia which is the main cause of disability in myotonic dystrophy.

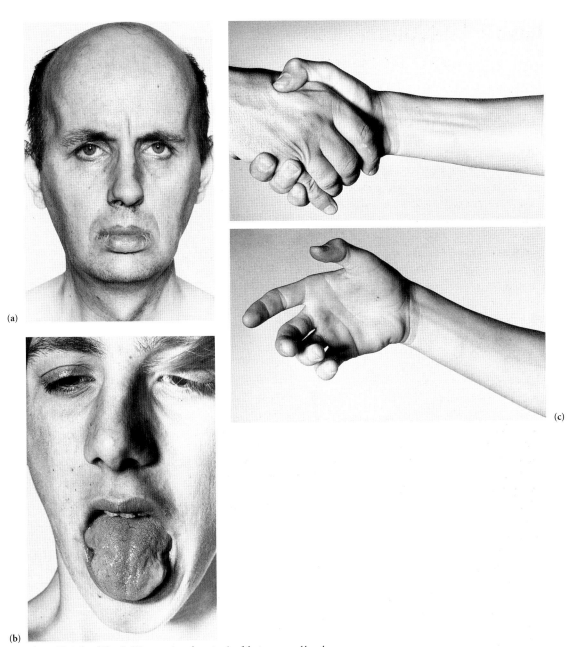

(a)

(b)

(c)

Figure C3.3 (a–c) Note balding, ptosis and myotonia of the tongue and hands.

Case 3 | Hemiplegia

Frequency in survey: main focus of a short case in 6% of attempts at PACES station 3, CNS. Additional feature in a further 2%.

Record

There is a R/L *upper motor neurone* weakness of the facial muscles.* The R/L *arm* and *leg* are *weak* (without wasting) with *increased tone* and *hyper-reflexia*. The R/L plantar is *extensor* and the *abdominal reflexes* are *diminished* on the R/L side.

This is a R/L hemiplegia.

There is also (may be) *hemisensory loss* on the R/L side. Visual field testing reveals (may be) a R/L homonymous hemianopia. The most likely causes are:

1 Cerebrovascular accident due to cerebral
   (a) thrombosis (?hypertension)
   (b) haemorrhage (?hypertension)
   (c) embolism (?atrial fibrillation, murmurs, bruits)

2 Brain tumour (?insidious onset, papilloedema, headaches; ?evidence of primary, e.g. clubbing).

A right-sided hemiplegia associated with dysphasia would suggest (in a right-handed patient) that the causative lesion is affecting the speech centres in the dominant hemisphere (see p. 240) as well as the motor cortex (precentral gyrus) and if there are sensory signs, the sensory cortex (postcentral gyrus). If cerebrovascular in origin the causative lesion is likely to be in the *carotid* distribution.

The presence of signs such as nystagmus, ocular palsy, dysphagia (?nasogastric or PEG feeding tube) and cerebellar signs suggest that the hemiparesis is due to a brainstem lesion. If cerebrovascular in origin the lesion is likely to be in *vertebrobasilar* distribution (see p. 273 for the eponymous syndromes†).

Parietal lobe and related signs‡

Agnosia. Though peripheral sensation is intact (tactile, visual, auditory) the patient fails to appreciate the significance of the sensory stimulus without the aid of other senses.

Tactile agnosia or astereognosis (contralateral posterior parietal lobe) — inability to recognize a familiar object placed in the hand (e.g. pen, keys) with the eyes closed. Opening the eyes or hearing the keys rattle may allow recognition

Visual agnosia (parieto-occipital lesions — especially in the left hemisphere of right-handed patients) — the patient is not able to identify the familiar object by sight (e.g. a pen, surroundings) but may do at once when he is allowed to handle it

Auditory agnosia (temporal lobe of dominant hemisphere) — the patient may only be able to recognize the sound of a voice, telephone or music when he is allowed to use the senses of vision or touch

Autotopagnosia (usually a left hemiplegia in a right-handed person) — difficulty in perceiving or identifying the various parts of the body; the patient may be unaware of the left side of his body. It may be associated with anosognosia in which case there is no appreciation of a disability (e.g. hemiplegia, blindness) on the same side.

---

* In an upper motor neurone lesion, the lower face is much weaker than the upper because the muscles frontalis, orbicularis oculi and corrugator superficialis ('raise your eyebrows', 'screw your eyes up tight', 'frown') are bilaterally innervated from the corticobulbar fibres and are all only minimally impaired.

† These are in fact rarely used in everyday practice.
‡ These did not occur in our survey of MRCP short cases.

Apraxia. Whereas in agnosia the difficulty is in recognition, in apraxia it is in execution. Though power, sensation and coordination are all normal, the patient is unable to perform certain familiar activities. It may affect:

The upper limbs—e.g. difficulty using a pen, comb or toothbrush, winding a watch, dressing or undressing ('dressing apraxia'*)

The lower limbs—may mimic ataxia or weakness†—the patient may appear unable to lift one foot in front of the other (gait apraxia)

The trunk—the patient may have difficulty seating himself on a chair or lavatory seat, getting on to his bed, or in turning over in bed

The face—the patient may be unable to whistle, put out his tongue or close his eyes.

The lesions (tumours or atrophy) tend to be in the corpus callosum, parietal lobes and premotor areas. Dominant lobe lesions may produce bilateral apraxia. Unilateral left-sided apraxia may be caused by a lesion in the right posterior parietal region or in the corpus collosum of a right-handed patient. The lesion in 'dressing apraxia' is usually in the right parieto-occipital region. In 'constructional apraxia' (most often seen in patients with hepatic encephalopathy) the patient is unable to construct simple figures such as triangles, squares or crosses from matchsticks.

Dyslexia (impairment of reading ability), *dysgraphia* (impairment of writing ability) and *dyscalculia* (difficulty with calculating) usually represent lesions in the posterior parietal lobe.

---

* Some authorities consider this to be a visuospatial right hemisphere disorder and not a true apraxia.

† A parietal lobe lesion may cause ataxia, hemiparesis or marked astereognosis. In hemiparesis of parietal origin, the limbs are often hypotonic with an absent plantar response, rather than spastic. The limb muscles may even waste (like a lower motor neurone lesion). Often the patient is disinclined to move the limb rather than being actually paralysed.

Case 4 | Cerebellar syndrome

Frequency in survey: main focus of a short case in 6% of attempts at PACES station 3, CNS. Additional feature in a further 6%.

Record 1

There is nystagmus to the R/L and there is ataxia with the eyes open as shown by impairment of rapid alternate motion on the same side (*dysdiadochokinesis*). The *finger–nose test* is impaired on the R/L with *past pointing* to that side and an *intention tremor* (increases on approaching the target). The *heel–shin test* is impaired on the R/L and the *gait* is *ataxic* with a tendency to fall to the R/L. There is *ataxic dysarthria* with explosive speech (staccato).

The patient has a R/L cerebellar lesion.

Causes include

1 Multiple sclerosis (?internuclear ophthalmoplegia, optic neuritis or atrophy, etc. — p. 209)
2 Brainstem vascular lesion
3 Posterior fossa space-occupying lesion (?papilloedema; e.g. tumour or abscess*)
4 Paraneoplastic cerebellar syndrome (?clubbing, cachexia, etc.)
5 Alcoholic cerebellar degeneration (nutritional†)
6 Friedreich's ataxia (?scoliosis, pes cavus, pyramidal and dorsal column signs, absent ankle jerks, etc. — p. 220).

Other causes of cerebellar ataxia include

Hypothyroidism (?facies, pulse, reflexes, etc. — p. 438)
Anticonvulsant toxicity (especially phenytoin which can cause gross multidirectional nystagmus)
Ataxia–telangiectasia (recessive; from childhood onwards progressive ataxia, choreoathetosis and oculomotor apraxia; later telangiectases on conjunctivae, ears, face and skin creases; low IgA leads to repeated respiratory tract infections; lymphoreticular malignancies are common; death is usually in the second or third decade of life)
Other cerebellar degeneration syndromes.‡

Other cerebellar signs

Ipsilateral hypotonia and reduced power
Ipsilateral pendular knee jerk
Skew deviation of the eyes (ipsilateral down and in, contralateral up and out)
Failure of the displaced ipsilateral arm to find its original posture (ask the patient to hold his arms out in front of him and keep them there. If you push the ipsilateral arm down it will fly past the starting point on release without reflex arrest).

---

* NB Otitis media may underlie a cerebellar abscess. Intracranial abscesses may result from direct spread from the upper respiratory passages (nasal sinuses, middle ear, mastoid). Less often the cause is haematogenous spread (e.g. intrathoracic suppuration), congenital heart disease or fracture of the base of the skull. Abscesses secondary to otitis occur in the temporal lobe about twice as often as they do in the cerebellum.

† Other causes of nutritional deficiency such as pellagra, amoebiasis and protracted vomiting may cause a similar syndrome.
‡ The names associated with these other rare hereditary ataxias apart from Friedreich are Charcot, Marie, Déjérine, Alajouanine, André Thomas, Gowers and Holmes. These have now been superseded by a genetic classification: spinocerebellar ataxia types 1–7.

Record 2 (vermis lesion)

There is a wide-based *cerebellar ataxia* (ataxic gait and rombergism more or less the same with eyes open and closed; cf. sensory ataxia—worse with eyes closed), but there is little or no abnormality of the limbs when tested separately on the bed. This suggests a lesion of the cerebellar vermis.

Case 5 | Charcot–Marie–Tooth disease (hereditary motor and sensory neuropathy)*

Frequency in survey: main focus of a short case in 5% of attempts at PACES station 3, CNS.

Record

There is *distal wasting* of the *lower limb* muscles with relatively well-preserved thigh muscles.† The feet show *pes cavus* and clawing of the toes, and there is weakness of the extensors of the toes and feet. The *ankle jerks* are *absent* and the plantar reflexes show no response. There is only slight *distal involvement* of *superficial* modalities of *sensation* (though occasionally marked sensory loss may lead to digital trophic ulceration). The lateral popliteal (?and ulnar) nerves are palpable (in some families only). The patient has a *steppage gait* (bilateral foot-drop). There is (may be) *wasting of the small muscles of the hand*.

The diagnosis is Charcot–Marie–Tooth disease.*

Patterns of inheritance are variable.

The degree of disability in this condition is commonly surprisingly slight in spite of the remarkable deformities. Toe retraction and talipes equinovarus may occur and fasciculation (much less apparent than in motor neurone disease) is sometimes seen.

The degeneration is mainly in the motor nerves. It is sometimes also found in the dorsal roots and dorsal columns, and slight pyramidal tract degeneration is often seen (however, in classic cases extensor plantars are not found). The condition usually becomes arrested in mid-life. Other members of the patient's family may have a *formes fruste* and show just minor signs such as pes cavus and absent ankle jerks only.

---

* Charcot–Marie–Tooth disease, which in the past has been called peroneal muscular atrophy, is now called *hereditary motor and sensory neuropathy* (HMSN) and is subdivided into HMSN type I (the demyelinating (and remyelinating) form of Charcot–Marie–Tooth disease), HMSN type II (the axonal (degeneration) form of Charcot–Marie–Tooth disease), HMSN type III (previously called Déjérine–Scotas disease), and four other subtypes.

† In classic descriptions, as the disease progresses, the wasting creeps very slowly up the limb, inch by inch, involving all muscles. According to the stage of the disease, the characteristic appearances have been described as 'stork' or 'spindle' legs, 'fat bottle' calves, and 'inverted champagne bottles'. The same process may occur in the arms; wasting of the small muscles of the hands is common with a tendency for the fingers to curl and the patient to have difficulty in straightening and abducting them. Classically, Charcot–Marie–Tooth wasting was described as stopping *abruptly* part of the way up the leg. In practice it is not usually so clear-cut and can be considered to be an example of neuromythology.

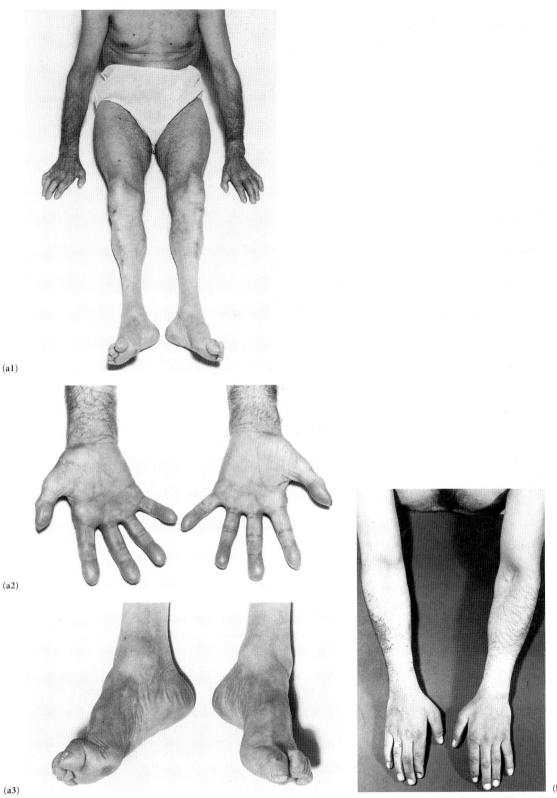

Figure C3.4 (a1–3) Note that the muscle wasting stops in the thighs, foot-drop, pes cavus, and wasting of the small muscles of the hand all in the same patient. (b) Distal wasting in the upper limbs .

(a1)

(a2)

(a3)

(b)

Case 6 | Motor neurone disease

Frequency in survey: main focus of a short case in 5% of attempts at PACES station 3, CNS. Additional feature in a further 1%.

Record

This patient has *weakness, wasting* and *fasciculation* of the muscles of the hand (p. 226), arms and shoulder girdle (***progressive muscular atrophy*** in its pure form is characterized by minimal pyramidal signs), but the upper limb reflexes are exaggerated (reflexes in motor neurone disease may be increased, decreased or absent depending on which lesion is predominant). There is upper motor neurone *spastic weakness* with *exaggerated reflexes* in the legs (***amyotrophic lateral sclerosis****). There is ankle clonus and the patient has bilateral *extensor plantar* responses. The patient also has (may have) indistinct *nasal speech*, a *wasted fasciculating tongue* and *palatal paralysis* (***progressive bulbar palsy***—p. 238). There are *no sensory signs*.

The diagnosis is motor neurone disease.

Other conditions in which fasciculation may occur

Cervical spondylosis (see below)

Syringomyelia (fasciculation less apparent, dissociated sensory loss, etc.—p. 249)

Charcot–Marie–Tooth disease (fasciculation less apparent, atrophy which stops abruptly part of the way up the legs, pes cavus, sometimes palpable lateral popliteal and ulnar nerves, etc.—p. 188)

Acute stages of poliomyelitis (and rarely also in old polio; see below)

Neuralgic amyotrophy (pain, wasting and weakness of a group of muscles in a limb, sometimes following a viral infection; usually C5,6 innervated muscles—shoulder)

Thyrotoxic myopathy (tachycardia, tremor, sweating, goitre with bruit, lid lag, etc.—p. 432)

Syphilitic amyotrophy (see below)

Chronic asymmetrical spinal muscular atrophy (see below)

After exercise in fit adults

After the Tensilon test (p. 242)

Benign giant fasciculation.

Differential diagnosis of motor neurone disease

Cervical cord compression (p. 236) is the most important condition to be excluded in the diagnosis of motor neurone disease. Bulbar palsy and sensory signs should be carefully sought, but a cervical MRI scan is often required to exclude it. *Syphilitic amyotrophy* (slowly progressing wasting of the muscles of the shoulder girdle and upper arm with loss of reflexes and no sensory loss; fasciculation of the tongue may occur) should always be excluded in the investigation of motor neurone disease as it is amenable to treatment. Occasionally patients with *old polio*, after many years, develop a progressive wasting disease (with prominent fasciculation) which is indistinguishable from progressive muscular atrophy motor neurone disease.

Another condition that needs to be considered is *spinal muscular atrophy of juvenile onset* type 3 (Kugelberg–Welander disease). This is due to a mutation in the survival motor neurone gene on chromsome 5. The onset is in childhood or in the teen years. It is a milder form of spinal muscular atrophy affecting mostly proximal muscles, but the patients can stand and walk unaided. It can be distinguished from chronic inflammatory demyelinating polyneuropathy by the presence of normal CSF protein and normal nerve conduction studies.

* Glutamate toxicity has been implicated as a factor leading to neuronal damage in amyotrophic lateral sclerosis. Trials suggest riluzole may retard progression and lengthen survival.

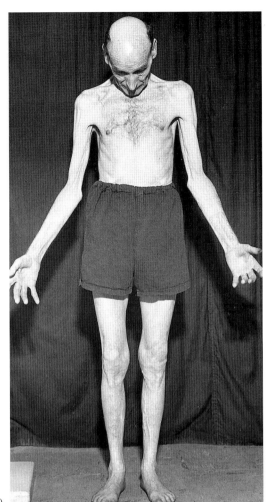

(a1)

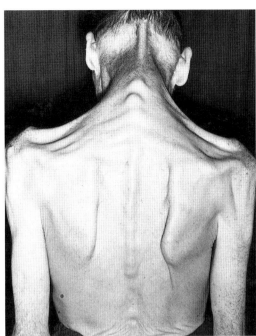

(a2)

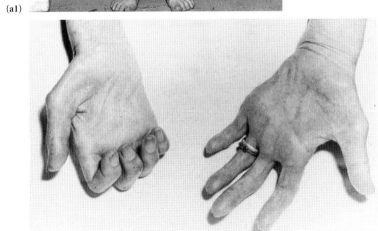

(b)

Figure C3.5 (a1,2) Generalized muscle wasting (note weakness of the extensors of the neck). (b) Wasting of the small muscles of the hand.

Case 7 | Ulnar nerve palsy

Frequency in survey: main focus of a short case in 5% of attempts at PACES station 3, CNS.

Record

The hand shows *generalized muscle wasting** and *weakness* which *spares* the *thenar eminence*. There is sensory loss over the *fifth finger*, the *adjacent half* of the *fourth finger* and the dorsal and palmar aspects of the *medial side* of the *hand*.† (Look for hyperextension at the metacarpophalangeal joints with flexion of the interphalangeal joints in the fourth and fifth fingers — the *ulnar claw hand*.)‡

The patient has an ulnar nerve lesion. (Now examine the elbow for a cause.)

Likely causes

1 Fracture or dislocation at the elbow (?scar or deformity; history of injury)
2 Osteoarthrosis at the elbow with osteophytic encroachment on the ulnar nerve in the cubital tunnel ('filling in' of the ulnar groove due to palpable enlargement of the nerve; limitation of elbow movement is often seen; certain occupations predispose to osteoarthrosis at the elbow — see below).

Other causes

Occupations with constant leaning on elbows (clerks, secretaries on telephone, etc.)

Occupations with constant flexion and extension at the elbow (bricklayer, painter/decorator, carpenter, roofer — shallow ulnar groove will predispose; these occupations may also lead to osteoarthrosis — see above)

Excessive carrying angle at elbow (malunited fracture of the humerus or disturbance of growth leading to cubitus valgus and, over the years, 'tardy ulnar nerve palsy')

Injuries at the wrist or in the palm (different degrees of the syndrome depending on which branches of the nerve are damaged; e.g. occupations using screwdrivers, drills, etc.)

The causes of mononeuritis multiplex (diabetes, polyarteritis nodosa and Churg–Strauss syndrome, rheumatoid, SLE, Wegener's, sarcoid, carcinoma, amyloid, leprosy, Sjögren's syndrome, Lyme disease).

NB Other causes of wasting of the small muscles of the hand (p. 226) may sometimes resemble ulnar nerve palsy. The major features pointing to ulnar nerve palsy as the cause are *sparing of the thenar eminence* and the characteristic sensory loss pattern. The main distinguishing features of the differential

---

*(i) The *hypothenar eminence wastes*, though in the manual worker with thickened skin the hand contour may be preserved and the wasting may only be detected on palpation. Loss of other small muscles is seen from (ii) *loss of the first dorsal interosseous* in the dorsal space between the first and second metacarpals, and (iii) *guttering of the dorsum* of the hand — which becomes more prominent as the lesion advances.

† *Record* (continuation): there is *weakness of abduction and adduction of the fingers*, and *adduction of the extended thumb* against the palm (inability to hold a piece of paper between the thumb and index finger without pinch-flexing the affected thumb (using the flexor pollicis longus, the median nerve) —

Froment's 'thumb sign' — now usually referred to as the journal sign). Flexion of the fourth and fifth fingers is weak. When the proximal portions of these fingers are held immobilized, flexion of the terminal phalanges is not possible. There is also *wasting of the medial aspect of the forearm* (flexor carpi ulnaris and half of the flexor digitorum profundus). When the hand is flexed to the ulnar side against resistance the tendon of flexor carpi ulnaris is not palpable.

‡ The ulnar claw hand or partial *main-en-griffe* is due to the unopposed action of the long extensors and is only seen in the fourth and fifth fingers because the radial lumbricals are supplied by the median nerve.

diagnoses which may mimic the muscle wasting of ulnar paralysis are:

Syringomyelia—dissociated sensory loss extending beyond the ulnar zone; loss of arm reflexes; ? Horner's

C8 lesion (e.g. Pancoast's syndrome)—sensory loss involves radial side of fourth finger, ?Horner's

Cervical rib—objective sensory disturbances are usually slight or absent and without characteristic ulnar distribution.

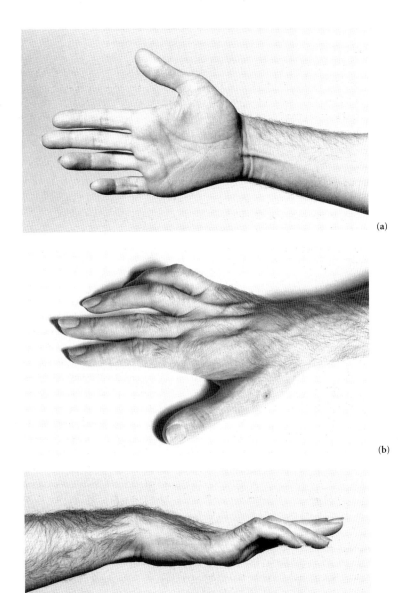

(a)

(b)

(c)

Figure C3.6 (a) Loss of hypothenar eminence. (b) Dorsal guttering. (c) Typical ulnar claw hand.

Case 8 | Visual field defect

Frequency in survey: main focus of a short case in 5% of attempts at PACES station 3, CNS. Additional feature in a further 2%.

Record 1

There is an *homonymous hemianopia*. This suggests a lesion of the *optic tract* behind the optic chiasma (with sparing of the macula and hence normal visual acuity).

Likely causes

1 Cerebrovascular accident (?ipsilateral hemiplegia, atrial fibrillation, heart murmurs or bruits, hypertension)
2 Tumour (?ipsilateral pyramidal signs, papilloedema).

Record 2

There is a *bitemporal* visual field defect worse on R/L side. This suggests a lesion at the *optic chiasma*. (NB There may be optic atrophy, sometimes with a central scotoma, on the R/L side due to simultaneous compression of the optic nerve by the lesion.)

Possible causes

1 Pituitary tumour (?acromegaly, hypopituitarism, gynaecomastia, galactorrhoea, menstrual disturbance, etc.)
2 Craniopharyngioma (?calcification on skull X-ray)
3 Suprasellar meningioma
4 Aneurysm.
Rarer causes are glioma, granuloma and metastasis.

Record 3

The visual fields are considerably constricted, the central field of vision being spared. This is *tunnel vision*.* I would like to examine the fundi, looking for evidence of retinitis pigmentosa, glaucoma (pathological cupping) or widespread choroidoretinitis. (Hysteria may occasionally be a cause; papilloedema causes enlargement of the blind spot and peripheral constriction.)

Record 4

There is a *central scotoma*. (NB The discs may be pale (atrophy), swollen and pink (papillitis), or normal (retrobulbar neuritis).)

Causes to be considered

Demyelinating diseases (?nystagmus, cerebellar signs, etc.; however, multiple sclerosis frequently causes retrobulbar neuritis without other signs)

---

* The Committee on the Safety of Medicine has received reports of visual field defects associated with the anti-epileptic drug *vigaba-* *trin* including three cases of severe, symptomatic, persistent visual field constriction (tunnel vision).

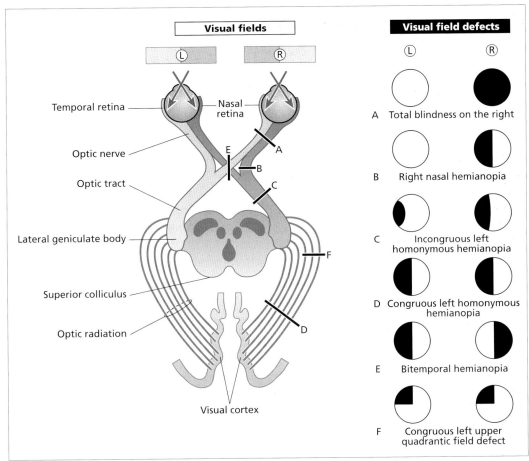

Visual fields

L   R

Temporal retina

Nasal retina

Optic nerve

E

A

B

Optic tract

C

Lateral geniculate body

F

Superior colliculus

Optic radiation

D

Visual cortex

Visual field defects

L   R

A   Total blindness on the right

B   Right nasal hemianopia

C   Incongruous left homonymous hemianopia

D   Congruous left homonymous hemianopia

E   Bitemporal hemianopia

F   Congruous left upper quadrantic field defect

Figure C3.7 The visual pathways and visual field defects resulting from different lesions. If there is exact overlap of the field defects from both eyes the defect is said to be congruous. If not, it is incongruous. The defects in B and E above are incongruous. Though the complete homonymous hemianopia in D is congruous, lesions of the optic tract (C), which are comparatively rare, produce characteristic incongruous visual changes. The fibres serving identical points in the homonymous half fields do not fully co-mingle in the anterior optic tract so lesions encroaching on this structure produce incongruous and usually incomplete homonymous hemianopias. Lesions of the geniculate ganglia, visual radiations or visual cortex produce congruous visual field defects. F represents a lesion of the temporal loop of the optic radiation.

Compression*
Ischaemia
Leber's optic atrophy (males : females = 6 : 1)
Toxins (e.g. methyl alcohol)
Macular disease
Nutritional (famine, etc., tobacco–alcohol amblyopia, vitamin B$_{12}$ deficiency, diabetes mellitus).

* There may be clues as to the site of the compression. (i) A lesion in the frontal lobe which compresses the optic nerve may cause dementia. (ii) It may also cause contralateral papilloedema (the *Foster–Kennedy syndrome* due to a frontal tumour or aneurysm, e.g. olfactory groove meningioma). (iii) A lesion in front of the chiasma involving crossing fibres that loop forward

Record 5
There is *homonymous upper quadrantic visual field loss.* This suggests a lesion in the temporal cortex.

NB Field defects may sometimes originate from retinal damage, e.g. occlusion of a branch of the retinal artery or a large area of choroidoretinitis.

into the opposite optic nerve may cause a contralateral upper temporal quadrantic field defect. (iv) A lesion at the chiasma may cause a bitemporal field defect. (v) A lesion at the lateral chiasma (pituitary tumour, aneurysm, meningioma) involving the terminal optic tract as well as the optic nerve may cause an homonymous hemianopia.

Case 9 | **Spinal cord compression***

Frequency in survey: main focus of a short case in 5% of attempts at PACES station 3, CNS.

Record 1

This patient (who complains of difficulty in walking) has a *monoparesis* of the R/L leg with *hypertonia, muscular weakness without wasting, hyper-reflexia* and an *extensor plantar* response. There is loss of *joint position* and *vibration* senses on the side of the monoparesis and loss of *pain* and *temperature* senses on the opposite side below the level (determine the upper limit of the sensory loss) of (e.g.) T8/9 segments.

These features suggest a diagnosis of the Brown–Séquard syndrome resulting from hemisection of the spinal cord. Among the causes are injury, tumour, late myelopathy from radiation therapy and multiple sclerosis.

Record 2

There is *muscular weakness* in both legs, more on the R/L side with *hypertonia, hyper-reflexia* (?clonus) and bilateral *extensor plantars. Soft touch* and *pinprick* sensations are diminished in both legs extending upwards to the *level* of (e.g.) T8 segment.† *Joint position* and *vibration* senses are intact. There is *no neurological abnormality in the upper limbs.*

These findings, together with your opening statement that this patient has had a recent onset of back pain, suggest spinal cord compression, possibly from a tumour at T7/8 level. This will need to be urgently investigated.

Record 3

The skin over the R/L buttock is *loose* and *droopy* due to *wasting* of the underlying *glutei.* The corresponding *calf muscles* are *flabby*, with *weakness* of *extension* and *abduction* at the hip joint and *plantar flexion* at the ankle joint. The patient is unable to stand on his toes and the *ankle jerk* is *absent* on the affected side. The sensation is *impaired* along the *outer border* of the *foot* and the *outer half* of the sole. The patient walks with a Trendelenburg's limp as the pelvis shifts to the normal side due to weak abductors on the affected side.

Since you said that the patient has a spinal disc problem, I would suggest that he has had herniation of the fifth lumbar disc compressing the S1 root.

---

* See also cervical myelopathy, p. 236.

† Spinal pain, progressive muscular paralysis and a sensory level are the cardinal features of spinal cord compression. Since the entire examination of the motor and sensory systems cannot be accomplished in the permitted time, the examiners may ask you to examine the sensory system only, and a sensory loss level on the trunk should alert you to the possibility of spinal cord compression. During this examination you should also be able to detect if there is any motor weakness.

Causes of spinal cord and root compression

Diseases of the vertebrae and discs:

Fracture and/or dislocation (trauma)

Prolapsed intervertebral disc

Spondylosis

Osteoporotic vertebral collapse

Paget's disease

Atlantoaxial dislocation (trauma, rheumatoid arthritis)

Ankylosing spondylitis

Sickle cell disease

Tumours:

Extradural:

Metastasis (lung, breast, prostate, kidney, GI tract, etc.)

Lymphoma

Primary bone tumours

Intradural but extramedullary (neurofibroma, meningioma, sarcoma, etc.)

Intramedullary (ependymoma, astrocytoma and rarely secondaries)

Haemorrhage/haematomyeloma:

Trauma

Spinal vascular malformation

Intradural spinal neoplasms

Coarctation of the aorta

Ruptured spinal artery aneurysm

Blood dyscrasias

Anticoagulants

Inflammatory disorders:

Spinal osteomyelitis

TB and Pott's disease of the spine

Spinal arachnoiditis

Introduction of blood and foreign substances in the intrathecal space

Acute disseminated encephalomyelitis

Multiple sclerosis

Devic's disease

Progressive necrotizing myelopathy (in young adults often after an acute illness, and in patients with a known malignancy, e.g. small cell carcinoma of the lung or a lymphoma)

Transverse myelitis.

Diagnosis

The diagnosis depends on the history (trauma, malignancy, pain in the spine, sometimes with a radicular distribution and aggravated by straining and coughing, weakness of the legs and arms and sphincter disturbance), a neurological examination, and plain X-ray of the spine and in urgent cases CT or MRI. Diseases of the vertebrae and discs can be diagnosed from history, examination and a plain film of the spine.

Back pain or neck pain should be taken seriously in a patient with a known malignancy. The pain of intraspinal lesions is exacerbated by straining, sneezing, coughing and movement. Unless investigated and treated early, midline pain progresses to radicular pain and is followed by weakness, sensory loss and sphincter disturbance. Patients who have neurological signs of cord compression require immediate treatment with dexamethasone and emergency evaluation. About 60–80% of patients with spinal cord compression will show erosion or loss of the pedicles, vertebral body destruction or collapse or a paraspinal mass on plain film.

All patients with neurological and/or plain film evidence of spinal metastases should have MRI with gadolinium enhancement. Myelography, previously an investigation of choice for suspected spinal cord compression, should be considered in those patients who either do not tolerate MRI or in whom an MRI is contraindicated (e.g. intracranial clips, intra-auricular implants, cardiac pacemakers, implantable cardiodefibrillators, 6000 Starr–Edwards prostheses). Patients with lymphoma suspected of having spinal cord compression but with no neurological or plain film abnormalities should also have an MRI, since an epidural tumour in such patients may not show up on a plain X-ray. All other patients with no neurological findings and no plain film abnormalities should have a bone scan and MRI as outpatients and should be monitored closely.

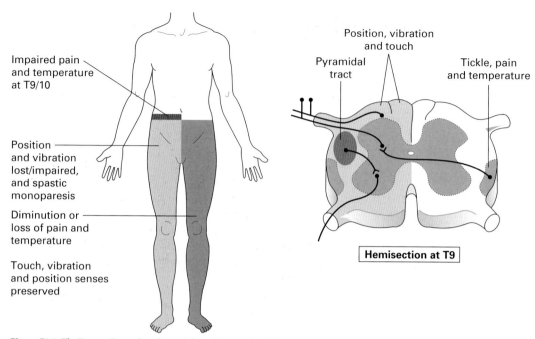

Figure C3.8 The Brown–Séquard syndrome (after Mir MA. *Atlas of Clinical Skills*, 1997, by kind permission of the author and the publisher, WB Saunders.).

Case 10 | **Spastic paraparesis**

Frequency in survey: main focus of a short case in 4% of attempts at PACES station 3, CNS. Additional feature in many others.

Record

The *tone* in the legs is *increased* and they are *weak* (in chronic immobilized cases there may be some disuse atrophy, and in severe cases there may be contractures). There is bilateral *ankle clonus*, patellar clonus and the *plantar* responses are *extensor*. (?Abdominal reflexes; consider testing gait if the patient can walk.)

The patient has a spastic paraparesis.* The most likely causes are:

1 Multiple sclerosis (?obvious nystagmus, incoordination or staccato speech from the end of the bed; ?impaired rapid alternate motion of arms when you check at the end of your leg examination—p. 209)

2 Cord compression (?sensory level; root, back or neck pain; no signs above the level of lesion. NB Cervical spondylosis—see p. 236)

3 Trauma (?scar or deformity on back)

4 Birth injury (cerebral palsy—Little's disease)

5 Motor neurone disease (?no sensory signs, muscle fasciculation, etc.—p. 190).

Other causes

Syringomyelia (?kyphoscoliosis, wasted hands, dissociated sensory loss, Horner's syndrome, etc.—p. 249)

Anterior spinal artery thrombosis (sudden onset, ?dissociated sensory loss up to the level of the lesion)

Friedreich's ataxia (?pes cavus, cerebellar signs, kyphoscoliosis, etc.—p. 220)

Hereditary spastic paraplegia

Subacute combined degeneration of the cord† (?posterior column loss, absent ankle jerks,‡ peripheral neuropathy, anaemia—p. 223)

Parasagittal cranial meningioma

Human T-cell lymphotrophic virus type 1 (HTLV-1) infection§ (Afro-Caribbean populations—tropical spastic paraparesis)

AIDS myelopathy (late phase—direct HIV CNS involvement, p. 351)

General paralysis of the insane (?dementia, vacant expression, trombone tremor of the tongue, etc.—see p. 265)

Taboparesis (?Argyll Robertson pupils, posterior column loss, etc.—p. 265).

---

* A clue to the underlying cause of spastic paraparesis may be:
Cerebellar signs: multiple sclerosis
         Friedreich's ataxia (?pes cavus)
Wasted hands: cervical spondylosis (?inverted reflexes)
         syringomyelia (?Horner's)
         motor neurone disease (?prominent fasciculation).

† Stocking sensory loss (with or without absent ankle jerks) in association with a spastic paraplegia, i.e. extensor plantars, is strongly suggestive of SACD.

‡ Absent ankle jerks and upgoing plantars—p. 259.

§ The other HTLV-1 associated disease is *adult T-cell leukaemia/lymphoma* which is especially found in southern Japan

and the Caribbean Islands. The clinical course is often associated with a high white count, *hypercalcaemia* and cutaneous involvement. Measurement of HTLV-1 antibodies should always be considered in the patient with unexplained hypercalcaemia. Other HTLV-1 associated diseases include polymyositis, infective dermatitis—a chronic generalized eczema of the skin—and B-cell chronic lymphocytic leukaemia.

HTLV-2 has been found in some patients with T-cell hairy cell leukaemia and in parenteral drug abusers but remains a true orphan virus without, at the time of writing, clear disease association.

Case 11 | Abnormal gait

Frequency in survey: main focus of a short case in 4% of attempts at PACES station 3, CNS. Additional feature in a further 4%.

Survey note: relative frequencies in the survey were cerebellar ataxia 45%, spastic paraplegia 27%, sensory ataxia 9%, Parkinson's disease 9% and Charcot–Marie–Tooth (steppage gait) 9%. Neither hemiplegia, waddling gait nor gait apraxia occurred in our survey.

Record 1

The gait is *wide-based* and the arms are held wide (both upper and lower limbs tend to tremble and shake). The patient is *ataxic* and tends to fall to the R/L, especially during the *heel-to-toe* test which he is unable to perform. Romberg's test is negative.

This suggests *cerebellar disease* which is predominantly R/L sided. (Now, if allowed, examine for other cerebellar signs: finger–nose, rapid alternate motion, nystagmus, staccato dysarthria, etc. —p. 186.)

Possible causes

1 Demyelinating disease (?pale discs, pyramidal signs, etc. —p. 209)
2 Tumour (primary or secondary—? evidence of primary, e.g. bronchus, breast, etc.)
3 Non-metastatic syndrome of malignancy (?evidence of primary, especially bronchus—clubbing, cachexia, etc.)
4 Alcoholic cerebellar degeneration
5 Other cerebellar degenerations (?pes cavus, kyphoscoliosis, absent ankle jerks and extensor plantars, etc. of Friedreich's ataxia).

Record 2

The patient has a *stiff*, awkward 'scissors' or 'wading through mud' gait.

This suggests *spastic paraplegia.* (Now, if allowed, examine tone, reflexes, plantars, sensation, etc. —p. 199)

Possible causes

1 Demyelinating disease (?impaired rapid alternate motion in arms, pale discs, etc. — p. 209)
2 Cord compression (?sensory level with no signs above)
3 Hereditary spastic paraplegia (rare)
4 Cerebral diplegia (rare).

Record 3

The gait is ataxic and *stamping* (his feet tend to 'throw'; both the heels and the toes slap on the ground). The patient walks on a wide base, *watching his feet and the ground* (to some extent he can compensate for lack of sensory information from the muscles and joints by visual attention). He has difficulty walking heel to toe and the ataxia becomes much worse when he closes his eyes; *Romberg's* test is *positive*.

He has *sensory ataxia* (now look for Argyll Robertson pupils and for clinical anaemia).

Possible causes

1 Subacute combined degeneration of the cord (?pyramidal signs, absent ankle jerks plus peripheral neuropathy; anaemia, spleen, etc.; no Argyll Robertson pupils—p. 223)

2 Tabes dorsalis (?facies, pupils, pyramidal signs if taboparesis, etc.—p. 265)

3 Cervical myelopathy (?mid-cervical reflex pattern in the arms; pyramidal signs in legs—p. 236)

4 Diabetic pseudotabes (?fundi)

5 Friedreich's ataxia (pes cavus, scoliosis, cerebellar signs, etc.—p. 220)

6 Demyelinating disease (ataxia in multiple sclerosis is usually mainly cerebellar).

Record 4

This (depressed, expressionless, unblinking and stiff) patient *stoops* and his gait, initially *hesitant*, is *shuffling* and has lost its spring. The *arms* are held flexed and *do not swing*. The hands show a *pill-rolling tremor*. His gait is *festinant*, i.e. he appears to be continually about to fall forward as if chasing his own centre of gravity.

He has *Parkinson's disease.* (Now examine the wrists for cog-wheel rigidity, elbows for lead-pipe rigidity, and for the glabellar tap sign, etc.—p. 207)

Record 5

The patient has a *steppage* gait. He lifts his R/L foot high to avoid scraping the toe because he has a R/L *foot-drop*. He is unable to walk on his R/L heel.

Possible causes

1 Lateral popliteal nerve palsy (?evidence of injury just below and lateral to the knee—p. 260)

2 Charcot–Marie–Tooth disease (?pes cavus, atrophy which stops abruptly part of the way up the leg, wasting of the small muscles of the hand, palpable lateral popliteal ± ulnar nerve—p. 188)

3 Old polio (?affected leg short due to polio in childhood—p. 234)

4 Heavy metal poisoning such as lead (rare).

Record 6

The R/L leg is stiff and with each step he tilts the pelvis to the other side trying to keep the toe off the ground; the R/L leg describes a *semicircle* with the toe scraping the floor and the forefoot flops to the ground before the heel. The R/L arm is flexed and held tightly to his side and his fist is clenched. †

The patient has a *hemiplegic gait*.

Record 7

The patient has a lumbar lordosis and walks on a wide base with a *waddling gait*, his trunk moving from side to side and his pelvis dropping on each side as his leg leaves the ground. At each step his toes touch the ground before his heel. (This is a description of the typical gait of a patient with Duchenne muscular dystrophy—the commonest cause of a waddling gait. Other conditions

---

* In the mild case, tell-tale signs are (i) the lesser swing of one arm compared to the other; (ii) the tremor which is often unilateral.

† Should not be seen these days with good physiotherapy care!

causing wasting or weakness of the proximal lower limb and pelvic girdle muscles also cause it — e.g. polymyositis, rickets/osteomalacia.)

Record 8

The patient (an elderly person) walks with a broad-based gait, taking short steps and placing his feet flat on the ground like a person 'walking on ice' — so-called 'sticky feet'. This is probably why this gait is also referred to as magnetic gait. Neither turning nor straight walking is fluent. (There is a tendency to retropulsion which increases the danger of falling.) The patient cannot hop on one foot.

This is *gait apraxia* (a common but little recognized disorder of the elderly; frontal lobe signs including dementia and grasp and suck reflexes will confirm the diagnosis). The commonest cause is a degenerative process similar to Alzheimer's disease. Other causes include subdural haematoma, tumour, normal pressure hydrocephalus, or a lacunar state.

Case 12 | Ocular palsy

Frequency in survey: main focus of a short case in 3% of attempts at PACES station 3, CNS. Additional feature in a further 1%.

Record 1

The patient has a *convergent strabismus* at rest. There is *impairment* of the *lateral movement* of the R/L eye and *diplopia* is worse on looking to the R/L (the outermost image comes from the affected eye).

The patient has a *VIth nerve palsy*.

Possible causes

1 The causes of mononeuritis multiplex*
2 Multiple sclerosis (?ipsilateral facial palsy because the VIth and VIIth nuclei are very close in the pons; ?nystagmus, cerebellar signs, pyramidal signs, pale discs, etc. — p. 209)
3 Raised intracranial pressure (?papilloedema) causing stretching of the nerve (a false localizing sign) during its long intracranial course
4 Neoplasm (?papilloedema; associated ipsilateral facial palsy if pontine tumour)
5 Myasthenia gravis (see below)
6 Vascular lesions (probably common as a cause of 'idiopathic' VIth nerve palsy)
7 Compression by aneurysm (ectatic basilar artery — uncommon)
8 Subacute meningitis (carcinomatous; lymphomatous; fungal (NB AIDS); tuberculous; meningovascular syphilis — see p. 265).

Record 2

There is *ptosis*. Lifting the eyelids reveals *divergent strabismus* and a *dilated pupil*. The eye is fixed in a *down and out position* (and there is *angulated diplopia*).

The diagnosis is complete (NB the condition is often partial) *IIIrd nerve palsy*.

Possible causes

1 Unruptured aneurysm† of posterior communicating (or internal carotid) artery (painful)
2 The causes of mononeuritis multiplex*
3 Vascular lesion† (if there is a contralateral hemiplegia the diagnosis is Weber's syndrome — p. 273)
4 Midbrain demyelinating lesion‡ (?cerebellar signs, staccato speech, pale discs, etc. — p. 209)
5 Myasthenia gravis (see below).

---

* The causes of mononeuritis multiplex include diabetes mellitus, polyarteritis nodosa and Churg–Strauss syndrome, rheumatoid disease, SLE, Wegener's granulomatosis, sarcoidosis, carcinoma, amyloidosis, leprosy, Sjögren's syndrome and Lyme disease.
† If the ophthalmoplegia is predominant compared to the ptosis/pupil dilatation, the cause is likely to be vascular (intrinsic).

If the ophthalmoplegia is minimal compared to the ptosis/pupil dilatation, the cause is more likely to be extrinsic compression by aneurysm, pituitary tumour, meningioma, etc.
‡ Third nerve palsy is rare in demyelinating disease; internuclear ophthalmoplegia (pp. 229 and 209) is a much commoner result of this condition.

Other causes of a IIIrd nerve palsy

Subacute meningitis (carcinomatous; lymphomatous; fungal (NB AIDS); tuberculous; meningovascular syphilis—at one time the commonest cause, now very rare—p. 265)

Ophthalmoplegic migraine (similar to posterior communicating artery aneurysm except that it begins in childhood or adolescence, recovery is more rapid and is always complete; recovery is never complete with an aneurysm)

Parasellar neoplasms†

Sphenoidal wing meningiomata†

Carcinomatous lesions of the skull base.†

Other causes of ocular palsy

Internuclear ophthalmoplegia (*adduction impaired bilaterally* but abduction normal or vice versa; no strabismus in the primary position; ataxic nystagmus is present and distinguishes it from bilateral VIth nerve palsy—see p. 229; ?cerebellar signs)

Exophthalmic ophthalmoplegia (exophthalmos and diplopia—upward and outward gaze most often reduced)

Myasthenia gravis (?ptosis, variable strabismus, facial weakness with a snarling smile, proximal muscle weakness, weak nasal voice, all of which worsen with repetition—p. 242. The key finding is fatiguable weakness and this should be explored by testing eye movements with the eyes held in one position in between the movements, and by getting the patient to count up to, say, 50. NB It may superficially resemble IIIrd or VIth nerve palsy)

Cavernous sinus and superior orbital fissure syndromes (total or subtotal ophthalmoplegia which is often painful, together with sensory loss over the first division of the Vth nerve—absent corneal reflex; it is due to a tumour or carotid aneurysm affecting the IIIrd, IVth, Vth and VIth nerves as they travel together through the cavernous sinus into the superior orbital fissure—see Fig. C5.64d, p. 437)

Fourth nerve palsy (adducted eye cannot look downwards—the patient experiences 'one above the other' diplopia when attempting to do this; angulated diplopia occurs when looking down and out; the diplopia is worse when reading and going down stairs; skew deviation of the two images should be enquired about and, if present, is strongly suggestive of a IVth cranial nerve palsy, though it may also be seen with brainstem lesions.)

Ocular myopathy (see p. 224 and footnote, p. 262).

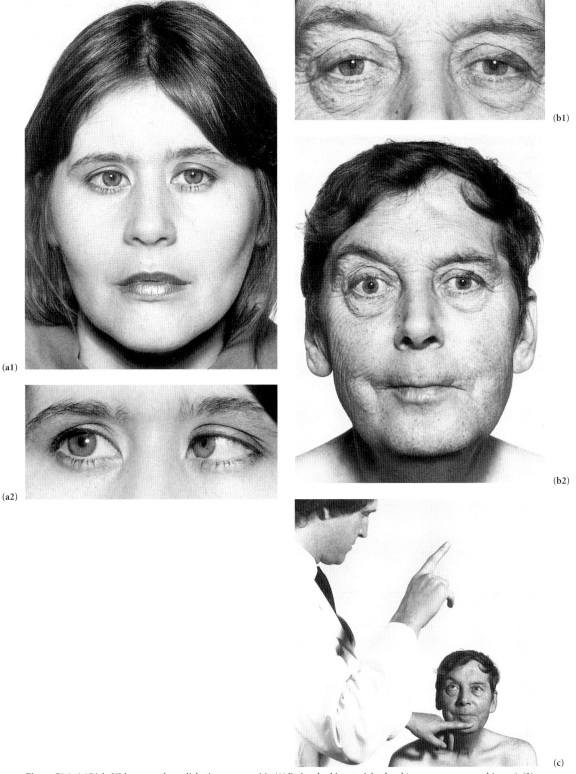

Figure C3.9 (a)Right VIth nerve palsy — diabetic mononeuritis. (1) Patient looking straight ahead (note convergent strabismus); (2) looking to the right. (b1,2) Left IIIrd nerve palsy (note ptosis and mydriasis of the left pupil). The patient had had surgery for a pituitary tumour (note scar on upper forehead and left frontal alopecia). (c) Upward gaze being tested (note the failure of the left eye to follow the examiner's finger).

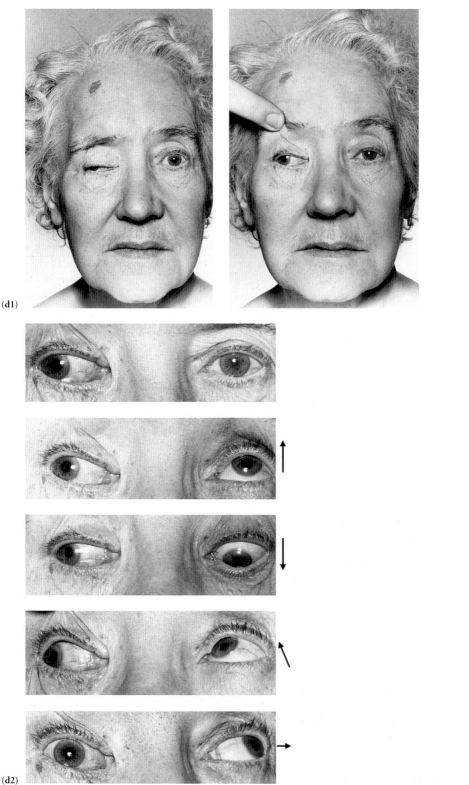

(d1)

(d2)

Figure C3.9 (*continued*) (d) Complete right IIIrd nerve palsy: (1) note mydriasis of the right pupil and the down and outward deviation of the right eye (due to the unopposed action of the superior oblique and lateral rectus muscles innervated by the IVth and VIth nerves, respectively); (2) testing eye movements (note the failure of the right eye to look straight, upwards, downwards, upwards and laterally, and medially).

Case 13 | Parkinson's disease

Frequency in survey: main focus of a short case in 3% of attempts at PACES station 3, CNS.

Record

This man has an *expressionless, unblinking face* and slurred *low volume monotonous speech.* He is drooling (due to excessive salivation and some dysphagia) and there is *titubation.* He has difficulty starting to walk ('freezing') but once started, progresses with quick shuffling steps as if trying to keep up with his own centre of gravity. As he walks he is *stooped* and he *does not swing his arms* which show a continuous *pill-rolling tremor.* (He has poor balance and tends to fall, being unable to react quickly enough to stop himself.) His arms show a *lead-pipe rigidity* at the elbow but *cog-wheel rigidity* (combination of lead pipe rigidity and tremor—i.e. worse with anxiety) at the wrist. He has a positive glabellar tap sign (an unreliable sign) and his signs generally are *asymmetrical*—note the greater tremor in the R/L arm. (The tremor is decreased by intention but hand-writing may be small*, tremulous and untidy.) There is *blepharoclonus* (tremor of the eyelids when the eyes are gently closed).

The diagnosis is Parkinson's disease.

Male to female ratio is 3 : 1.

The features of Parkinson's disease are

1 Tremor
2 Rigidity
3 Bradykinesia.
Bradykinesia (the most disabling) can be demonstrated by asking the patient to touch his thumb successively with each finger. He will be slow in the initiation of the response and there will be a progressive reduction in the amplitude of each movement and a peculiar type of fatiguability. He will also have difficulty in performing two different motor acts simultaneously.

Other causes of the parkinsonian syndrome

Drug-induced (p. 214)
Postencephalitic (increasingly rare; definite history of encephalitis—encephalitis lethargica pandemic 1916–1928; there may be ophthalmoplegia, pupil abnormalities and dyskinesias; poor response to L-dopa)

Brain damage from anoxia (e.g. cardiac arrest), carbon monoxide or manganese poisoning (dementia and pyramidal signs are likely with all)
Neurosyphilis
Cerebral tumours affecting the basal ganglia.

Other conditions which may have some extrapyramidal features

Arteriosclerotic Parkinson's (stepwise progression, broad-based gait, pyramidal signs; may be no more than simply two common conditions occurring in the same patient—cerebral arteriosclerosis and idiopathic parkinsonism)
Normal pressure hydrocephalus (may have a number of causes including head injury, meningitis or subarachnoid haemorrhage, though in many instances the cause cannot be determined; the classic triad is *urinary incontinence, gait apraxia* and *dementia;* diagnosed by CT or MRI scan; important to diagnose because it may respond to ventriculosystemic shunting)
Steele–Richardson–Olszewski syndrome (supranuclear

---

* When present this is often the earliest sign to appear.

gaze palsy, axial rigidity, a tendency to fall backwards, pyramidal signs, subtle dementia or frontal lobe syndrome)

Striatonigral degeneration as part of multiple system atrophy, which often comprises autonomic failure and olivopontocerebellar atrophy

Alzheimer's disease (severe dementia, mild extrapyramidal signs)

Wilson's disease (Kayser–Fleischer rings, cirrhosis, chorea, psychotic behaviour, dysarthria, dystonic spasms and posturing; leading, if untreated, to dementia, severe dysarthria and dysphagia, contractures and immobility)

Jakob–Creutzfeldt disease (prion protein encephalopathy leading to rapidly progressive dementia with myoclonus and multifocal neurological signs including aphasia, cerebellar ataxia, cortical blindness and spasticity)

Hypoparathyroidism (basal ganglia calcification).

NB A condition which is often misdiagnosed as Parkinson's disease in the elderly is *benign essential tremor* (often autosomal dominant, intention tremor worse with stress, no other neurological abnormality; usually improves when alcohol is taken and sometimes with diazepam or propranolol).

Stiff-man syndrome (SMS)

This is a rare disease of severe progressive muscle stiffness of the spine and lower extremities with superimposed muscle spasms triggered by external stimuli or emotional stress. When stiffness and spasms are present together patients have difficulty ambulating and are prone to unprotected falls, i.e. falls like a tin soldier. When in spasm the muscles are hard to palpation. Typically symptoms begin between the age of 30 and 50 and respond to benzodiazepines. EMG shows a characteristic abnormality and anti-GAD (glutamic acid decarboxylase) antibodies* are present in 60%. In GAD antibody positive SMS there is a strong association with other autoimmune diseases such as Type 1 diabetes, hyperthyroidism, hypothyroidism, pernicious anemia and vitiligo (see page 293).

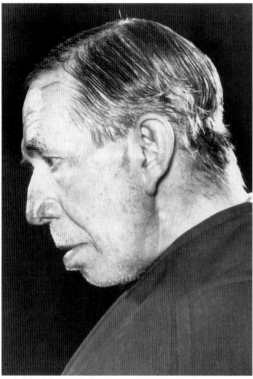
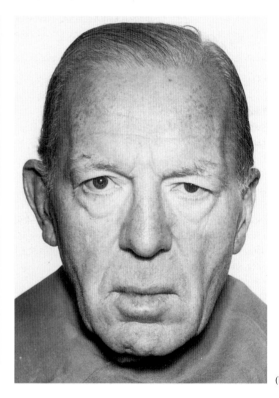

(a) (b)

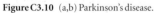

Figure C3.10 (a,b) Parkinson's disease.

* GAD antibodies are found in about 70% of patients with type 1 diabetes at the time of diagnosis. These antibodies appear early in the disease process and can be used to predict who will develop Type 1 diabetes.

Case 14 | Multiple sclerosis

Frequency in survey: main focus of a short case in 3% of attempts at PACES station 3, CNS. Additional feature in many others.

Record 1

The patient (?a young adult) has *ataxic nystagmus* (p. 229), *internuclear ophthalmoplegia* (p. 204), *temporal pallor of the discs* (p. 477), and *slurred speech* (p. 239) with *ataxia* (p. 200) and widespread *cerebellar* signs (p. 186). There are *pyramidal* signs and *dorsal column* signs.

The likely diagnosis is demyelinating disease* (a useful euphemism for multiple sclerosis).

Record 2

The legs of this (?middle-aged) patient have increased tone, they are bilaterally spastic and weak. There is bilateral *ankle clonus* and patellar clonus and the *plantars* are *extensor*. The *abdominal reflexes* are absent. The heel–shin test suggests some *ataxia* in the legs and there is slight *impairment of rapid alternate motion* in the upper limbs.

These features suggest that this *spastic paraplegia* is due to demyelinating disease. An examination of the fundi may show involvement of the discs.†

Male to female ratio is 2 : 3.

Features of multiple sclerosis

Rare in tropical climates

Euphoria despite severe disability (not invariable—the patient may be depressed)

Unpredictable course

May present acutely, subacutely, remittently or insidiously

Relapses and remissions (occurring in two-thirds of patients) are often a useful diagnostic pointer

May very closely imitate other neurological conditions (including neurosis)

Fatigue or a rise in temperature may exacerbate symptoms (the patient may be able to get into, but not out of, a hot bath)

Paroxysmal symptoms (e.g. trigeminal neuralgia) may occur and may respond to carbamazepine

Lhermitte's phenomenon may occur (see p. 223)

Benign course more likely if:

pure sensory presentation

infrequent relapses and long remissions

onset with optic neuritis, or sensory or motor symptoms—in contrast to those of brainstem or cerebellar lesions

benign condition 5 years after onset

The visual evoked response (VER) test is useful in a patient with an isolated lesion which may be due to multiple sclerosis—e.g. spastic paraparesis,† VIth nerve palsy, trigeminal neuralgia, facial palsy, postural vertigo

Cerebrospinal fluid examination may show an increase in total protein up to $1 \, gl^{-1}$ or an increase in lymphocytes up to 50 cells mm^{-3} in 50% of patients. Oligoclonal bands in the gamma region on immunoelectrophoresis that are unique to CSF only

---

* The features in this *record* are some of those which are commonly seen in a case of MS. There are, of course, few neurological signs which it may not produce.

† Multiple sclerosis may present in middle age with insidious spastic paraplegia mimicking cord compression. Signs above the level of the cord lesion may point clinically to demyelination as the

cause. In this case the slight cerebellar signs are highly suggestive of MS. However, syringomyelia or a tumour at the foramen magnum could also be the cause. If the diagnosis is of a tumour there may be papilloedema. If the diagnosis is MS the discs may show global or temporal pallor (and the VERs may be delayed—even if, as is often the case, the discs are normal).

(i.e. are not found in serum) are found in over 95% of patients with MS. CSF oligoclonal bands are also found in some patients with CNS infection, and occasionally in patients with strokes or brain tumours.

MRI scans often detect many more MS lesions than are suspected clinically (CT scans can also detect lesions but are much less sensitive than MRI).

Case 15 | Lower motor neurone VIIth nerve palsy

Frequency in survey: main focus of a short case in 2% of attempts at PACES station 3, CNS.

Record

On the R/L side there is *paralysis* of the *upper** and *lower face,* so that the *eye cannot be closed* (or it can easily be opened by the examiner; the patient cannot bury the eyelashes); the eyeball turns up on attempted closure (*Bell's phenomenon*) and the patient is unable to raise his R/L eyebrow. The corner of the *mouth droops,* the *nasolabial fold* is *smoothed out,* and the voluntary and involuntary (i.e. including emotional) movements of the mouth are paralysed on the R/L side (the lips may be drawn to the opposite side and the tongue may deviate as well—not necessarily hypoglossal involvement—see footnote, p. 184).

This is a R/L lower motor neurone VIIth nerve lesion (now check the ipsilateral ear for evidence of *herpes zoster*).

Causes of a lower motor neurone VIIth nerve lesion

1 Bell's palsy†
2 Ramsay Hunt syndrome (herpes zoster on the external auditory meatus and the geniculate ganglion—taste to the anterior two-thirds of the tongue is lost; there may be lesions on the fauces and palate).

Other differential diagnoses

Cerebellopontine angle compression (acoustic neuroma or meningioma; Vth, VIth, VIIth, VIIIth nerve palsy, cerebellar signs and loss of taste to the anterior two-thirds of the tongue—p. 258)
Parotid tumour (?palpable; taste not affected)
Trauma
A pontine lesion (e.g. MS, tumour or vascular lesion)
Middle ear disease (deafness)
The causes of mononeuritis multiplex (diabetes, polyarteritis nodosa and Churg–Strauss syndrome, rheumatoid, SLE, Wegener's, sarcoid, carcinoma, amyloid and leprosy)

Causes of bilateral lower motor neurone VIIth nerve paralysis‡

Guillain–Barré syndrome (occasionally only VIIth nerves affected)
Sarcoidosis (parotid gland enlargement not always present)
Bilateral Bell's palsy
Myasthenia gravis (?ptosis, variable strabismus, proximal muscle weakness, etc.—p. 242)
Congenital facial diplegia
Some forms of muscular dystrophy
Motor neurone disease (rarely)
Lyme disease (may be bilateral, alone or with signs of meningoencephalitis or peripheral radiculoneuropathy, knee effusion, Baker's cyst rupture, heart block, etc.).

---

* That is, including frontalis ('raise eyebrows'), corrugator superficialis ('frown') and orbicularis oculi ('close your eyes tight').
† In the mild case of Bell's palsy taste over the anterior two-thirds of the tongue is usually preserved, because the lesion is due to swelling of the nerve in the confined lower facial canal. In cases with more extensive involvement this taste is lost and the patient may also show increased susceptibility to high-pitched or loud sounds (hyperacusis due to stapedius paralysis).
‡ Bilateral lower motor neurone VIIth nerve lesions are easily missed because there is no asymmetry.

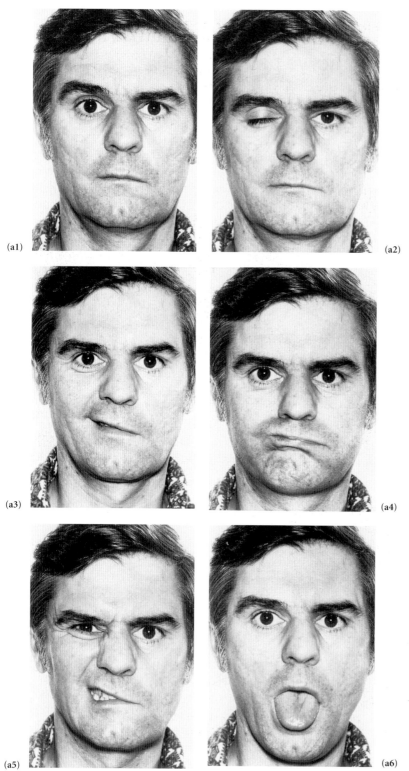

(a1)   (a2)

(a3)   (a4)

(a5)   (a6)

Figure C3.11   (a) Left Bell's palsy: (1) 'Look straight ahead'; (2) 'Close your eyes'; (3) 'Smile'; (4) 'Puff out your cheeks'; (5) 'Show me your teeth'; (6) 'Put out your tongue'.

The chorda tympani leaves the facial nerve in the middle ear to supply taste to the anterior two-thirds of the tongue. The superficial petrosal branch to supply the lachrymal glands, and the nerve to stapedius both leave higher in the facial canal than the chorda tympani. The level of the lesion in the facial canal can sometimes be assessed (very unlikely to be required in the examination) by assessing the relative involvement of these nerves.

Variation of the Ramsay Hunt syndrome

Occasionally facial palsy is associated with trigeminal, occipital or cervical herpes with or without auditory involvement (see anecdote 31, vol. 2, p. 364). In some of these cases the geniculate ganglion may be spared — see p. 342.

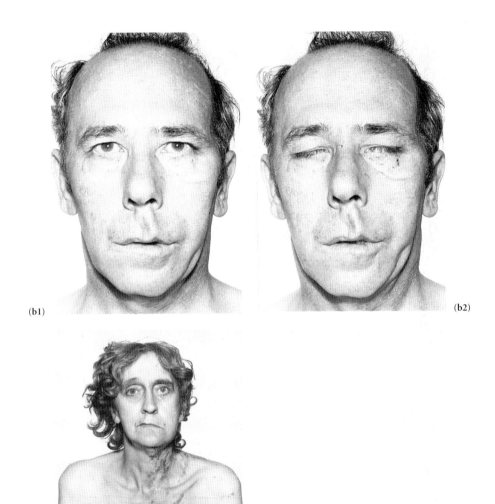

(b1)

(b2)

(c)

Figure C3.11 (*continued*) (b1) Bilateral lower motor neurone VIIth nerve palsy (Guillain–Barré syndrome); (2) 'Close your eyes'. (c) Ramsay Hunt syndrome.

Case 16 | Drug-induced extrapyramidal syndrome

Frequency in survey: main focus of a short case in 2% of attempts at PACES station 3, CNS.

Record

There are (in this ?elderly, chronic schizophrenic) stereotyped tic-like *orofacial dyskinesias* (involuntary movements) including *lip-smacking, chewing, pouting* and *grimacing*. There is (may be) *choreoathetosis* of the limbs and trunk.

The diagnosis is tardive dyskinesia.* (It is likely that the patient has been on sustained phenothiazine treatment for at least 6 months. The condition often persists when the drug is withdrawn, in which case tetrabenazine may help.)

Neuroleptics which may cause abnormal involuntary movements (by inhibiting dopamine function)
Phenothiazines (e.g. chlorpromazine)
Butyrophenones (e.g. haloperidol)
Substituted benzamides (e.g. metoclopramide)
Reserpine
Tetrabenazine.

Other neuroleptic-induced extrapyramidal adverse reactions (apart from tardive dyskinesia)
Acute dystonias (soon after starting the drug; e.g. oculogyric crises)
Akathisia (uncontrollable restlessness with an inner feeling of unease)
Parkinson's syndrome (indistinguishable from Parkinson's disease though tremor is less common; tends to respond to anticholinergics rather than L-dopa).

---

* Called tardive (late) because it does not appear until at least 3 months, or more often a year, after the start or withdrawal of long-term treatment with neuroleptic drugs. This distinguishes tardive dyskinesia from acute dystonias and parkinsonism which develop early. The latter respond to anticholinergic drugs, while tardive dyskinesia responds poorly, or not at all.

Case 17 | **Choreoathetosis**

Frequency in survey: main focus of a short case in 2% of attempts at PACES station 3, CNS. Additional feature in a further 3%.

Survey note: often hemichorea associated with a hemiplegia.

Record

There are *brief, jerky, abrupt, irregular, quasi-purposeful, involuntary movements* (which never integrate into a coordinated act but may match it in complexity). The movements *flit* from one part of the body to another in a random sequence; they are *present at rest* and *accentuated by activity* (at rest the movements prevent the patient's relaxation and they interrupt and distort voluntary movement). The patient has a general air of restlessness. He is *unable* to keep his *tongue protruded* (it darts in and out). There is *abnormal posturing* of the *hands* in which the wrist is flexed and the fingers are hyperextended at the metacarpophalangeal joints. When the upper limbs are raised and extended there is *pronation of the forearm*.

This is chorea.*

Causes of chorea

Sydenham's chorea (usually between age 5 and 15; ?heart murmur; one-third have a history of rheumatic fever; it may recur during pregnancy and when on the oral contraceptive pill)

Huntington's chorea (affects the lower limbs more often than the upper, producing a dancing sort of gait; chorea may precede dementia; onset age 35–50; family history)

Drug-induced chorea (e.g. neuroleptics, L-dopa)

Senile chorea (idiopathic orofacial dyskinesia; no dementia).

Other causes of chorea include epidemic encephalitis, the encephalopathies occurring with exanthema, idiopathic hypocalcaemia, thyrotoxicosis, SLE, carbon monoxide poisoning and Wilson's disease.

Causes of hemichorea/hemiballism†

Cerebrovascular accident† (?hemiplegia, homonymous hemianopia)

Intracerebral tumour (?pyramidal signs on the side of the chorea, papilloedema)

Trauma

Post-thalamotomy.

Other types of involuntary movement (dyskinesias)

Athetosis‡ (slow, coarse, irregular, writhing muscular distortion most commonly of the hands, feet and digits, though the face and tongue may be affected—many choreic and dystonic movements are indistinguishable from athetosis)

Dystonia‡ (sustained spasm of some portion of the body; the movements are powerful and deforming,

---

* In choreoathetosis (cerebral palsy, tumours involving the pallidum, vascular insufficiency, Wilson's disease, carbon monoxide poisoning, etc.) the movements mainly involve the under limbs and cranial nerves (grimacing, writhing movements of the tongue, etc.). The hands are repeatedly brought in front of the chest shaped like cups with flexion at the MCP joints and extension at the interphalangeal joints.

† Hemiballism is wild irregular flinging or throwing movements of whole limbs on one side. Vascular lesions are the commonest

cause. The lesion is in the contralateral subthalamic nucleus. The ballistic movements often begin as the other neurological signs of the cerebrovascular accident start to clear (i.e. after an interval). They disappear during sleep. Though initially they may exhaust the patient, they usually die out gradually over 6–8 weeks.

‡ The common causes of the two closely linked dyskinesias, dystonia and athetosis, are drugs (neuroleptics, L-dopa) and post-hypoxia. There are many rare causes.

torticollis is a common example of torsion dystonia; lordosis and scoliosis may also be caused)

Myoclonus (rapid shock-like muscular jerks often repetitious and sometimes rhythmic—most common causes include epilepsy, essential (familial), physiological (sleep, exercise, anxiety), metabolic disorders (renal, respiratory or hepatic failure), subacute encephalitis)

Tremors (e.g. Parkinson's, anxiety, thyrotoxicosis, drugs (e.g. alcohol, caffeine, salbutamol), MS, spino-cerebellar degeneration, cerebrovascular accident, essential/familial)

Tics.

Case 18 | Carpal tunnel syndrome

Frequency in survey: main focus of a short case in 2% of attempts at PACES station 3, CNS. Additional feature in a further 3%.

Record

There is (in this ?stout, ?middle-aged lady who complains of pain, numbness or paraesthesiae in the palm and fingers, which is particularly bad in the night*) *sensory loss* over the *palmar* aspects of the *first three and a half fingers* and *wasting of the thenar eminence*. There is weakness of *abduction, flexion* and *opposition of the thumb*.

The diagnosis is median nerve palsy. The non-involvement of the flexor muscles of the forearm (i.e. can flex the distal interphalangeal joint of the thumb) suggests that the cause is carpal tunnel syndrome (now check the facies for underlying *acromegaly* or *myxoedema*; underlying *rheumatoid arthritis* should be obvious). *Tinel's sign†* is positive to confirm this.

Though in early cases there may be no abnormal physical signs, usually some impairment of sensation over the affected fingers can be detected. Tenderness on compression of the nerve at the wrist† and thenar atrophy are relatively rare. If the story is characteristic the absence of physical signs should not deter one from advising treatment with intracarpal tunnel steroid injection or carpal tunnel decompression. Investigation with nerve conduction studies may be helpful in cases of doubt. In advanced, unrecognized cases, the patient may present with burns on one or more of the first three fingers.

Causes of carpal tunnel syndrome

Idiopathic (almost entirely in females, middle-aged, often obese; or younger women with excessive use of hands; may occur in males after unaccustomed hand use—e.g. house painting)

Pregnancy
Contraceptive pill
Myxoedema (?facies, hoarse croaking voice, pulse, ankle jerks, etc.—p. 438)
Acromegaly (?facies, large spade-shaped hands, bitemporal hemianopia, etc.—p. 429)
Rheumatoid arthritis of the wrists (?spindling of the fingers, ulnar deviation, nodules, etc.—p. 384)
Osteoarthrosis of the carpus (perhaps related to an old fracture)
Tuberculous tenosynovitis
Primary amyloidosis (?peripheral neuropathy, thick nerves, autonomic neuropathy; heart, joint and gut (rectal biopsy) involvement may occur—see also footnote, p. 180)
Tophaceous gout (p. 399).

---

* The nocturnal discomfort may be referred to the whole forearm with paraesthesiae extending beyond the cutaneous distribution of the median nerve in the hand. The sensory *signs* however, are confined to the classic median nerve distribution (Fig. B.4, p. 51).
† *Tinel's sign* is tingling in the distribution of a nerve produced by percussion of that nerve. Percussion over the carpal tunnel sometimes produces a positive Tinel's sign in carpal tunnel syndrome.

Other signs are *Phalen's sign* (the patient flexes both wrists for 60 seconds and this produces a prompt exacerbation of paraesthesia which is rapidly relieved when the flexion is discontinued) which is positive in half the patients, as is the *tourniquet test* (a sphygmomanometer is pumped above systolic pressure for 2 minutes and this produces the paraesthesia). Symptoms may sometimes be induced by *hyperextension* at the wrist.

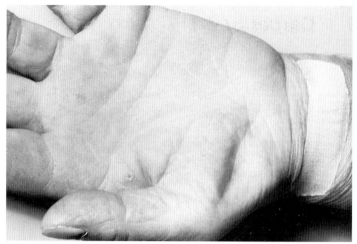

Figure C3.12 Wasting of the thenar eminence.

Case 19 | **Diabetic foot**

Frequency in survey: main focus of a short case in 1% of attempts at PACES station 3, CNS. Additional feature in a further 1%.

Diabetic foot is dealt with on p. 396.

Case 20 | Friedreich's ataxia

Frequency in survey: main focus of a short case in 1% of attempts at PACES station 3, CNS.

Record

There is *pes cavus, (kypho)scoliosis* and (may be) a deformed and high-arched palate. The patient is *ataxic* and clumsy with an *intention tremor* and his *head shakes*. There is *nystagmus* (often slow and coarse and observed before formal examination) and *dysarthria* (slow and slurred or scanning and explosive). There is (?gross) bilateral impairment of rapid alternate motion, finger–nose and heel–shin tests. Knee and *ankle jerks* are *absent* and the *plantar responses* are *extensor. Position and vibration* sense are diminished in the feet.
The diagnosis is Friedreich's ataxia.

Other features (if asked)

1 Cardiomyopathy (may cause sudden death)
2 Optic and retinal atrophy
3 Diabetes mellitus
4 Mild dementia.

The condition is one of the hereditary spinocerebellar degenerations. It is an autosomal recessive trinucleotide repeat disorder with a GAA unstable expansion in the long arm of chromosome 9. The fully-fledged syndrome is rare among affected family members who more commonly show slight signs of abnormality in the lower limbs, chiefly pes cavus and absent reflexes (*formes fruste*).

The major classic ataxic conditions which may need to be differentiated from Friedreich's ataxia, particularly if the latter is mild and presents late, are MS and tabes dorsalis (rare). Typical features which may help to differentiate these conditions are shown in Table C3.4.

Other conditions which may have features of Friedreich's ataxia (all are recessive)
Bassen–Kornzweig syndrome (abetalipoproteinaemia*)—steatorrhoea, acanthosis, pigmentary retinal

Table C3.4 Features which may help to differentiate the major ataxic conditions

	Friedreich's ataxia	Multiple sclerosis	Tabes dorsalis
Family history	Major	Minor	None
Onset before age 15	Usual	Rare	Rare
Knee and ankle jerks	Absent	Usually exaggerated	Absent
Spine	(Kypho)scoliosis	Normal	Normal
Feet shape	Pes cavus	Normal	Normal
Pupils	Normal	Normal	Argyll Robertson
Plantars	↑	↑	↓ or → (unless taboparesis)
Pain and deep pressure	Normal	Normal	Absent
Romberg's sign	±	−	+

* LDL, VLDL and chylomicra are absent from the serum, cholesterol is very low and triglycerides are barely detectable.

degeneration and a spinocerebellar degeneration which resembles Friedreich's ataxia

Refsum's disease (elevated serum phytanic acid due to defective lipid α-oxidase) — pupillary abnormalities, optic atrophy, deafness, pigmentary retinal degeneration, cardiomyopathy, icthyosis and a Friedreich-like ataxia

Roussy–Lévy syndrome (this is a variant of type I hereditary motor and sensory neuropathy and its features are intermediate between Charcot–Marie–Tooth disease and Friedreich's ataxia) — ataxia, areflexia, pes cavus and kyphoscoliosis but absence of nystagmus, dysarthria, extensor plantar responses and posterior column signs.

Case 21 | Proximal myopathy

Frequency in survey: main focus of a short case in 1% of attempts at PACES station 3, CNS.

Record 1 (patient lying on a bed)

There is considerable *proximal muscular weakness*, particularly in abduction at the shoulder joints and extension as well as flexion at the hip joints. The patient is *unable* to *sit up* with the upper limbs outstretched in front.

This patient has a proximal myopathy.

Record 2 (patient sitting in a chair)

The patient has *proximal muscular weakness* in both *upper* and the *lower limb girdle groups*. I can overcome his abduction of the arms and he has considerable difficulty *standing up* from the chair. He is unable to *stand up from a squatting position*. (In both cases you should ask the examiner's permission to examine the gait.)

This patient has a proximal myopathy.

Causes of proximal myopathy

Polymyalgia rheumatica — usually occurs over the age of 50 years, male to female ratio 1:3. The predominant features are fatigue, morning stiffness in the limb girdles and/or neck, weight loss, proximal pain at rest and during movement and tenderness of the muscles. There is a sense of weakness but on careful testing muscle strength is found to be normal or nearly normal. The apparent weakness is due to pain and stiffness. The ESR is elevated. Closely related to temporal arteritis. Responds dramatically to corticosteroids

Cushing's syndrome (?moonface, acne, axial obesity, hirsutism, evidence of rheumatoid arthritis, etc. — p. 441)

Thyrotoxicosis (?eye signs, goitre, fidgety, tachycardia, etc. — p. 432); the proximal muscular weakness is particularly severe in upper limb muscles

Polymyositis (?tender muscles — p. 415)

Dermatomyositis (?heliotrope rash around the eyes, on the knuckles, the hands and over the knee joints, tender muscles, etc. — p. 288)

Drugs — alcohol, corticosteroids, amiodarone, chloroquine, β-blockers, lithium, isoniazid, labetalol, methadone, etc.

Carcinomatous myopathy — the muscular weakness may precede the neoplasia. The lower limb girdle is much more adversely affected than the upper limb girdle muscles. The onset is usually between the age of 50 and 60 years and men are more often affected than females. At times there may be many myasthenic features (Lambert–Eaton syndrome — p. 242) and the weakness is often improved after a short muscular contraction. The malignancy is often small cell carcinoma of the lung. The neurological symptoms may precede the neoplasia by 1–2 years

Osteomalacia (?ethnic origin — mostly females, waddling gait, bone pain — p. 418)

McArdle's syndrome (myophosphorylase deficiency; ?stiffness and cramps after exercise, exercising muscles feel hard, pain on movement)

Mitochondrial myopathy (a group of biochemical disorders involving the mitochondrial enzymes. Muscle biopsy may show 'ragged red fibres'. Typically there is slowly progressive weakness of limbs and/or external ocular (see footnote, p. 262) and other cranial muscles, abnormal fatiguability on sustained exertion, and lactic acidaemia on exertion or even at rest. Sometimes the myopathy is but one facet of a multisystem disease)

Endstage renal failure — (?uraemic facies).

Case 22 | Subacute combined degeneration of the cord

Frequency in survey: main focus of a short case in 1% of attempts at PACES station 3, CNS. Additional feature in a further 1%.

Record

There is (in this patient who may complain of burning paraesthesiae in the feet) loss of *light touch, vibration* and *joint position* sensation over the feet (*stocking,* may also be *glove*), and *Romberg's* sign is positive. The legs are (may be) weak, and though the knee (may be brisk) and *ankle jerks* are *lost* (due to peripheral neuropathy) the *plantar responses* are *extensor*.

The pupils are normal, there are no cerebellar signs or pes cavus (p. 259) and though the patient is not (may not be) clinically anaemic* (having checked conjunctival mucous membranes) and the tongue and complexion are normal (glossitis and classic 'lemon yellow' pallor are now rarely seen in SACD), these findings suggest the diagnosis of subacute combined degeneration of the cord. (Findings in the abdomen might be splenomegaly, carcinoma of the stomach as this is commoner in pernicious anaemia, or a laparotomy scar from a previous gastrectomy.)

Although vitamin B_{12} neuropathy usually starts with peripheral neuropathy followed by posterior column signs, and signs of pyramidal disturbances are seldom marked in the early stages (progressive spasticity may occur), vitamin B_{12} deficiency should always be excluded in a patient in whom any of the following are unexplained:

Peripheral sensory neuropathy

Spinal cord disease

Optic atrophy (rare)

Dementia (frank dementia is rare; progressive enfeeblement of intellect and memory, or episodes of confusion or paranoia may be seen; more commonly the patient is simply difficult and uncooperative).

Causes of severe vitamin B_{12} deficiency

Addisonian pernicious anaemia (NB associated organ-specific autoimmune diseases, especially autoimmune thyroid disease, diabetes mellitus, Addison's, vitiligo and hypoparathyroidism — see also p. 293)

Partial or total gastrectomy

Stagnant loop syndrome

Ileal resection or Crohn's disease

Vegan diet

Fish tapeworm

Chronic tropical sprue

Congenital intrinsic factor deficiency.

Lhermitte's phenomenon: the patient describes a 'tingling' or 'electric feeling' or 'funny sensation' which passes down his spine, and perhaps into lower limbs, when he bends his head forward.† The most common cause is MS but it can also occur in cervical cord tumour, cervical spondylosis and SACD.

---

* Although the patient may be anaemic, vitamin B_{12} neuropathy may develop without anaemia and with normal blood film and bone marrow (see p. 518). Serum vitamin B_{12} level may be required to confirm the diagnosis.

† A similar sensation provoked by neck *extension* is termed 'reversed Lhermitte's phenomenon' and strongly suggests cervical spondylosis.

Case 23 | Muscular dystrophy

Frequency in survey: main focus of a short case in 0.4% of attempts at PACES station 3, CNS.

Survey note: all cases in the original, pre PACES, survey were of facioscapulohumeral except one possible case of limb-girdle type.

Record 1

The patient has a dull, unlined, expressionless face (*myopathic facies*) with lips that are (usually) open and slack. There is *wasting* of the *facial* and *limb-girdle muscles*, and the superior margins of the scapulae (viewed from the front) are (may be) visible above the clavicles. The movements of smiling, whistling and closing the eyes are impaired. There is *winging of the scapulae* (when the patient leans against a wall with arms extended). There is (may be) involvement of the trunk and legs (anterior tibials may cause bilateral foot-drop) now or in the future.

The diagnosis is *facioscapulohumeral* muscular dystrophy* (autosomal dominant, course variable but usually relatively benign).

Record 2

There is *limb-girdle wasting* and *weakness* which affects some groups of muscles more than others (e.g. deltoid and spinati are usually spared), and the *face* is *spared*. There is (not uncommonly) enlargement of the calf muscles.

These features suggest *limb-girdle* muscular dystrophy (autosomal recessive, both sexes affected equally, more benign if the upper limb is involved first, usually begins in the second or third decade, sometimes arrests but usually patients are severely disabled within 20 years of onset).

Other muscular dystrophies

Duchenne or pseudohypertrophic—X-linked, severe, onset age 3–4 years, initially enlargement of calves, buttocks and infraspinati (this disappears later) while other muscles (especially the proximal lower limb) waste; waddling lordotic gait; usually confined to wheelchair by age of 10 years; cardiac muscle involved; face spared; death from respiratory infection and/or cardiac failure commonly at about age of 20

Benign X-linked (Becker) muscular dystrophy—similar to Duchenne but much less severe—onset 5–25 years; confined to wheelchair 25 years later

Distal muscular dystrophy—dominant; most cases occur in Sweden—eventually spreads to proximal muscles unlike peroneal muscular atrophy (p. 188) with which it is most often confused

Oculopharyngeal muscular dystrophy—sporadic or dominant—first ptosis, then ophthalmoplegia, face and neck muscles are often mildly involved. Dysphagia is usually the most prominent symptom and ptosis often complete. It has been shown to be due to a mutation in the PABP gene.

---

*There may be an inflammatory component in the aetiology of facioscapulohumeral muscular dystrophy, as perivascular inflammation may be seen on muscle biopsy and *retinal microvascular abnormalities* (sparse and dilated (telangiectatic) peripheral retinal vessels which leak causing exudate to track to the posterior pole with consequent retinal detachment and blindness) also characterize the disorder. *Sensorineural deafness* may occur but clinical cardiomyopathy is rare.

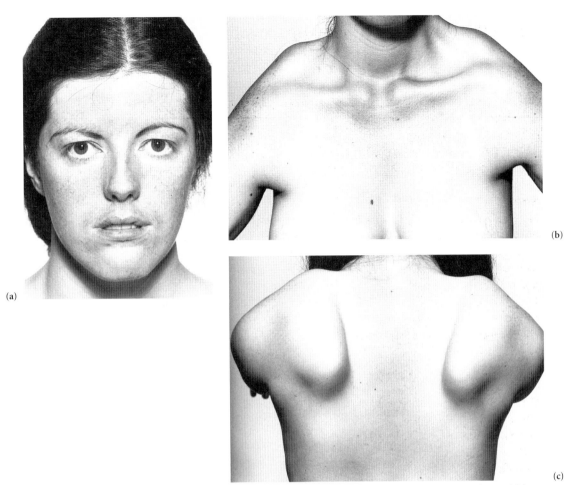

Figure C3.13 (a) Myopathic facies (facioscapulohumeral muscular dystrophy). (b) The superior margins of the scapulae are visible from the front (same patient as (a)). (c) Winging of the scapulae (same patient).

Case 24 | Wasting of the small muscles of the hand

Frequency in survey: did not occur in the small initial survey of PACES station 3, CNS.

Predicted frequency from older, more extensive MRCP short case surveys: main focus of a short case in 4% of attempts at PACES station 3, CNS. Additional feature in many others.

Record

There is *wasting* (and weakness) of the *thenar* and *hypothenar* eminences and of the other small muscles of the hand so that *dorsal guttering* is seen. There is (may be) hyperextension at the metacarpophalangeal joints and flexion at the interphalangeal joints (due to the action of the long extensors of the fingers being unopposed by the lumbricals. In the advanced case a claw hand or *main-en-griffe* is produced).

Generalized wasting of the small muscles of the hand suggests a lesion affecting the lower motor neurones which originate at the level C8, T1 (unless there is arthropathy leading to disuse atrophy).

Causes

A lesion affecting the anterior horn cells at the level C8, T1 such as:

Motor neurone disease (?prominent fasciculation, spastic paraparesis, wasted fibrillating tongue, no sensory signs—p. 190)

Syringomyelia (fasciculation not prominent, ?dissociated sensory loss, burn scars, Horner's, nystagmus—p. 249)

Charcot–Marie–Tooth disease (?distal wasting of the lower limb, pes cavus, etc.—p. 188)

Other causes are old polio, tumour, meningovascular syphilis and cord compression.

A root lesion at the level C8, T1 such as:

Cervical spondylosis affecting the C8, T1 level (usually affects higher roots—C6,7, and therefore significant wasting of the small muscles of the hand is uncommon—see p. 236, ?pyramidal signs in the legs, no signs above the level of the lesion, cervical collar)

Tumour at the C8, T1 level (e.g. neurofibroma).

A lesion damaging the brachial plexus (especially lower trunk and medial cord) such as:

Cervical rib (symptoms provoked by a particular posture or movement, e.g. sleeping on the limb, cleaning windows, etc.; ?supraclavicular bruit though Raynaud's and other vascular manifestations are rare in the presence of prominent neurological features)

Pancoast's tumour (?Horner's, clubbing, chest signs, lymph nodes, cachexia, etc.)

Damage caused by violent traction of arm (e.g. the patient who tried to stop himself falling from a tree by grabbing a passing branch; the same damage in obstetric practice produces Klumpke's paralysis).

Combined ulnar and median nerve lesions (see p. 192 and p. 217, respectively).

Arthritis leading to disuse atrophy* (wasting out of proportion to weakness).

Cachexia.

---

* E.g. rheumatoid arthritis. The factors which may contribute to small muscle wasting in the hand in rheumatoid arthritis are disuse atrophy, vasculitis, peripheral neuropathy, mononeuritis multiplex and entrapment neuropathy (median nerve at wrist, ulnar at elbow, and branches—e.g. the deep palmar branch of the ulnar nerve damaged by subluxation of the carpal bones on the radius and ulna).

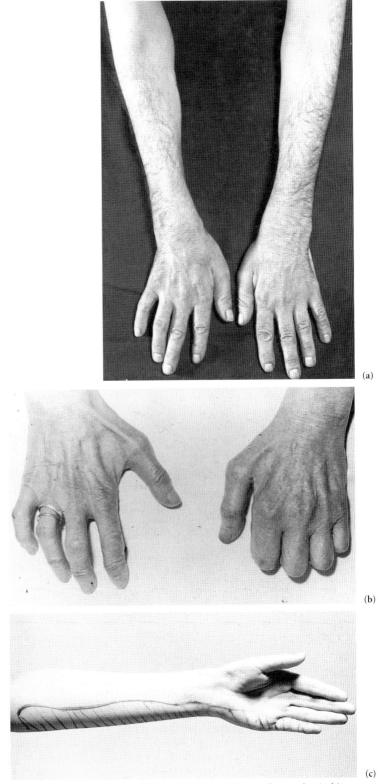

Figure C3.14 (a) Charcot–Marie–Tooth disease. (b)Motor neurone disease. (c) Cervical rib (showing the area of sensory loss in this case T1 and part of C8. See Fig. B.2, p. 32).

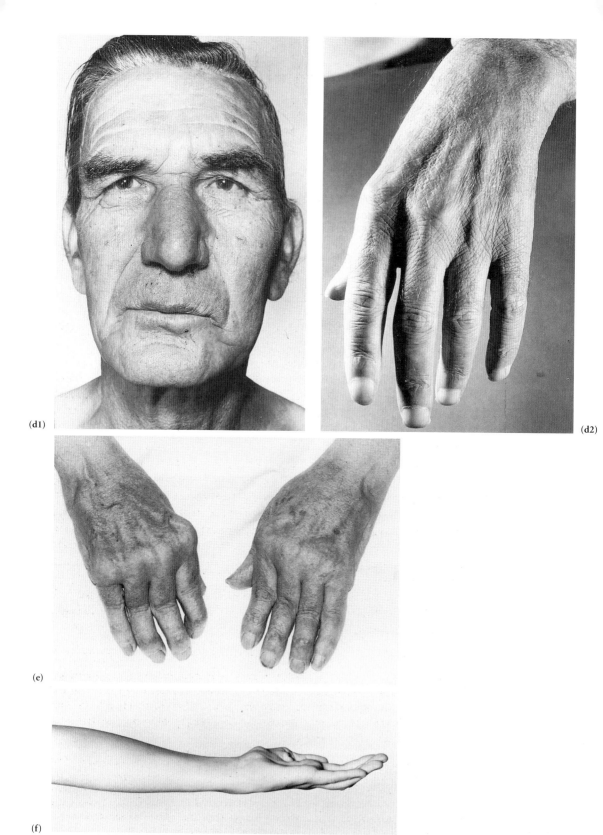

(d1)

(d2)

(e)

(f)

Figure C3.14 (*continued*) (d1,2) Pancoast's tumour (note left Horner's syndrome and clubbing). (e) Rheumatoid arthritis.
(f) *Main-en-griffe* (cervical rib).

Case 25 | Nystagmus

Frequency in survey: did not occur in the small initial survey of PACES station 3, CNS.

Predicted frequency from older, more extensive MRCP short case surveys: main focus of a short case in 3% of attempts at PACES station 3, CNS. Additional feature in a further 2%

Survey note: in most cases nystagmus was cerebellar in origin—usually due to multiple sclerosis.

Record 1

There is nystagmus, greater on the R/L with the fast component to the same side. This suggests:

1 an ipsilateral cerebellar lesion (?cerebellar signs—p. 186), *or*

2 a contralateral vestibular lesion (?vertical nystagmus, ?vertigo—see below). (Now, if allowed, *look for cerebellar signs*; occasionally there will be signs of a lesion in the brainstem, e.g. infarction—p. 273, syringobulbia*—p. 249)

Record 2

The nsystagmus is *ataxic* in that the *abducting eye has greater nystagmus* than the adducting eye.† With this there is dissociation of conjugate eye movements. There is (may be) a divergent strabismus at rest. On looking to the right, the right eye abducts normally, but there is *impairment of adduction*† of the left eye. On looking to the left, the left eye abducts normally but there is *impairment of adduction*† of the right eye (occasionally the reverse may occur with weakness of abduction on each side but adduction remains normal). When the abducting eye is covered, however, the medial movement of the other eye occurs normally.

The diagnosis is *internuclear ophthalmoplegia*. It suggests multiple sclerosis‡ with a lesion in the medial longitudinal fasciculus. (Now, if allowed, *look for cerebellar signs*, pyramidal signs, pale discs, etc. —pp. 186 and 209)

Causes and types of nystagmus

A simplified diagrammatic representation of conjugate gaze and its various connections is depicted in Fig C3.15. As can be seen from the multiplicity of these pathways a disorder within the end-organs (i.e. eye, labyrinth, semicircular canals), or in the medial longitudinal fasciculus anywhere through its long course, or in its nuclear connections (i.e. cerebellar,

---

* As can be seen from Fig. C3.15, the medial longitudinal bundle extends into the spinal cord so that syringomyelia confined to the spinal cord, if extending above C5, may also cause nystagmus.
† The key sign of internuclear ophthalmoplegia is the *failure of adduction*—the nystagmus is not essential.

‡ Internuclear ophthalmoplegia is highly characteristic of MS though rarely it may be caused by brainstem gliomata or vascular lesions, or Wernicke's encephalopathy (ocular palsy, nystagmus, loss of pupillary reflexes, ataxia, peripheral neuropathy, Korsakoff's psychosis or other disturbance of mentation; dramatic response to thiamine in the early stages).

vesibular nuclei, etc.), can cause nystagmus. Nystagmus can be divided into:

Physiological nystagmus (a few brief jerks can occur in the normal eye at the extreme lateral gaze)

Ocular nystagmus (in patients with a congenital visual defect in one eye a pendular movement of the eye occurs while gazing straight — fixation nystagmus)

Vestibular nystagmus (see below)

Cerebellar nystagmus (record 1)

Ataxic nystagmus (record 2)

Vestibular nystagmus

This may arise in the periphery (labyrinth or vestibular nerve) or in the central vestibular nuclei and its connections.

Peripheral The fast component is towards the contralateral side (except with an early irritative lesion when it can be on the side of the lesion) and the nystagmus is fatiguable — it becomes less and less intense on repetition of the test. The patient tends to be unsteady on the ipsilateral side (contralateral to the fast component) as can be revealed whilst assessing Romberg's test (the patient cannot stand on a narrow base even with the eyes open in this situation, whereas the patient with sensory ataxia becomes more unsteady when the eyes are closed) and gait (tends to reel on the affected side). Cochlear function is usually affected (diminishes leading to deafness, e.g. Menière's syndrome) and the patient may have vertigo.

Causes of peripheral vestibular nystagmus:

Labyrinthitis (probably viral and self-limiting; nystagmus may be absent and only positional and provoked by movements of the head — often it can be elicited by bending the head backwards about 45° — the nystagmus, as well as the vertigo, may appear but fades with repeated testing)

Menière's syndrome (progressive deafness and tinnitus, with recurrent attacks of vertigo)

Acoustic neuroma (progressive tinnitus and nerve deafness; neighbouring nerves — Vth, VIth and VIIth may be involved and there may be cerebellar signs, etc. — p. 258)

Vestibular neuronitis (acute vertigo without deafness or tinnitus which usually improves within 48 h; full recovery may take weeks or months; may be viral).

Other causes include degenerative middle ear disease, hypertension and head injury.

Central Lesions affecting vestibular nuclei (cerebrovascular accident, MS, encephalitis, tumours, syringobulbia, alcoholism,* anticonvulsants, etc.) cause nystagmus which is spontaneous but may be brought on or increased by head movements. It is not adaptable and usually has a vertical component. *Downbeat nystagmus* with the eyes looking straight ahead is characteristic of an Arnold–Chiari malformation.† Downbeat nystagmus on lateral gaze normally indicates a lesion at the foramen magnum level (tumour, syringomyelia, cerebellar degeneration).

---

* Acute alcohol toxicity may cause nystagmus. Nystagmus is also almost always present in Wernicke's encephalopathy. Paradoxically alcohol may reduce congenital nystagmus — a condition which may be gross but symptomless.

† *Arnold–Chiari malformation* may be asymptomatic until adult life when the patient gradually develops cerebellar symptoms and signs. There is cerebellar herniation through the foramen magnum. There may be coexisting syringomyelia of the cervical cord and medulla (p. 249). Commonly there is radiographic evidence of fusion of the cervical vertebrae, platybasia or basilar impression. MRI (CT may miss it) establishes the diagnosis when there are no coexisting bony abnormalities. Surgical intervention may benefit selected cases.

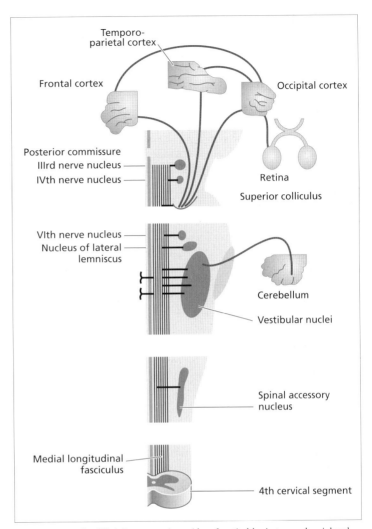

Figure C3.15 A simplified diagram to give an idea of cortical, brainstem and peripheral control of conjugate gaze. The medial longitudinal bundle starts just below the posterior commissure and ends in the upper cervical spinal cord. During its long course it receives fibres from various nucleii (and the lateral pontine gaze centre) which are concerned with the control of conjugate gaze. Interruption in the cortical or midbrain connections often produces a disorder of conjugate gaze rather than nystagmus. Lesions in the brainstem or below result in nystagmus.

Case 26 | Horner's syndrome

Frequency in survey: did not occur in the small initial survey of PACES station 3, CNS.

Predicted frequency from older, more extensive MRCP short case surveys: main focus of a short case in 3% of attempts at PACES station 3, CNS.

Record

There is *miosis,** *enophthalmos* and slight *ptosis* on the R/L side (the other features are ipsilateral *anhydrosis* and vasodilatation of the head and neck).

This is a R/L-sided Horner's syndrome—now examine the *neck* (scars, nodes, aneurysms), *hands* (wasting of the small muscles) and *chest* (ipsilateral apical signs).

Causes of Horner's syndrome

1 Neck surgery or trauma (?scars)

2 Carotid‡ and aortic aneurysms

3 Brainstem vascular disease (e.g. Wallenberg's syndrome†)

4 Pancoast's syndrome (?wasting of ipsilateral small muscles of the hand, T1 and sometimes C7/8 sensory loss and pain, clubbing, tracheal deviation, lymph nodes, ipsilateral apical signs)

5 Enlarged cervical lymph nodes especially malignant (?evidence of primary)

6 Idiopathic (common in neurological practice)

7 Syringomyelia (?bilateral wasting of the small muscles of the hand, dissociated sensory loss, scarred hands, bulbar palsy, pyramidal signs, nystagmus—p. 249)

8 Brainstem demyelination (?nystagmus, cerebellar signs, pyramidal signs, pale discs, etc.).

The syndrome can be caused by any other lesion in the sympathetic nervous system as it travels from the sympathetic nucleus, down through the brainstem to the cord, out of the cord at C8, T1,2, to the sympathetic chain, stellate ganglion and carotid sympathetic plexus (see Fig. C3.16b). Some cases of Horner's are idiopathic (usually females).

* NB Argyll Robertson pupils in neurosyphilis are usually bilateral, irregular and very small.

† Ipsilateral Vth, IXth, Xth, XIth nerve lesions, cerebellar ataxia and nystagmus. Contralateral pain and temperature loss (see p. 273).

‡ Horner's syndrome may be the only manifestation of *carotid dissection.* An urgent carotid and head MRI scan should be performed in newly presenting Horner's syndrome of uncertain cause. Carotid dissection is an important cause of ischaemic stroke in young and middle-aged patients. Spontaneous dissection of carotid and vertebral arteries may affect all age groups, including children, but there is a distinct peak in the fifth decade. A history of a minor precipitating event is frequently elicited in spontaneous dissection of the carotid or ventebral artery, particularly associated with hyperextension or rotation of the neck (e.g. painting a celling, coughing, vomiting, sneezing, the receipt of anaesthesia are all described). The typical patient with carotid artery dissection presents with pain on one side of the head, face or neck accompanied by a partial Horner's syndrome and followed hours or days later by cerebral or retinal ischemia. However, this classic triad is found in less than one third of patients and there may be just one or two of the features. The priority in management is to avoid thromboembolic complications. Although no randomized trials have been reported, anticoagulation has been recommended for acute dissections of the carotid or vertebral artery unless there are contraindications such as intracranial extension of the dissection. Following this approach there is a high rate of recanalization within the first three months. The fear that anticoagulant therapy will extend the dissection appears to be unfounded.

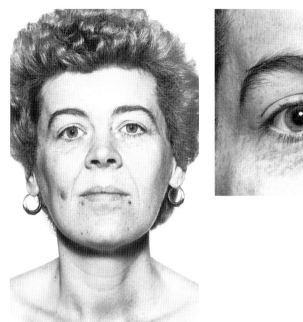
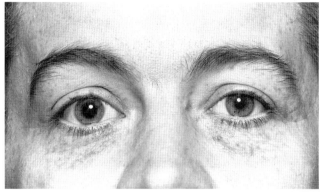

(a1)

(a2)

(b)

Midbrain

Medulla

Demyelination

Vascular disease

Syringomyelia

T1

T2

Parasympathetic
efferent fibres

Short ciliary nerve
to ciliary muscle

Ciliary ganglion

Long ciliary nerve
to dilator pupillae

Carotid plexus

Aneurysm

Postganglionic fibres

Superior cervical ganglion

Cervical lymph nodes

Surgery or trauma

Pancoast's tumour

T1 ganglion

Short ciliary nerve
to sphincter pupillae

Sympathetic efferent
(preganglionic) fibres

Figure C3.16 (a1,2) Left Horner's syndrome (note the scar over the left clavicle). (b) Sympathetic and parasympathetic nerve supply to dilator and sphincter pupillae. The diagram shows the sympathetic pathway and the sites where it may be interrupted to produce Horner's syndrome. (Pathways diagram adapted from *Gray's Anatomy of the Human Body* by kind permission of the publisher, Lea & Febiger.)

Case 27 | Old polio

Frequency in survey: did not occur in the small initial survey of PACES station 3, CNS.

Predicted frequency from older, more extensive MRCP short case surveys: main focus of a short case in 3% of attempts at PACES station 3, CNS. Additional feature in a further 1%.

Record

The R/L leg is *short, wasted, weak* and *flaccid* with *reduced (or absent) reflexes* and a normal plantar response. There is *no sensory defect*. The disparity in the length of the limbs suggest growth impairment in the affected limb since early childhood. The complete absence of sensory and pyramidal signs point to a condition affecting only lower motor neurones.*

    The diagnosis is old polio affecting the R/L leg.

If you see one limb smaller than the other a possible differential diagnosis to consider is infantile hemiplegia. In this there is usually hypoplasia of the whole of that side of the body and the neurological signs will reflect a contralateral hemisphere lesion (i.e. upper motor neurone).

---

* Fasciculation is only occasionally seen in old polio. Very rarely patients with old polio for many years develop a progressive wasting disease (with prominent fasciculation) which is indistinguishable from progressive muscular atrophy and motor neurone disease (see p. 190).

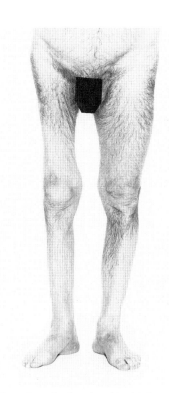

Figure C3.17 Generalized wasting of the right lower limb due to old poliomyelitis.

Case 28 | Cervical myelopathy

Frequency in survey: did not occur in the small initial survey of PACES station 3, CNS.

Predicted frequency from older, more extensive MRCP short case surveys: main focus of a short case in 2% of attempts at PACES station 3, CNS. Additional feature in a further 2%.

Survey note: cervical collar may be a clue.

Record

The legs (of this middle-aged or elderly patient) show *spastic weakness,** the *tone* being *increased,* the *reflexes brisk* (?clonus) and the *plantar responses extensor. Vibration* and joint position senses are (may be) lost in the lower limbs (spinothalamic loss may also occur but is less common). In the upper limbs† there is (often asymmetrical) *inversion‡* of the biceps and supinator jerks.

These features suggest cervical myelopathy as the cause of the spastic paraparesis. *Cervical spondylosis* is the commonest cause though a *spinal cord tumour* cannot be excluded clinically.

In the upper limbs there may be segmental muscle wasting and weakness, particularly if there is an associated radiculopathy. Gross wasting of the small muscles of the hand due to cervical spondylosis is uncommon because the latter usually affects C5/6 or C6/7 and the small muscles are supplied by C8/T1. Mild wasting of the small muscles does sometimes occur probably due to vascular changes in the cord below the lesion.

There is often no sensory loss in the hand. Sometimes in the elderly a complaint of numb, useless hands may be accompanied by constant unpleasant parasthesiae and writhing ('sensory wandering' or 'pseudoathetosis') of the fingers when the eyes are closed. Position and vibration senses are lost in such hands.

Neck pain is surprisingly rare in cervical spondylosis causing cervical myelopthy, and sphincter function is seldom disturbed. Among patients with cervical spondylosis (which is very common) those with a narrow cervical canal are most likely to develop cervical myelopathy. Lhermitte's phenomenon may occur (see p. 223).

---

* In this condition signs often exceed symptoms and spasticity often exceeds weakness.
† The myelopathy hand sign may be present; see footnote, p. 31).
‡ When attempts are made to elicit the normal biceps and supinator tendon reflexes, there is a brisk finger flexion despite little or no response of the biceps and supinator jerks themselves. This is because the lower motor neurones and pyramidal tracts are damaged at the C5/6 level producing lower motor neurone signs at that level and upper motor neurone signs below. The combination of inverted biceps and supinator jerks (the C5/6 jerks) and a brisk triceps jerk (C7/8) is termed the 'mid-cervical reflex pattern'.

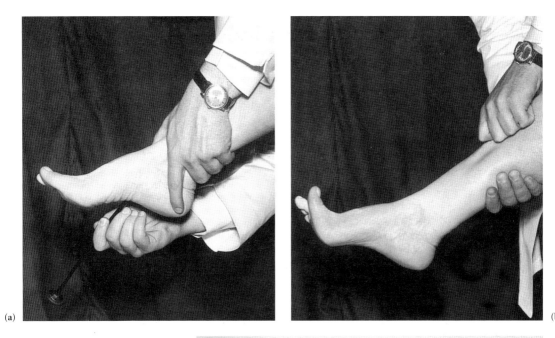

(a)

(b)

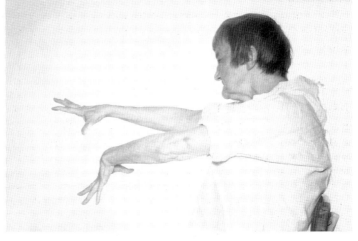

(c)

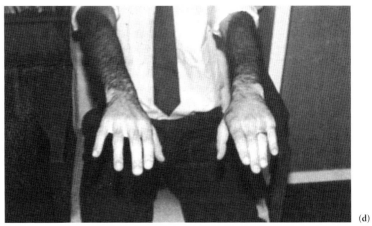

(d)

Figure C3.18 (a) Babinski's sign. (b) Oppenheim's sign (see p. 35). (c) Pseudoathetosis. (d) The myelopathy hand sign (in the right arm).

Case 29 | Bulbar palsy

Frequency in survey: did not occur in the small initial survey of PACES station 3, CNS.

Predicted frequency from older, more extensive MRCP short case surveys: main focus of a short case in 0.9% of attempts at PACES station 3, CNS.

Record

The *tongue* is *flaccid* and *fasciculating* (it is wasted, wrinkled, thrown into folds and increasingly motionless). The *speech is indistinct* (flaccid dysarthria), lacks modulations and has a *nasal twang*, and *palatal movement is absent*. There is (may be) saliva at the corners of the mouth (and while the patient talks he may be seen to pause periodically to gulp the secretions that have accumulated meanwhile in the pharynx; there may be dysphagia and nasal regurgitation).

This is bulbar palsy.

Possible causes

1 Motor neurone disease (?muscle fasciculation, absence of sensory signs, etc. — p. 190)

2 Syringobulbia (?nystagmus, Horner's, dissociated sensory loss, etc. — p. 249)

3 Guillain–Barré syndrome (?generalized including facial flaccid paralysis, absent reflexes, peripheral neuropathy or widespread sensory defect; monitor peak flow rate — p. 246)

4 Poliomyelitis

5 Subacute meningitis (carcinoma, lymphoma, etc.)

6 Neurosyphilis.

Case 30 | Dysarthria

Frequency in survey: did not occur in the small initial survey of PACES station 3, CNS.

Predicted frequency from older, more extensive MRCP short case surveys: main focus of a short case in 0.9% of attempts at PACES station 3, CNS. Additional feature in a further 1%.

Survey note: the only dysarthria used as a short case in our survey was cerebellar (ataxic) dysarthria.

Record

There is dysarthria with *slurred*, *jerky* and *explosive* (slow, lalling, staccato, scanning) speech. (There may be inspiratory whoops indicating the lack of coordination between respiration and phonation.)

This suggests cerebellar disease (?nystagmus, dysdiadochokinesis, finger–nose test, etc.—p. 186).

Other varieties of dysarthria

Spastic dysarthria
Conditions in which all or some of the articulatory parts are rigid or spastic:

Pseudobulbar palsy (indistinct, suppressed, without modulations, high-pitched, 'hot potato', 'Donald Duck' speech due to a tight, immobile tongue—?bilateral spasticity with extensor plantars—p. 248)

Parkinson's disease (monotonous without accents or emphasis, somewhat slurred speech—?expressionless unblinking face, glabellar tap sign, tremor, etc.—p. 207)

Myotonic dystrophy (slurred and suppressed speech—?ptosis, frontal balding, etc.—p. 182)

Huntington's chorea (slurred and monotonous—?chorea, dementia)

General paresis of the insane—very rare (slurred, hesitant or feeble voice—?dementia, vacant expression, trombone tremor of tongue, brisk reflexes, extensor plantars, etc.—p. 265).

Flaccid dysarthria
Bulbar palsy (nasal, decreased modulation, slurring of labial and lingual consonants—?lingual atrophy, fasciculations, etc.—p. 238)

Paralysis of the VIIth, IXth, Xth or XIIth nerves (cerebrovascular accident).

Myopathic dysarthria
Myasthenia gravis (weak hoarse voice with a nasal quality, pitch unsustained, soft accents—?ptosis, variable strabismus, facial and proximal muscle weakness all of which worsen with repetition, etc.—p. 242).

Variegated dysarthria
Hypothyroidism (low-pitched, catarrhal, hoarse, croaking, gutteral voice as if the tongue is too large for the mouth—?facies, pulse, ankle jerks, etc.—p. 438)

Amyloidosis—large tongue (rolling and hollow, hardly modulated)

Multiple ulcers or thrush in the mouth (some parts of the speech indistinct)

Parotitis or temporomandibular arthritis (monotonous, suppressed, badly modulated).

Case 31 | **Dysphasia**

Frequency in survey: did not occur in the small initial survey of PACES station 3, CNS.

Predicted frequency from older, more extensive MRCP short case surveys: main focus of a short case in 0.9% of attempts at PACES station 3, CNS. Additional feature in a further 1%.

Survey note: where the type of dysphasia was reported by the candidate, it was always expressive.

Record 1

The patient's speech *lacks fluency*. He has *difficulty finding certain words* and sometimes produces the *wrong word* and makes grammatical errors. *Comprehension*, however, is *well preserved* (as are the higher cerebral functions and general intellect — the prognosis for eventual adaptation of the patient to his disability is good). His ability to repeat and to name objects is impaired.

The patient has Broca's (*expressive*, motor, non-fluent) *dysphasia* (?associated *right hemiplegia*). The brain damage causing this condition is believed to disconnect the dominant* inferior frontal gyrus (Broca's area).

Record 2

Though the patient *speaks fluently* (often rapidly) with normal intonation, his speech is completely *unintelligible*. He puts words together in the wrong order and mixes them with non-existent words† and phrases (*jargon dysphasia*). Attempts to repeat result in paraphasic† distortions and irrelevant insertions. *Comprehension* is severely *impaired* (and the patient may seem unaware of his dysphasia).

The patient has Wernicke's (*receptive*, fluent) *dysphasia* (?associated *homonymous visual field defect* and/or *sensory diminution* down the right side of the body). The brain damage causing this condition is believed to disconnect the posterior part of the dominant* superior temporal gyrus (Wernicke's area).

Record 3

The patient shows combined expressive and receptive dysphasia. There is marked disturbance in comprehension (and inability to read or write).

The patient has *global dysphasia*‡ (?dense right hemiplegia with sensory loss, homonymous visual field defect and general intellectual deterioration). The common cause of this is infarction of the territory supplied by the

---

* The left hemisphere is dominant in right-handed and in 50% of left-handed people.

† Paraphasia: an incorrect syllable in a word (usually there is some phonemic relationship to the original word, e.g. 'tooth spooth' for 'toothbrush') or an incorrect word in a phrase (often with a semantic relationship to the correct word, e.g. 'hand' for 'foot').

Neologism: paraphasia with slight or no relationship to the original syllable/word.

‡ Global dysphasia is sometimes confused with Broca's dysphasia but the speech defects are severe in this condition affecting fluency, repetition, naming and comprehension. Some stereotypes may be preserved and the patient may be able to recite automatic sequences of prayer or popular songs (*speech automatism*).

left middle cerebral artery. The prognosis for recovery is poor.

Record 4

The patient has difficulty naming objects though he knows what they are (e.g. hold up some keys: 'What is this?' — patient does not answer. 'Is this a spoon?' — 'No'. 'Is it a pen?' — 'No'. 'Is it keys?' — 'Yes'). Despite this, comprehension and other aspects of speech production are relatively normal.

This is *nominal dysphasia* (uncommon in its pure form — usually part of a wider dysphasia). The underlying brain damage is believed to be in the most posterior part of the superior temporal gyrus and the adjacent inferior parietal lobule.

Case 32 | Myasthenia gravis

Frequency in survey: did not occur in the small initial survey of PACES station 3, CNS.

Predicted frequency from older, more extensive MRCP short case surveys: main focus of a short case in 0.9% of attempts at PACES station 3, CNS. Additional feature in a further 1%.

Record

There is *ptosis* (one or both sides) accentuated by upward gaze, *variable strabismus* (with *diplopia*) and when she tries to screw her eyes up tight, the eyelashes are not buried. The face shows a *lack of expression*, the mouth is slack and there is generalized *facial weakness*. The patient *snarls* when she tries to smile, she cannot whistle, and her *voice* is *weak* and *nasal* (if you ask the patient to count aloud, speech may become progressively less distinct and more nasal). There is *proximal muscle weakness*. Repetitive movements cause an increase in the muscle weakness (myasthenia = abnormal muscular fatiguability).

The diagnosis is myasthenia gravis. A tensilon (edrophonium) test will confirm it.

Male to female ratio is 1:2.

Other features of myasthenia gravis

Difficulty with swallowing, chewing and nasal regurgitation

Symptoms worsen as the day progresses

Tendon reflexes are normal or exaggerated (cf. Eaton–Lambert syndrome)

The *jaw-supporting sign*, if present, is pathognomonic — the patient puts her hand under her chin to support both the weak jaw and neck; may only become obvious after prolonged conversation

Antiacetylcholine receptor antibodies are present in 90%

In long-standing cases there may be an element of permanent irreversible myopathic change

Breathlessness is a sinister symptom requiring urgent attention (respiratory deterioration may develop rapidly and should be watched for by monitoring the FVC or peak flow rate)

Pathological changes are present in the thymus in 70–80% and some patients are improved by thymectomy; thymomata occur in 10% (mostly males) and give a worse prognosis.

Associated immune disorders include thyrotoxicosis (5% of patients), hypothyroidism, rheumatoid arthritis, diabetes mellitus, polymyositis, SLE, pernicious anaemia, Sjögren's syndrome, pemphigus and sarcoidosis.

Crisis

Signs of *cholinergic crisis* are collapse, confusion, abdominal pain and vomiting, sweating, salivation, lachrymation, miosis and pallor. The features which distinguish *myasthenic crisis* are response to edrophonium and absence of cholinergic phenomena. Occasionally it is exceptionally difficult to determine whether the collapsed myasthenic has been under- or overtreated. Temporary withdrawal of all drugs and assisted positive pressure respiration is then indicated.

Myasthenic crisis may be provoked by:

Infection

Emotional upset

Undue exertion*

Drugs (streptomycin, gentamicin, kanamycin, neomycin, viomycin, polymyxin, colistin, curare, quinine, quinidine, procainamide).

---

* Childbirth requires careful management.

Eaton–Lambert syndrome (myasthenic-myopathic syndrome) is often associated with oat-cell carcinoma of the bronchus. There is proximal muscle wasting, weakness and fatiguability. Often, however, power is initially increased by brief exercise (reversed myasthenic effect). The tendon reflexes are depressed (but increased soon after activity; this can be demonstrated dramatically by showing the depressed biceps reflex and then by repeating it after getting the patient to flex the forearm against resistance). The electromyographic response to ulnar nerve stimulation shows a characteristic increase in amplitude (it declines in myasthenia gravis). Cholinergic drugs have no effect.

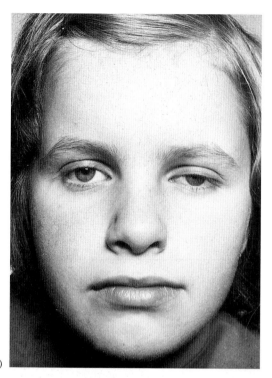

(a)

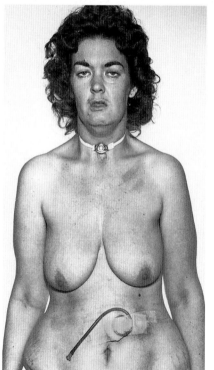

(b1)

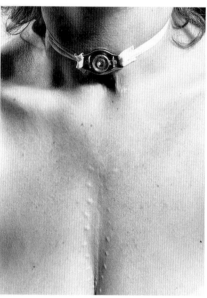

(b2)

Figure C3.19 (a) A mild case with unilateral ptosis. (b1,2) A severe case (note myasthenic facies, thymectomy scar, gastrostomy feeding tube and tracheostomy).

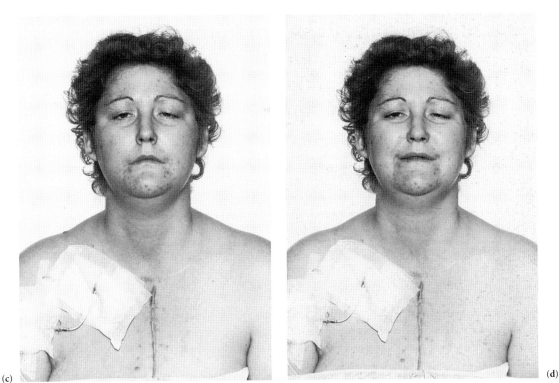

(c)

(d)

Figure C3.19 (*continued*) (c) Myasthenic facies (note the subclavian line which was being used for plasmapheresis). (d) 'Smile'.

Case 33 | Guillain–Barré syndrome (acute inflammatory demyelinating polyradiculopathy)

Frequency in survey: did not occur in the small initial survey of PACES station 3, CNS.

Predicted frequency from older, more extensive MRCP short case surveys: main focus of a short case in 0.9% of attempts at PACES station 3, CNS.

Record

This (most commonly) young adult has a predominantly *motor neuropathy*. The weakness is more marked distally* and there is generalized *hyporeflexia*. There is a lower motor neurone *facial weakness* (often bilateral) and evidence of bulbar palsy. There is (may be) mild impairment of distal position and vibration perception and slight loss of pinprick sensation over the toes.† The patient has a tachycardia.‡

These features suggest Guillain–Barré syndrome (acute inflammatory demyelinating polyradiculopathy — AIDP).

Features of AIDP

There is an antecedent upper respiratory tract infection or gastrointestinal illness (e.g. *Campylobacter jejuni*) within 1 month in 60%§ of cases.

There is a bimodal age distribution — main peak in young adults, lesser peak in 45–64-year age group.

Cerebrospinal fluid protein is usually normal during the first 3 days; it then steadily rises and may continue to rise even though recovery has begun; it may exceed $5\,g\,l^{-1}$.

A few mononuclear cells may be present in the CSF ($<10\,mm^{-3}$).

Mortality is 5%. The apparently mild case may worsen rapidly and unpredictably. *Vital capacity* (peak flow rate measurement on its own is insufficient), blood gases, blood pressure and ability to cough and swallow should be closely monitored; if mechanical ventilation is anticipated from the results then it should be instituted early, before decompensation.

---

* Though the weakness classically begins in the distal lower limbs and spreads upwards (*ascending paralysis*) it may be more marked proximally or uniform throughout the limbs.

† The mild case may just have slight foot-drop which never progresses, while the severe case may have quadraplegia and inability to breathe, speak, swallow or close the eyes. The facial involvement helps to distinguish AIDP from other neuropathies except for that related to sarcoidosis. Complaints of numbness and paraesthesiae are common but are usually mild and transient and objective sensory loss is slight.

‡ Autonomic involvement is common with a relative tachycardia almost always present; orthostatic hypotension and hypertension are frequent and difficult to treat. Pupillary disturbances, neu-roendocrine disturbance, peripheral pooling of blood, poor venous return and low cardiac output may all occur. *Sudden death* can occur following unexplained fluctuations in blood pressure or cardiac dysrhythmias. Pharmacological interventions to control blood pressure are risky and should be avoided unless absolutely necessary. Patients who are unable to swallow or gag are given nasogastric feeding and should be sitting when food is given and for 30–60 minutes thereafter to reduce the risk of aspiration.

§ Predisposing factors that have been implicated include infectious mononucleosis, viral hepatitis, Epstein–Barr virus, rabies, swine flu, HIV infection, surgery, pregnancy and malignancy (especially lymphoma).

Paralysis is maximum within 1 week in more than 50% of cases and by 1 month in 90%. Recovery usually begins 2–4 weeks later.* Rate of recovery is variable, occasionally rapid even after quadraplegia. Eighty-five per cent of patients are ambulatory within 6 months. Residual peripheral nervous system damage occurs in >50%.

Plasmapheresis in the first 2 weeks shortens the clinical course and reduces morbidity. *Intravenous immunoglobulin* in the first 2 weeks is an alternative therapy that has equivalent efficacy to plasmapheresis, and is now the treatment of choice.

Some patients present with rapid onset of symmetrical, multiple cranial nerve palsies, most notably bilateral facial palsy (polyneuritis cranialis). Occasionally, there may be a combination of an external ophthalmoplegia, ataxia and areflexia (*Miller–Fisher syndrome*) associated with high CSF protein and some motor weakness. Serum IgG antibodies to GQ1b ganglioside are found in acute phase sera of over 90% of Miller–Fisher syndrome patients. They disappear during recovery.

Most patients achieve good recovery from AIDP. The importance of fastidious supportive care during the acute stage cannot be overstressed.

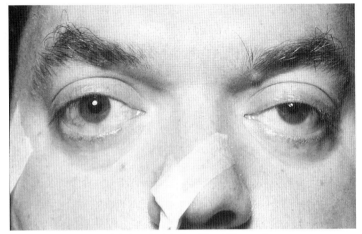

Figure C3.20 External ophthalmoplegia in the Miller–Fisher syndrome.

* Pathologically, inflammatory cell infiltration followed by segmental demyelination is the hallmark, especially in spinal roots, limb girdle plexuses and proximal nerve trunks. Axons are relatively spared and blood vessels are normal. Within 2–3 weeks of onset, Schwann cell proliferation occurs as a prelude to remyelination and recovery.

Case 34 | **Pseudobulbar palsy**

Frequency in survey: did not occur in the small initial survey of PACES station 3, CNS.

Predicted frequency from older, more extensive MRCP short case surveys: main focus of a short case in 0.8% of attempts at PACES station 3, CNS.

Record

There is monotonous, slurred, high-pitched 'Donald Duck' *dysarthria* and the patient *dribbles persistently* from the mouth (he has dysphagia and may have nasal regurgitation). He *cannot protrude his tongue* which lies on the floor of the mouth and is *small and tight. Palatal movement* is *absent*, the *jaw jerk* is *exaggerated* and he is *emotionally labile*.

The diagnosis is pseudobulbar palsy (?bilateral generalized spasticity and extensor plantar responses).

Commonest cause	**Other causes**
Bilateral cerebrovascular accidents of the internal capsule.	Multiple sclerosis
	Motor neurone disease
	High brainstem tumours
	Head injury.

Case 35 | Syringomyelia

Frequency in survey: did not occur in the small initial survey of PACES station 3, CNS.

Predicted frequency from older, more extensive MRCP short case surveys: main focus of a short case in 0.8% of attempts at PACES station 3, CNS.

Record

This patient (with *kyphoscoliosis*) shows *wasting* and weakness of the *small muscles* of the *hands* (sometimes there is curling of the fingers), flattening of the muscles of the ulnar border of the forearm and the upper limb *reflexes are absent* (conspicuous fasciculation is uncommon). There is *dissociated sensory loss** over (one or both of) the upper limbs and the upper chest† and there are *scars* (from painless burns and cuts) on the hands. The lower limb reflexes are exaggerated and the plantars are extensor. A *Horner's syndrome* is (may be) present (involvement of sympathetic neurones especially at C8/T1).

These findings suggest syringomyelia (?*nystagmus*, which may occur with lesions from C5 upwards—i.e. involving the medial longitudinal bundle—see Fig. C3.15, p. 231).

Syringobulbia. Syrinx may involve upper cervical and bulbar segments (usually an extension of syringomyelia but it may begin in the brainstem) and cause:
Nystagmus
Ataxia
Facial dissociated sensory loss (initially onion skin loss over the outer part of the face, from involvement of the lower part of the Vth nucleus in the cord, may occur before the syrinx reaches the medulla)
Bulbar palsy (wasted fasciculating tongue, palatal paralysis, nasal dysarthria, dysphasia, weakness of sternomastoids and trapezius from XIth nerve involvement, etc.—p. 238).

Trophic and vasomotor disturbances are common in syringomyelia, e.g.:
Areas of loss of, or excessive, sweating
La main succulente (ugly, cold, puffy, cyanosed hands with stumpy fingers and podgy soft palms)
Coarse, thickened skin over the hands with callosities over the knuckles and scars from old injuries
Slow healing and indolent ulceration of digits.

Charcot's joints may occur, usually at the elbow or shoulder. Tabes dorsalis (knees, hips) and diabetes mellitus (toes, ankles) are the other causes of Charcot's joints (see also p. 396).

Skeletal abnormalities which may be associated with syringomyelia
(Kypho)scoliosis (mild, very common)
Short neck (e.g. fusion of the cervical vertebrae; Klippel–Feil syndrome—p. 520)
Asymmetrical thorax
Sternal depression or prominence
Cervical ribs (may cause diagnostic difficulty).

---

* Analgesia and thermoanaesthesia, but light touch and proprioception intact. In the early stages cold stimuli may be perceived but not warm stimuli.
† Due to destruction by the syrinx of crossing axons carrying pain and temperature sensation. The area affected depends on the length of the syrinx—e.g. lower cervical and upper thoracic. Separate from this effect on crossing axons, the syrinx may also involve one or both spinothalamic tracts producing dissociated sensory loss in one or both lower limbs.

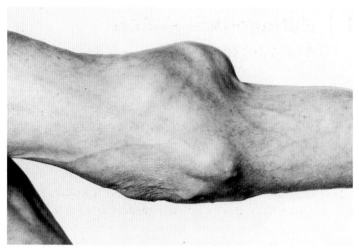

Figure C3.21 Charcot's joint at the elbow.

Case 36 | Holmes–Adie–Moore syndrome

Frequency in survey: did not occur in the small initial survey of PACES station 3, CNS.

Predicted frequency from older, more extensive MRCP short case surveys: main focus of a short case in 0.7% of attempts at PACES station 3, CNS.

Record
This young lady has a unilateral *dilated pupil* which *fails* (or almost fails) *to react to light.* There is no ptosis or diplopia and eye movements are otherwise normal (i.e. not IIIrd nerve palsy).

The patient has a myotonic pupil. Her tendon reflexes may be lost (check if allowed).

If exposed to light for prolonged periods the pupil may constrict slowly. If then exposed to darkness for a long period it will again dilate very slowly. During accommo- dation–convergence, after a delay, the abnormal pupil constricts slowly until it may become smaller than the normal pupil. The reaction to mydriatics is normal (Argyll Robertson pupil dilates poorly with mydriatics) and the pupil may be hyper-reactive to weak cholinergic substances, e.g. 0.1% pilocarpine.

The condition is usually chronic and symptomless but in some cases onset is acute with associated blurring of vision and photophobia. Syphilitic serology will be negative. Differential diagnosis from neurosyphilis may be difficult in the chronic stages of this disorder, when the pupil may be chronically constricted, and especially when both pupils are affected (bilateral involvement is rare with Holmes–Adie pupils but invariable with syphilitic Argyll Robertson pupils—p. 255).

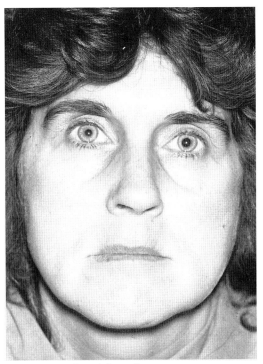

Figure C3.22 Holmes–Adie pupil.

Case 37 | Jugular foramen syndrome

Frequency in survey: did not occur in the small initial survey of PACES station 3, CNS.

Predicted frequency from older, more extensive MRCP short case surveys: main focus of a short case in 0.6% of attempts at PACES station 3, CNS.

Record

The patient has an *absent gag reflex* on the R/L side (and will have ipsilateral impaired taste over the posterior third of the tongue). *Palatal movements* on that side are *reduced* and the *uvula* is *drawn* to the *opposite side*. The R/L *sternomastoid* muscle is *wasted* and there is weakness in rotating the head to the opposite side. The *shoulder* is *flattened* and there is weakness of elevation of that shoulder.

There is therefore a lesion affecting the *IXth, Xth and XIth cranial nerves* on the R/L side.

This suggests a jugular foramen syndrome (to exclude a brainstem lesion* check carefully for evidence of ipsilateral wasting, fasciculation and deviation of the tongue — XIIth nerve, ipsilateral Horner's and, if allowed, for evidence of brainstem compression, e.g. spastic paraparesis).

An isolated lesion of the glossopharyngeal nerve is rare. It is usually damaged with the vagus and accessory nerves near the jugular foramen which all three nerves traverse (Fig. C3.23). A lesion inside the skull is more likely to cause a syndrome restricted to the IXth, Xth and XIth nerves only (syndrome of Vernet†). An internal lesion may cause brainstem compression.* A lesion outside the skull is more likely to involve the XIIth nerve as well (syndrome of Collet–Sicard†) — this nerve exits through the hypoglossal foramen near the external opening of the jugular foramen. An external lesion may also involve the cervical sympathetic* (syndrome of Villaret†). Other combinations of associated lower cranial lesions are vagus and accessory (syndrome of Schmidt†), and vagus, accessory and hypoglossal (syndrome of Hughlings Jackson†).

Causes of jugular foramen syndromes

Neurofibroma of IXth, Xth or XIIth nerves (especially left XIIth in young females)

Meningiomata

Epidermoid tumours (cholesteatomata)

Glomus or carotid body tumours

Metastases

Cerebellopontine angle lesions (p. 258—may also extend down and involve the last four cranial nerves in numerical order)

Infection from the middle ear spreading into the posterior fossa

Granulomatous meningitis.

---

* Intrinsic brainstem disease may cause lower cranial nerve palsies and Horner's syndrome (e.g. pp. 249 and 273), but when the pathology is in the brainstem there is nearly always spinothalamic sensory loss on the opposite side of the body to the lesion.

† Though the age of such neurological eponyms is undoubtedly passing, their usage may still impress!

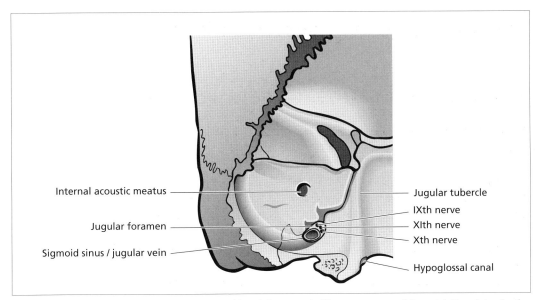

Internal acoustic meatus
Jugular foramen
Sigmoid sinus / jugular vein
Jugular tubercle
IXth nerve
XIth nerve
Xth nerve
Hypoglossal canal

Figure C3.23 The posterior aspect of the posterior cranial fossa (after removal of the squamous part of the occipital bone) showing the jugular foramen and the nerves passing through it (note the position of the hypoglossal canal which conducts the XIIth nerve).

Case 38 | Polymyositis

Frequency in survey: did not occur in the small initial survey of PACES station 3, CNS.

Predicted frequency from older, more extensive MRCP short case surveys: main focus of a short case in 0.5% of attempts at PACES station 3, CNS.

Record

There is *symmetrical,** *proximal* muscle *weakness* (the patient may be unable to sit up from lying or stand up from squatting position) with associated muscle *wasting*. The muscles are *tender* (in 50% of cases—suggesting an inflammatory myopathy). The patient is (may be) unable to flex his neck against resistance. The tendon reflexes are present though reduced.† There is (may be) dysphonia (and/or dysphagia) due to involvement of the bulbar muscles.

The diagnosis is polymyositis.

Male to female ratio is 1 : 2.

Features of polymyositis

A rash may occur (dermatomyositis—p. 288)

Features and associations similar to dermatomyositis (p. 288)

Association with malignancy‡

Onset of muscle weakness is usually insidious (with difficulty in running, climbing stairs, getting up from a chair, and combing hair)

Lower limb-girdle more often affected than shoulder-girdle

Ocular involvement is rare (if present, think of myasthenia gravis)

Respiratory muscle weakness can lead to respiratory failure—monitor peak flow rate and vital capacity

Cardiac muscle may be involved.

Other causes of proximal muscle weakness

(See also p. 222)

Carcinomatous neuromyopathy (including Eaton–Lambert syndrome—p. 242)

Diabetic amyotrophy (?fundi, peripheral neuropathy)

Muscular dystrophies (?long-standing, familial—p. 224)

Dystrophia myotonica (?frontal balding, cataracts, myotonia, etc.—p. 182)

Alcoholism

Thyrotoxicosis (?eye signs, hypermobile, goitre, etc.—p. 432)

Corticosteroid treatment (?cushingoid facies, underlying disorder, etc.—p. 441)

Familial periodic paralysis

Osteomalacia

Hyperparathyroidism

Insulinoma.

Polymyalgia rheumatica is characterized by pain and stiffness of proximal muscles, especially the shoulder-girdle, in a patient who is usually elderly. The ESR is high. Significant objective weakness is not common. There is a relationship with temporal (giant cell) arteritis (see also p. 222).

---

* In general, if muscle weakness is symmetrical it suggests myopathic disease, and if asymmetrical neurogenic disease.

† If very reduced or absent it suggests underlying carcinoma causing polyneuropathy and polymyositis.

‡ There is an increased risk of malignancy (lungs, breast, ovary, GI tract, nasopharynx, prostate, blood) in older patients with dermatomyositis; the risk is lower in polymyositis. Current wisdom is that a search for malignancy should be made in older patients (>40 years old) with dermatomyositis and polymyositis, and in those with atypical or intractable lesions. A reasonable approach in this direction would constitute a thorough clinical assessment, including a per rectum examination in males and pelvic examination in females, and some baseline investigations (full blood count, stool occult blood, chest X-ray, USS abdomen/pelvis, prostate specific antigen (PSA) and mammogram in women).

Case 39 | **Argyll Robertson pupils**

Frequency in survey: did not occur in the small initial survey of PACES station 3, CNS.

Predicted frequency from older, more extensive MRCP short case surveys: main focus of a short case in 0.4% of attempts at PACES station 3, CNS. Additional feature in occasional others.

Record

The pupils are *small* and *irregular* and react to *accommodation but not to light.**

The likely diagnosis is tabes dorsalis (?wrinkled forehead with ptosis, stamping ataxia, Romberg's test positive, loss of joint position and vibration sense, absent ankle jerks, Charcot's knee joint and aortic incompetence — see p.265).

The exact site of the lesion is not known. It is generally believed to be in the tectum of the midbrain proximal to the oculomotor nuclei. The classic Argyll Robertson pupil is very small. However, pupils affected by neurosyphilis are not always small and may even be dilated. They may be unequal in size. Though the signs may be more advanced in one eye than the other, pupillary abnormalities occurring in neurosyphilis are invariably bilateral. The characteristic features of Argyll Robertson pupils are that they are *irregular* (may be subtle and should be looked for with an ophthalmoscope), and that even though they may react to light this is always *less* than their reaction to accommodation. Argyll Robertson-like pupils occasionally occur in diabetes mellitus.

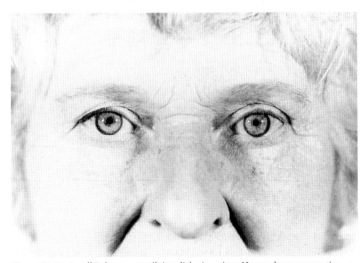

Figure C3.24 Argyll Roberston pupils in a diabetic patient. Her serology was negative.

* The light reflex may be present (before it becomes increasingly sluggish and then disappears), but the accommodation reflex is always *brisker* than the light.

Case 40 | **Congenital syphilis**

Frequency in survey: did not occur in the initial small survey of PACES station 3, CNS.

Predicted frequency from older, more extensive MRCP short case surveys: main focus of a short case in 0.4% of attempts at PACES station 3, CNS.

Record
There is flattening of the bridge of the nose (*saddle nose*), the superior maxilla is under-developed which makes the mandible appear prominent (*bull-dog jaw*), and there is frontal bossing. There are *rhagades* at the corners of the mouth and there are *Hutchinson's teeth* (widely spaced peg-shaped upper incisors with a crescentic notch at the cutting edge) and *Moon's molars* (dome-shaped deformity of the first lower molars with underdeveloped cusps). The tibiae have a wide middle third with palpable irregularities (due to osteoperiostitis) along the anterior skin (*sabre tibiae*).

The diagnosis is congenital syphilis.

Other manifestations of late congenital syphilis*
VIIIth nerve deafness

Clutton's joints (effusions into the knee joints with no pain or difficulty with joint movement)

Interstitial keratitis (acute attacks;† may eventually lead to corneal opacities—ground-glass appearance of cornea; a closer look shows the underlying radiating, brush-like vascularization referred to as *salmon-patch* appearance).

Old choroidoretinitis (peripheral and bilateral—'salt and pepper fundus')

Optic atrophy

Perforations of the palate or nasal septum

Collapse of the nasal cartilage.

---

* Early congenital syphilis in the first few months of life resembles severe secondary syphilis in the adult. Features include rhinitis, a mucocutaneous rash, osteochondritis, dactylitis, hepatosplenomegaly, lymphadenopathy, anaemia, jaundice, thrombocytopenia and leucocytosis. Nephrotic syndrome may occur.

† May be due to hypersensitivity. Corticosteroids may sometimes help.

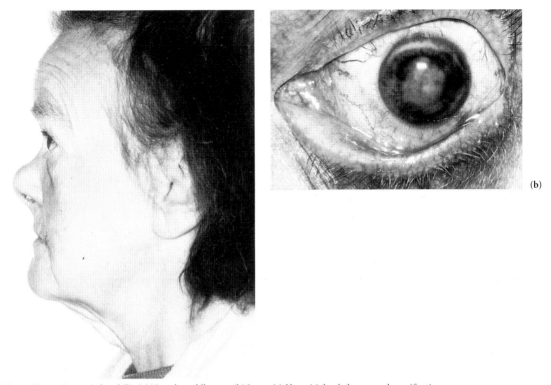

(a)

(b)

Figure C3.25 Congenital syphilis. (a) Note the saddle nose. (b) Interstitial keratitis has led to corneal opacification.

Case 41 | Cerebellopontine angle lesion

Frequency in survey: did not occur in the small initial survey of PACES station 3, CNS.

Predicted frequency from older, more extensive MRCP short case surveys: main focus of a short case in 0.4% of attempts at PACES station 3, CNS.

Record

On the R/L side there is evidence of *Vth* (may be absent corneal reflex only), *VIth* (p. 203) and *VIIth cranial nerve impairment* (both may be minimal), *perceptive deafness* (*VIIIth* nerve — the patient usually has tinnitus but may complain of vague unsteadiness or giddiness*) and *cerebellar* impairment (may be slightly impaired rapid alternate motion of the hands only). There is *nystagmus* (again may be just a few beats intermittently; it may be cerebellar and/or vestibular in origin).

These findings suggest a lesion at the cerebellopontine angle, *acoustic neuroma*† being the commonest cause (X-ray for evidence of expansion of the internal auditory meatus — not always seen†). Meningioma can give a similar picture (normal auditory meatus on X-ray).

The IXth and Xth cranial nerves may be involved and dysphagia and dysphonia may occur. In severe cases, with large tumours, there may be signs of raised intracranial pressure (?papilloedema) in addition to ipsilateral cerebellar involvement.

---

* Rotational vertigo in acoustic neuroma seldom occurs in the discrete attacks that are found in Menière's syndrome.

† Acoustic neuromata may cause symptoms even if extremely small, if confined within the acoustic canal. They are much commoner than all other cranial nerve tumours put together. MRI scans accurately detect even very small acoustic neuromata. Patients with hearing loss developing in middle age should be considered to have acoustic neuroma until proved otherwise. Audiometry is suggestive but not diagnostic. Caloric testing almost always shows abnormalities but the auditory evoked response is the most efficient physiological assessment. The CSF protein is elevated (may be $>3\,\mathrm{g\,l^{-1}}$) but cerebrospinal fluid assessment should not usually be necessary and might be dangerous.

Case 42 | Absent ankle jerks and extensor plantars

Frequency in survey: did not occur in the small initial survey of PACES station 3, CNS.

Predicted frequency from older, more extensive MRCP short case surveys: main focus of a short case in 0.4% of attempts at PACES station 3, CNS. Additional feature in a further 1%.

Record

The knee and *ankle jerks are absent* and the *plantar responses are extensor.*

Possible causes

1 Subacute combined degeneration of the cord (?posterior column signs, positive Romberg's sign, clinical anaemia, splenomegaly, etc.—p. 223)

2 Syphilitic taboparesis (?Argyll Robertson pupils, ptosis and wrinkled forehead, posterior column signs, positive Romberg's sign, etc.—p. 265)

3 Hereditary cerebellar ataxias, e.g. Friedreich's ataxia (?pes cavus, (kypho-)scoliosis, nystagmus, cerebellar ataxia, scanning speech, etc.—p. 220), spinocerebellar ataxia (ataxia, dysarthria, ophthalmoplegia, pyramidal and extrapyramidal signs, peripheral neuropathy, etc.)

4 Motor neurone disease (?fasciculation, absence of sensory signs, etc.—p. 190)

5 Common conditions in combination* (e.g. an elderly person with diabetes and cervical myelopathy—see experience 57, vol. 2, p. 332—or cervical and lumbar spondylosis causing a mixture of upper and lower motor neurone signs in the legs)

6 A lesion of the conus medullaris.

---

* Whilst the above order in which the possible causes are listed represents the traditional order in which the conditions are presented, in practice number 5 is by far the commonest.

Case 43 | Lateral popliteal (common peroneal) nerve palsy

Frequency in survey: did not occur in the small initial survey of PACES station 3, CNS.

Predicted frequency from older, more extensive MRCP short case surveys: main focus of a short case in 0.4% of attempts at PACES station 3, CNS.

Record

There is *wasting* of the *anterior tibial* and *peroneal* group of *muscles*, the patient *cannot dorsiflex* or *evert* the R/L foot,* and there is *impairment* of *sensation* over the *outer side* of the *calf*. He can stand on his toes but cannot stand on the R/L heel and the gait is altered as a result of *foot-drop* (there is an audible 'clop' of the foot as he walks). The ankle jerk is preserved.

The diagnosis is lateral popliteal (common peroneal) nerve palsy.

Injury to the nerve is usually at the head of the fibula where it can be involved in fractures or compressed by splints, tourniquets or bandages. Some individuals are particularly susceptible to temporary pressure palsy of this nerve (and in some cases other nerves such as the radial and ulnar as well), experiencing symptoms induced by crossing knees, squatting (strawberry picker's palsy) or unusual physical activity.

The nerve has two branches—the superficial and deep peroneal nerves. The superficial supplies sensation to the lateral calf and dorsum of the foot supplying the peroneus longus and brevis muscles. The deep branch supplies sensation to a triangular area of skin between the first and second toes dorsally and it innervates the anterior tibial muscles, the long extensors of the toes and the peroneus tertius muscle.

---

* Presentation of inversion of the ankle (tibialis posterior) distinguishes common peroneal nerve palsy from a L4/5 root lesion.

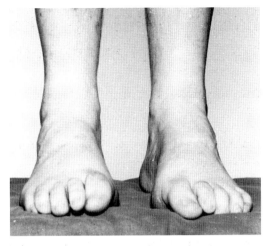

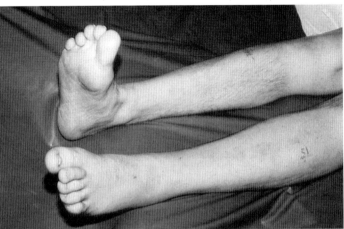

Figure C3.26 (a) Right common peroneal nerve palsy. Note failure of eversion. (b) Left common peroneal nerve palsy. Note failure of eversion and dorsiflexion on the left side.

Case 44 | **Ptosis**

Frequency in survey: did not occur in the small initial survey of PACES station 3, CNS.

Predicted frequency from older, more extensive MRCP short case surveys: main focus of a short case in 0.4% of attempts at PACES station 3, CNS. Additional feature in a further 4%.

Record 1

There is *unilateral* ptosis.*

Possible causes

1 Third nerve palsy (?dilated ipsilateral pupil, divergent strabismus, etc. — p. 203)
2 Horner's syndrome (?ipsilateral small pupil, etc. — p. 232)
3 Myasthenia gravis (may be the only sign of this condition; ?induced or worsened by upward gaze; variable strabismus, facial and proximal muscle weakness, weak nasal voice, all of which may worsen with repetition, etc. — p. 242)
4 Congenital/idiopathic† (may increase with age; there may be an associated superior rectus palsy)
5 Myotonic dystrophy (usually bilateral).

Record 2

There is *bilateral* ptosis.*

Possible causes

1 Myasthenia gravis
2 Myotonic dystrophy (?myopathic facies, frontal balding, wasting of facial muscles and sternomastoids, cataracts, myotonia, etc. — p. 182)
3 Tabes dorsalis (?Argyll Robertson pupils, etc. — p. 265)
4 Congenital† (may increase with age)
5 Bilateral Horner's (e.g. syringomyelia — ?wasting of small muscles of the hand, dissociated sensory loss, scars, extensor plantars, etc. — p. 249)
6 Chronic progressive external ophthalmoplegia‡ (CPEO) (?absence of soft tissue in the lids and periorbital region, ophthalmoplegia, mild facial and neck weakness). It is usually due to mitochondrial cytopathy, e.g. Kearns–Sayre syndrome (progressive ophthalmoplegia, retinopathy, cardiomyopathy and ataxia)
7 Oculopharangeal muscular dystrophy‡ (see p. 224).

---

* NB Overaction of frontalis with wrinkling of the forehead tends to be associated with ptosis due to non-myopathic conditions.
† There should be no response to a test dose of edrophonium before this diagnosis is accepted.
‡ Many of the ocular myopathies are associated with characteristic morphological features ('ragged red fibres') and mitochondrial myopathy and are now referred to as CPEO. The disorder lies in the cytochromes and the conditions are sometimes termed the mitochondrial cytopathies. Ocular myopathy and oculopharangeal muscular dystrophy may be manifestations of the same condition.

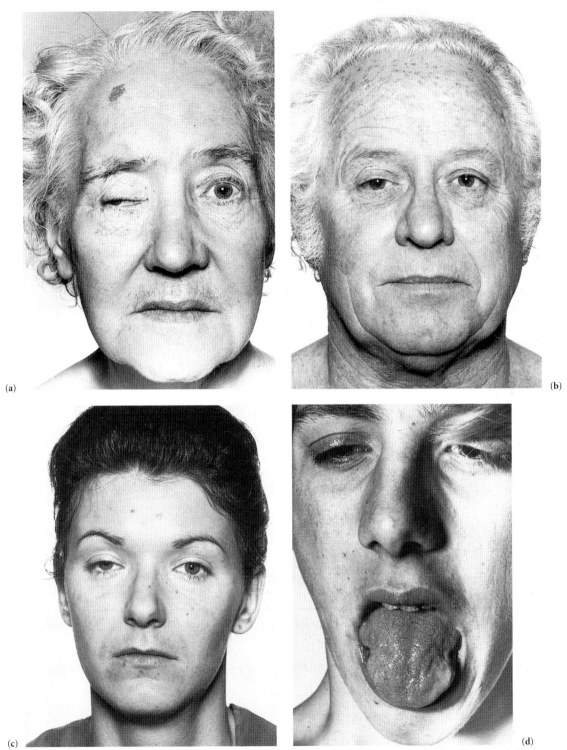

Figure C3.27 (a) Third nerve palsy: complete ptosis. (b) Right Horner's syndrome. (c) Myasthenia gravis: bilateral, asymmetrical ptosis. (d) Myotonic dystrophy: sustained contraction of the lingual muscles after percussion on the tongue plus bilateral ptosis.

Other causes of ptosis

Pseudoptosis (following recurrent inflammation or extreme thinning of lids after repeated angioneurotic oedema)

Voluntary ptosis (to suppress diplopia)

Apraxia of the eyelids (the patient may need to pull down the lower eyelids, tilt back the head or open the mouth to enable the eyes to be opened; there is usually evidence of basal ganglia involvement).

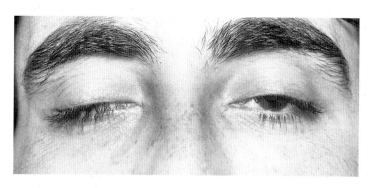

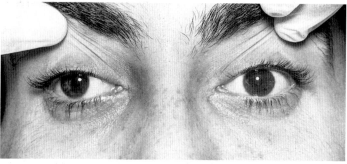

(e)

Figure C3.27 (*continued*) (e) Ocular myopathy.

Case 45 | Tabes

Frequency in survey: did not occur in the small initial survey of PACES station 3, CNS.

Predicted frequency from older, more extensive MRCP short case surveys: main focus of a short case in 0.3% of attempts at PACES station 3, CNS. Additional feature in a further 0.8%.

Record 1

There are (in this underweight patient who appears older than his years) *Argyll Robertson pupils* (see p. 255). There is bilateral *ptosis* with *wrinkling* of the *forehead* due to compensatory overaction of the frontalis, there is loss of *vibration* and *joint position* sense, loss of *deep pain* in the Achilles tendon, hypotonia, *absent reflexes* and plantar responses; the gait is ataxic and *Romberg's* test is *positive.*

The diagnosis is *tabes dorsalis.** The patient may have *optic atrophy* (may antedate other manifestations; centre of vision may be the last to be affected) and is at risk of developing a *Charcot's* neuropathic hip, knee or ankle joint.

Record 2

As appropriate from the above plus: the *plantars* are *extensor* (with or without other pyramidal signs and other signs of general paresis of the insane (GPI) — see below).

The diagnosis is *taboparesis.*

Other features of tabes dorsalis, though well known, are rarely seen now; features such as:

Wide-based, high, stepping gait

Zones of cutaneous analgesia with delayed perception of pain

Ligament laxity allowing extreme degrees of lower limb movement

Perforating foot ulcers

Lightening pains (a good reliable history is virtually pathognomonic and may antedate other symptoms)

Bladder insensitivity.

Other forms of neurosyphilis

GPI† (dementia which classically progresses to euphoria and delusions of grandeur though this is less common than simple dementia, epileptic fits, tremor of the hands, lips and tongue ('trombone' tremor — the tongue darts in and out of the mouth involuntarily), and spastic paraparesis of cortical origin)

Meningovascular syphilis‡ (may present in a wide variety of ways including: isolated cranial nerve palsies especially IIIrd and VIth, cerebral or spinal stroke, meningism, epilepsy. Rare syndromes include meningomyelitis, pachymeningitis, acute transverse myelitis, Erb's spastic paraplegia, and syphilitic amyotrophy which resembles motor neurone disease).

---

* Tabes dorsalis occurs 10–35 years after infection with syphilis and the prognosis is poor. There is atrophy of the posterior nerve root and (probably secondary) degeneration of the posterior columns (lumbosacral and lower thoracic worst affected).

† GPI occurs 10–15 years after infection and the prognosis is good if it is treated before the development of cortical atrophy (initially the patient may present simply with a change of temperament, slight pupillary abnormalities and brisk reflexes). There is meningeal thickening and degeneration of the cerebral cortex (especially frontal).

‡ Meningovascular syphilis (only 3% of syphilitic patients) occurs in the first 4 years after infection and shows a good response to treatment except where cerebral or spinal cord infarction has occurred. Fibrosed meninges may nip cranial nerves and endarteritis may produce areas of ischaemic necrosis.

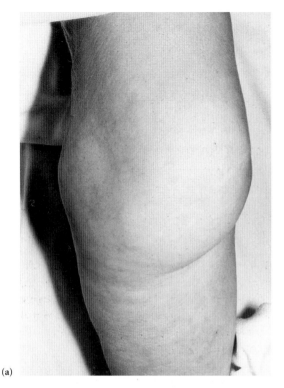

(a)

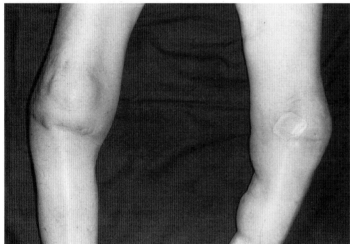

(b)

Figure C3.28 (a,b) Charcot's knee joints.

Case 46 | Subclavian-steal syndrome

Frequency in survey: did not occur in the small initial survey of PACES station 3, CNS.

Predicted frequency from older, more extensive MRCP short case surveys: main focus of a short case in 0.3% of attempts at PACES station 3, CNS.

Survey note: one candidate was told that the patient's arm got tired and that she felt faint whenever hanging out washing and he was asked what he would like to examine.

Record

The R/L arm (which gets easily tired on exercise) has a weaker pulse than the other side. The *tension* in the brachial artery (the ease with which the radial pulse can be obliterated by pressure in the brachial artery) is lower on the affected side and (ask to measure the blood pressure) the blood pressure is 100/70 compared with 140/80 in the normal side. There is a systolic bruit heard over the corresponding subclavian artery.

The features and the history suggest the subclavian-steal syndrome.

This rare syndrome occurs when there is stenosis of the subclavian artery near its origin, leading to a retrograde flow of blood down the ipsilateral vertebral artery, in order to supply the upper limb — subclavian steal. There is relative ischaemia of the arm during exercise. Symptoms are of cerebral ischaemia usually of vertebrobasilar insufficiency, e.g. vertigo, transient bilateral blindness, syncope, olfactory hallucination, diplopia and bilateral blurring of vision. Any combination of these symptoms may occur either spontaneously or after exercise in the affected arm. There may be features of vascular insufficiency elsewhere (e.g. legs, heart, etc.).

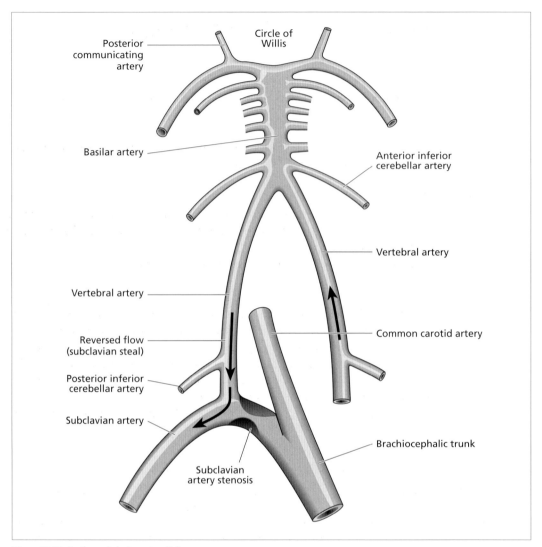

Figure C3.29 Basilar–subclavian artery link.

Case 47 | Infantile hemiplegia

Frequency in survey: did not occur in the small initial survey of PACES station 3, CNS.

Predicted frequency from older, more extensive MRCP short case surveys: main focus of a short case in 0.3% of attempts at PACES station 3, CNS.

Record 1

The R/L leg (in this patient with normal intelligence, normal speech and no history of epilepsy) is slightly *shorter* and thinner than the L/R, its *reflexes* are *brisk* and the R/L *plantar* response is *extensor*.

These features suggest mild infantile hemiplegia affecting the R/L leg.

Record 2

There is (in this patient with epilepsy and mental retardation) marked *hypoplasia* of the R/L arm and leg, with *spasticity* and *contractures*, R/L *homonymous hemianopia* and R/L *ankle clonus* and *extensor plantar* response. There is *asymmetry of the trunk*, smaller on the R/L and diffuse impairment of sensation on the R/L. There is asymmetry of the skull, smaller on the L/R (the other side to the hemiplegia), *jaw clonus* and *spastic dysarthria* (there may be a squint, e.g. convergent on the L/R).

These features suggest severe infantile hemiplegia with spasticity affecting the R/L side.

Infantile hemiplegia results from a lesion which develops during the first year of life; only rarely is it from prenatal lesions or birth trauma. The hemiplegia may occur as a complication of an infective disorder such as pertussis, measles or scarlet fever; more commonly, however, there is no obvious predisposing cause and the hemiplegia is probably a manifestation of an encephalitis or toxic encephalopathy. There is an arrest of growth on the affected side and the hemiplegic limbs may be the site of spontaneous involuntary movements of either a choreic or athetoid character. Epilepsy is common with convulsions beginning on the affected side. The extent and severity of the hemiplegia and the degree of cerebral retardation depend on the extent of the original involvement of the cerebral cortex. In some cases the abnormality may be very slight—a smallness of a hand or foot, a thinness of a forearm or calf, a clumsiness of the fingers or contracture of the Achilles tendon. There may be just an imperceptible degree of general body asymmetry. Focal convulsions in an otherwise healthy child or adolescent should always raise the possibility of a minimal infantile hemiplegia. Only by careful scrutiny of the undressed patient as a whole will such slight asymmetry be detected.

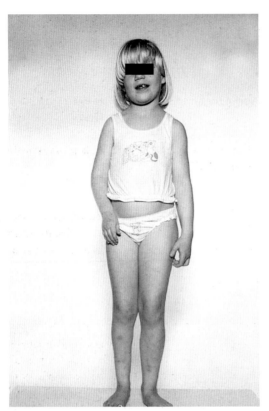

Figure C3.30 Infantile hemiplegia. The right arm and leg are smaller then the left. The features continue into adulthood and the patient may then appear in the MRCP PACES exam.

Case 48 | Thalamic syndrome

Frequency in survey: did not occur in the small initial survey of PACES station 3, CNS.

Predicted frequency from older, more extensive MRCP short case surveys: main focus of a short case in 0.3% of attempts at PACES station 3, CNS.

Record

The patient (who complains of *pain down one side of the body and head*) has (may have) a *hemiplegia* on the R/L side (the side of the pain), and on that side says that the *touch sensation is different* compared to the other side. Pinprick sensation was perceived as increased pain on the R/L.

These features suggest a thalamic syndrome.

Proximal occlusion of the posterior cerebral artery causes ischaemia of the penetrating branches to the thalamic and limbic structures.

Damage to the ventral posterolateral nucleus of the thalamus causes decreased sensation of all modalities on the contralateral side of the body and face. The sensory loss is often accompanied by dysaesthesiae. A thalamic syndrome often appears within weeks or months of the acute thalamic damage and has been attributed to denervation hypersensitivity of sensory neurones in the midbrain reticular formation. The patient develops spontaneous pain in the distribution of the sensory loss. The quality of the pain is difficult to define. It is often ex-acerbated by anxiety and tends to be rather diffuse but is most marked in one limb and rarely involves the face alone. The quality of sensation on the affected side is usually distorted with diminution to all modalities and hypoalgesia. Nevertheless stimuli exceeding the sensory threshold may produce an intense exacerbation of the background spontaneous pain. Occasionally there is frank hyperalgesia. With involvement of the subthalamic nucleus, hemiballismus (wild, uncontrolled, flailing limb movements) may develop. The thalamic syndrome is rare but causes a particularly unpleasant pain intractable to most therapeutic manoeuvres.

Case 49 | Radial nerve palsy

Frequency in survey: did not occur in PACES station 3, CNS. However, it does seem to have occurred in PACES station 5, locomotor (see experience 1, vol. 2, p. 282).

Record

There is *wrist-drop* and sensory loss over the first dorsal interosseous.*

The diagnosis is radial nerve palsy.

The hand hangs limply and the patient is unable to lift it at the wrist or to straighten out the fingers. If the wrist is passively extended he is able to straighten the fingers at the interphalangeal joints (because the interossei and lumbricals still work) but not at the MCP joints where the fingers remain flexed. The patient may feel that his grasp is weak in the affected hand because of lack of the wrist extension necessary for powerful grip. If the wrist is passively extended the power of grip improves. Abduction and adduction of the fingers may appear weak in radial nerve palsy unless they are tested with the hand resting flat on the table with the fingers extended.

The commonest cause (of this rare condition) is 'Saturday night paralysis' in which the patient, heavily sedated with alcohol, falls asleep with his arm hanging over the back of a chair. The nerve is compressed against the middle third of the humerus, and brachioradialis (flexion of the arm against resistance—with the arm midway between supination and pronation) and supinator are also paralysed as well as the forearm extensor muscles. Muscle wasting does not usually occur and complete recovery in a matter of weeks† is usual. If the nerve is injured by a wound in the axilla, paralysis involves the triceps so that extension at the elbow is lost as is the triceps reflex.

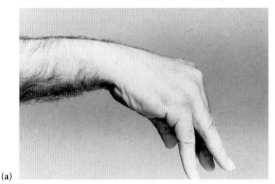

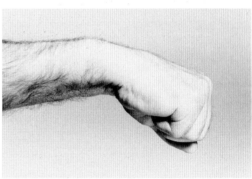

(a)   (b)

Figure C3.31 (a) Wrist-drop. (b) Weak grip due to the missing synergistic effect of an extended wrist.

---

* Though the cutaneous area supplied by the radial nerve is more extensive than this (Fig. B.4, p. 51) an overlap in supply by both the median and ulnar nerves usually means that only this small area over the first dorsal interosseous has detectable impaired sensation. If there is *no* sensory loss whatsoever, in a patient with symptoms of progressive radial nerve palsy, then a lesion of the posterior interosseous nerve (the main, purely motor, branch of the radial nerve) may be suspected and surgical exploration considered.

† Usually damage occurs to the myelin sheath only and the Schwann cells will repair the nerve rapidly. If the pressure is prolonged and causes axonal degeneration then the peripheral nerve regeneration rate is about 1 mm day^{-1} (from the undamaged proximal nerve).

Case 50 | Lateral medullary syndrome (Wallenberg's syndrome)

Frequency in survey: did not occur in any of the MRCP surveys.*

Record

(Assumes a lesion affecting the artery on the right.) On the right of the patient (who presented with acute vertigo†) there is (*ipsilateral*):

Horner's syndrome (descending sympathetic tract)

Cerebellar signs (cerebellum and its connections)

Palatal paralysis and diminished gag reflex (may be dysphagia and hoarseness due to a vocal cord paralysis—IXth and Xth nerves)

Decreased *trigeminal* pain and temperature sensation (descending tract and nucleus of the Vth nerve).

On the left of the patient the trunk and limbs (and sometimes the face) show (*contralateral*) decreased *pain and temperature* sensation‡ (spinothalamic tract).

The patient has a lateral medullary syndrome (produced by infarction of a small wedge of lateral medulla posterior to the inferior olivary nucleus—Fig. C3.32) classically due to a lesion of the right *posterior inferior cerebellar artery*.§

Involvement of the nucleus and tractus solitarius may cause loss of taste. Hiccup may occur. When occlusion of the posterior inferior cerebellar artery is isolated the pyramidal pathways escape and there is no hemiplegia. In the majority of cases of lateral medullary syndrome there is also an occlusion of the vertebral artery and pyramidal signs are present. Rarely, occlusion of the lower basilar artery, vertebral artery, or one of its medial branches produces the *medial medullary syndrome* (contralateral hemiplegia which spares the face, contralateral loss of vibration and joint position sense, and ipsilateral paralysis and wasting of the tongue).

Other eponymous brainstem infarction syndromes

Weber's syndrome (*midbrain*; ipsilateral IIIrd nerve palsy and contralateral hemiparesis)

Nothnagel's syndrome (*midbrain*; ipsilateral IIIrd nerve palsy and cerebellar ataxia)

Millard–Gubler syndrome (*pons*; ipsilateral VIth nerve palsy and facial weakness with contralateral hemiplegia)

Foville's syndrome (*pons*; as Millard–Gubler but with lateral conjugate gaze palsy).

These and a number of other eponymous brainstem syndromes (e.g. Claude, Benedict, Raymond–Cestau) were, in their classic descriptions, mostly related to tumours and other non-vascular diseases. The diagnosis of brainstem vascular disorders is facilitated more by knowledge of the neuroanatomy of the brainstem than of these

---

* It did not occur in our surveys but it has occurred in the exam. One candidate contacted us: 'Just my luck!—one of my short cases was lateral medullary syndrome: it was your penultimate short case (in the first edition of your book) and as, according to your book, it had not occurred in the exam, it was the only short case in your book I did not study!'

† Vestibular involvement may produce nystagmus, diplopia, oscillopsia, vertigo, nausea and vomiting.

‡ Involvement of the cuneate and gracile nuclei may cause numbness of the ipsilateral (right in this case) arm.

§ Occlusion of any one of five vessels may be responsible—vertebral, posterior inferior cerebellar, superior, middle or inferior lateral medullary arteries. The resulting clinical picture is variable and the rehabilitating patient may not show all features.

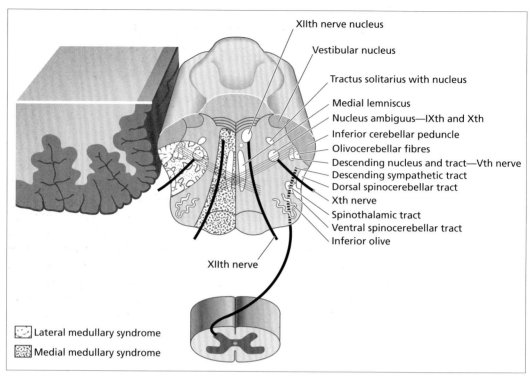

Figure C3.32 A cross-section through the medulla at the level of the inferior olivary nucleus showing the area infarcted in the lateral and medial medullary syndromes, respectively (adapted from Mohr J P *et al.* in *Harrison's Principles of Internal Medicine*, 1983, 10th edn, p. 2037, by kind permission of McGraw-Hill).

eponyms. In one analysis of 50 patients (Cornell–Bellevue series) with brainstem infarction, only two fitted into these syndromes as originally described. The rest had an extensive mixture of signs and symptoms indicating an overlap in the areas believed to be infarcted by occlusions in specific arteries.

Case 51 | **Psychogenic/factitious**

Psychogenic and factitious illnesses occur in everyday clinical practice and it would seem from the following anecdotes and the one on p. 380, from our pre PACES surveys, that it is possible that they have also occasionally appeared in the Membership!

Anecdote 1

A candidate was asked to examine a female patient's right hand neurologically. He found normal tone but decreased power in all groups of muscles in the wrist and hand. He said there was some wasting but the examiners disputed this. The candidate thought he had better not retract, even though he felt they were probably right so he said that he thought there was some. The examiners said, 'OK'. The candidate then asked for a pin, but at that moment the bell went. The examiners told him to ask about sensory loss. The patient pointed to various places in a pattern that did not suggest organic pathology saying, 'Here, here, here . . .'. The examiner said, 'You're having difficulty, aren't you?' The candidate responded in the affirmative, trying to offer some possible explanations, but the examiners moved away chuckling to themselves. The candidate (who passed) reports 'It obviously was psychogenic!'

Anecdote 2

A candidate reports that he was taken to see a gentleman who was lying on a couch smoking and was told that he complained of being numb down one side. He felt that 'this seemed most bizarre from the start'. He was asked to examine sensation and started with light touch; this seemed to show that the patient had a sharply demarcated hemianaesthesia. Pain and joint position sensation were similar. As the bell went he was asked what he thought could cause this. He initially mumbled something about 'vascular', but then said he thought it was 'factitious'. He reports 'I'm still not sure whether my findings were correct or what the true diagnosis was' (he did not pass until his next attempt).

As stated by Anderson and Trethowan,* hysterical behaviour or symptoms have a place in a spectrum at one end of which motivation, due to extreme capacity for the denial of inconvenient reality, is almost if not entirely hidden from the patient. This probably applies to no more than a tiny minority of patients. At the other end of the spectrum, and once again a minority, motivation is clear and purposive, amounting no more or less, to simulation.† The great bulk of hysterical disorders show various

shades of 'awareness' in between. Thus there is no 'either/or'—it is a question of how much of each. The capacity for self-deception and denial is a common human attribute which varies greatly between individuals. In deceiving himself the hysteric supposes he can deceive others. In some this belief is justified so that even the most experienced psychiatrist or clinician may err at times. The manifestations of hysteria are legion. The symptoms can be divided into:

* Anderson EW, Trethowan WH (1973) *Psychiatry*, 3rd edn. Baillière Tindall, London.
† Frank malingering with a motive such as avoiding work that is disliked. It might be thought that compensation neurosis would fall at the frank malingering end of the spectrum. It is believed,

however, that the power of human self-deception is far too strong to make this necessary. Patients suffer from complaints that they hope will bring compensation and at the same time retain their self-respect by believing in them themselves.

Physical symptoms

Pseudoneurological (including paralyses, contractures, anaesthesiae not corresponding to the sensory distribution of a nerve, hemianaethesia of the whole side of the body,* hysterical gaits,† tremors, fits, aphonia, hysterical deafness, tubular vision and many more)

Cardiovascular (pseudoanginal crises)

Respiratory (simulated asthma, hyperventilation until tetany occurs)

Gastrointestinal (globus hystericus, abdominal proptosis from downward pressure of the diaphragm and a lordotic posture, hysterical vomiting)

Gynaecological (exaggerated dysmenorrhoea; some female hysterical patients are sexually frigid and some may suffer from dyspareunia or from vaginismus).

Mental symptoms

Somnambulism (sleep walking)

Hysterical fugue

Hysterical amnesia

Pseudodementia (simulated dementia in a characteristic way — e.g. $2 + 2 = 5$, date before or after the actual one, elementary knowledge denied or given in a childishly perverted way)

Ganser's syndrome (disturbances of consciousness, hallucinations, somatic conversion symptoms, and a tendency to give approximate answers — as in pseudodementia; usually occurs in those in some kind of trouble — e.g. remand prisoners; it represents an attempt to escape from an intolerable situation)

Puerilism (patient regresses to childish level in an attempt to escape from a difficult situation, for manipulative purposes or as a form of attention seeking)

Twilight states (dream-like state of consciousness, visual pseudohallucinations, re-enactment of emotionally charged episodes; hysterical stupor, hysterical trance states; multiple personality — patient becomes at times 'a different person' claiming no knowledge of the other 'self').

Behavioural symptoms

Repeated spurious suicidal attempts (not intended to succeed; attempt to gain attention; may succeed by accident and must therefore be taken seriously)

Dermatitis artefacta‡ (self-inflicted lesions varying from redness to ulceration; absence of complete resemblance to any other disorder; lesions have an artificial and curiously bizarre appearance, possessing angles and edges not associated with lesions of any other disorder; severity depends on the agent used — e.g. carbolic acid, alkalis, cigarettes, matches, sandpaper — they may be ingeniously hidden — severe burns, deep scars and ragged ulcers may be seen; hospitalization may be required to definitely discover the diagnosis and cause)

Thermometer manipulation (spurious impression of fever)

Pseudohaemoptysis or pseudohaematemesis (extraction of blood from lips, gums or pharynx)

Swallowing objects (e.g. buttons, safety pins, even cutlery).

Munchausen's syndrome

First described and named by Richard Asher (as in Appendix 5, p. 545) in 1951. Patients travel from hospital to hospital telling dramatic but untruthful stories, simulating acute illnesses and submitting to countless unnecessary operations and investigations. A few days after admission they discharge themselves and resume their travels. Common varieties include laparotomophilia migrans (acute abdominal crises), neurologica diabolica (fits, blackouts, disturbances of consciousness, etc.) and haemorrhagica histrionica (haematemesis, etc.).

---

* Usually the left side; sometimes incongruously differential to different sensations, e.g. feel cold but not warm items.

† May mimic hemiparetic (usually an atypical dragging behind of the affected leg during a series of hops or supported steps), steppage or ataxic gait disorders. The diagnosis is obvious when the patient walks in a lurching, irregularly based, sometimes bent-forward manner, grasping anything in reach for support and reeling from side to side inconsistently. He may sink to the floor but does not usually endure a self-injuring fall.

‡ As with the other conditions mentioned, dermatitis artefacta is usually a manifestation of hysteria, with the usual minorities of cases at either end of the spectrum — at the one end the patient who not only denies knowing how the lesions developed but also may not in fact know their cause; and at the other end the frank malingerer. It should be remembered also that patients with psychotic illnesses may mutilate themselves without any obvious motive.

Case 52 | Normal central nervous system

Frequency in survey: did not occur in the initial small survey of PACES station 3, CNS.

The College has made it clear that 'normal' is an option in stations 1, 3 and 5 of PACES. Because of the change in the structure of the exam compared to the old short cases format, it is likely to occur more frequently than it did before. This is because in order for PACES to proceed there must be a neurological case in station 1, central nervous system. If, at the last minute, neither of the scheduled neuro cases turn up on the day; or if in the middle of a carousel the only one who did turn up decides not to continue or is too ill to continue, a substitute case has to be found at short notice. In the old, pre-PACES, days the exam would have proceeded without a neuro case whilst the wards were searched and one was found. In the case of PACES, if there is not time for this, one option is to proceed with a patient without any abnormality and make up an appropriate scenario. One simply has to imagine oneself as the invigilating registrar to think what that might be. One would first look amongst any surplus cases in the other stations for a volunteer or one might ask a member of the nursing, portering or other support staff and come up with a scenario such as:

'This . . . -year-old patient had a transient episode of weakness of the right leg. Please examine the legs neurologically . . .'.

There may thus be a clue in the case scenario and the fact that the scenario has been hurriedly hand-scribbled.

From the pre PACES surveys it was clear that the commonest reason for finding no abnormality is missing the physical signs that are present (probably the anecdote on p. 177, possibly anecdote 2, p. 135; see also experience 49, vol. 2, p. 331). Other reasons for cases of 'normal' will be either because the physical signs are no longer present by the time the patient comes to the examination (see anecdote below), or that the examiners and candidate disagree with the selectors of the cases about the presence of physical signs (may have happened in the anecdote on p. 508; see also experience 87b (p. 335) and anecdote 55 (p. 367), vol. 2). The following anecdote is from the original, pre PACES, surveys.

Anecdote

A candidate was asked to examine a patient's eye movements. He found no abnormality and said so. He reports that the examiners confirmed this and he passed. Apparently the patient had been included in the examination because she had had internuclear ophthalmoplegia, but this was no longer present at the time of this examination.

Station 5
Skin

1 Systemic sclerosis/CRST syndrome	**27** Vasculitis	
2 Neurofibromatosis (von Recklinghausen's disease)	**28** Ehlers–Danlos syndrome	
3 Osler–Weber–Rendu syndrome	**29** Livedo reticularis	
4 Psoriasis	**30** Pemphigus/pemphigoid	

1 Systemic sclerosis/CRST syndrome
2 Neurofibromatosis (von Recklinghausen's disease)
3 Osler–Weber–Rendu syndrome
4 Psoriasis
5 Rash of uncertain cause
6 Dermatomyositis
7 Xanthomata
8 Vitiligo
9 Tuberous sclerosis/adenoma sebaceum
10 Pseudoxanthoma elasticum
11 Lichen planus
12 Yellow nail syndrome
13 Gouty tophi
14 Alopecia
15 Eczema
16 Pretibial myxoedema
17 Clubbing
18 Necrobiosis lipoidica diabeticorum
19 Lupus pernio
20 Tinea
21 Koilonychia
22 Raynaud's phenomenon
23 Erythema nodosum
24 Sturge–Weber syndrome
25 Purpura
26 Peutz–Jeghers syndrome

27 Vasculitis
28 Ehlers–Danlos syndrome
29 Livedo reticularis
30 Pemphigus/pemphigoid
31 Radiation burn on the chest
32 Herpes zoster
33 Henoch–Schönlein purpura
34 Mycosis fungoides
35 Morphoea
36 Kaposi's sarcoma (AIDS)
37 Porphyria
38 Lupus vulgaris
39 Dermatitis herpetiformis
40 Urticaria pigmentosa (mastocytosis)
41 Tylosis
42 Secondary syphilis
43 Ectodermal dysplasia
44 Partial lipodystrophy
45 Fabry's disease
46 Reiter's syndrome/keratoderma blenorrhagica
47 Malignant melanoma
48 Acanthosis nigricans
49 Keratoacanthoma
50 Pyoderma gangrenosum
51 Psychogenic/factitious

Case 1 | Systemic sclerosis/CRST syndrome

Frequency in survey: main focus of a short case in 15% of attempts at PACES station 5, skin. Additional feature in a further 1%.

Survey note: also one case of mixed connective tissue disease.

Systemic sclerosis/CRST syndrome is dealt with on p. 393

Case 2 | Neurofibromatosis (von Recklinghausen's disease)

Frequency in survey: main focus of a short case in 13% of attempts at PACES station 5, skin. Additional feature in a further 4%.

Survey note: occurred as either a spot diagnosis, with or without a mention of the associated features, or as a case with an associated nerve pressure effect (such as one with an ulnar nerve/T1 lesion).

Record

There are multiple *neurofibromata* and *café-au-lait spots* (normal person allowed up to five of the latter).

The diagnosis is neurofibromatosis.*

or

There are multiple skin lesions: *sessile* and *pedunculated* cutaneous *fibromata*, as well as neurofibromata which are both *soft* and *firm*, *single* and *lobulated*, and felt both as mobile subcutaneous lumps† and *nodules* along the course of peripheral nerves. There are *café-au-lait* spots (especially in the axillae —axillary freckling occurs in two-thirds of affected individuals).

The diagnosis is neurofibromatosis.*

Autosomal dominant.

The condition is usually asymptomatic.

Complications

Kyphoscoliosis

Pressure effects of the neurofibromata on peripheral nerves and cranial nerves, especially:

(a) acoustic neuroma (?Vth, VIth, VIIth, VIIIth nerve lesions, nystagmus and cerebellar signs; may be bilateral—p. 258)*

(b) Vth nerve neuroma

Spinal nerve root involvement which may cause:

(a) cord compression

(b) muscle wasting

(c) sensory loss (Charcot's joints may occur)

Sarcomatous or other malignant change (5–16%)

Lung cysts (honeycomb lung)

Pseudoarthrosis and other orthopaedic abnormalities

Plexiform neuroma.‡

Other intracranial tumours which can occur

in this condition are:

Gliomata (optic nerve and chiasma; cerebral)

Meningiomata*

Medulloblastomata.

---

* The phakomatoses or neurocutaneous syndromes are characterized by disordered growth of neurocutaneous tissues. More than 20 syndromes have been described the most important of which are *neurofibromatosis 1 (von Recklinghausen's*—chromosome 17), neurofibromatosis 2 (chromosome 22), tuberous sclerosis (p. 297) and Sturge–Weber disease (p. 326). *Neurofibromatosis 2*, often called *central neurofibromatosis*, is rare and characterized by bilateral acoustic neuromata and often other intracranial tumours such as meningiomata or ependymomata. A few *café-au-lait* spots are present in about 40% of cases. At-risk family members should be screened regularly with hearing tests, etc.

† Neurofibromatosis should not be confused with lipomatosis with its characteristic soft subcutaneous lumps. In Dercum's disease (usually middle-aged females) subcutaneous lipomata may be painful and associated with marked obesity. These are easily recognized because, unlike neurofibromata, they are subcutaneous, soft, rounded or lobulated nodules that are moveable against the overlying skin.

‡ An entire nerve trunk and all its branches are involved in diffuse neurofibromatosis with associated overgrowth of overlying tissues leading to gross deformities (temporal and frontal scalp are favourite sites but it may occur anywhere); may grow to lemon or even melon size.

Other features of neurofibromatosis

An association with phaeochromocytoma — 5% of cases (?blood pressure)

Nodules of the iris — these are small, circular, pigmented hamartomata of the iris (Lisch nodules)

Hamartomata of the retina

Rib notching

Mental deficiency

Epilepsy

Renal artery stenosis.

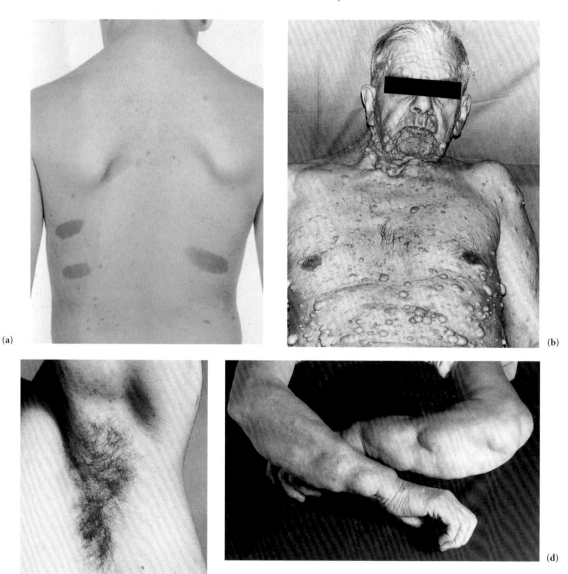

(a)

(b)

(c)

(d)

Figure C5.1 (a) *Café-au-lait* spots: multiple small and three large (>1 cm) dark macules with well-demarcated margins. (b) Myriads of skin-coloured and darkish neurofibromata. (c) Axillary freckling. (d) Lipomatosis: multiple, soft, easily moveable, subcutaneous nodules.

Case 3 | **Osler–Weber–Rendu syndrome**

Frequency in survey: main focus of a short case in 11% of attempts at PACES station 5, skin.

Record

There is *telangiectasia* on the face, around the *mouth*, on the lips, on the *tongue* (look under the tongue), the buccal and nasal mucosa and on the fingers, of this (?clinically anaemic) patient (who has none of the features of systemic sclerosis—p. 393).

The diagnosis is Osler–Weber–Rendu syndrome (hereditary haemorrhagic telangiectasia). The lesions may occur elsewhere, especially in the gastrointestinal tract, and may bleed. Patients may present with *epistaxis* (the most common and sometimes the only site of bleeding), *gastrointestinal haemorrhage*, chronic iron deficiency *anaemia* and occasionally with haemorrhage elsewhere (e.g. haemoptysis).

Usually considered to be autosomal dominant. In fact it is a family of disorders caused by mutations in various genes.

The telangiectasis consists of a localized collection of non-contractile capillaries and shows a prolonged bleeding time if punctured. The disease is frequently heralded by recurrent epistaxis in early childhood. In some cases, it presents as anaemia due to chronic blood loss from GI telangiectasia. In some variants (the pattern in individual families tends to be constant) pulmonary arteriovenous aneurysms are common and increase in frequency (as do the telangiectases) with advancing age. These cases may have *cyanosis* and *clubbing,* and *bruits* over the lung fields. The neurological complications include haemorrhage and the formation of bland or mycotic aneurysms. In the eye there may be bloody tears (conjunctival telangiectasia); retinal haemorrhage or detachment may occur. Cirrhosis* (due to telangiectasia or multiple transfusions) and massive intrahepatic shunting may occur.

Treatment

Chronic oral iron therapy may be required. Oestrogens (inducing squamous metaplasia of the nasal mucosa) may be helpful if epistaxis is the main symptom. Also for epistaxis, a low dose of the antifibrinolytic agent, aminocaproic acid, may be successful but should not yet be considered the standard approach. Individual lesions should not be cauterized. Pulse dye laser may be used to destroy cutaneous and accessible mucosal lesions.

---

* See experience 23, vol. 2, p. 313.

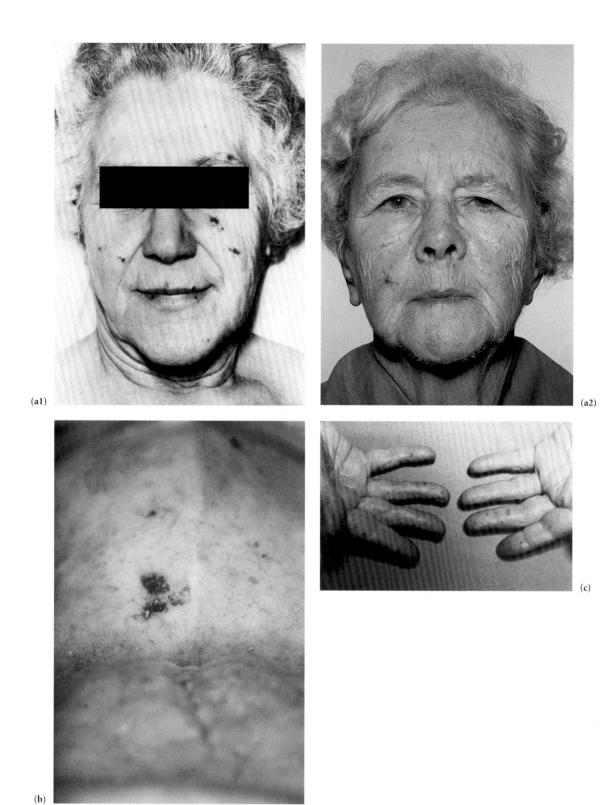

(a1)

(a2)

(b)

(c)

Figure C5.2 (a,b) Note palatal telangiectasia in (b). (c) Multiple, 1–2 mm, discrete, red macular and papular telangiectasiae on the fingers.

Case 4 | **Psoriasis**

Frequency in survey: main focus of a short case in 11% of attempts at PACES station 5, skin. Additional feature in a further 1%.

Record

There are patches of psoriasis over the *bony prominences*, particularly the *elbows* and *knees*, and also on the *trunk* and *scalp* and in the *intragluteal cleft* (the latter two areas are frequently overlooked). The plaques are circular with well-defined edges and they are *red* with a *silvery scaly* surface.

The patient has psoriasis.

I note also that there is an *asymmetrical arthropathy* involving mainly the *terminal interphalangeal joints*. There is *pitting* of the fingernails and *onycholysis*. Some of the nail plates (say which) are thickened and there is a thick scale (*hyperkeratosis*) under them.

The patient also has psoriatic arthropathy.*

Treatment

Treatments of the skin lesions include sunlight, ultraviolet light, coal tar, dithranol, local steroids, calipotriol, PUVA (psoralen and UVA light). Systemic treatment with acitretin (a retinoid) or antimetabolites (methotrexate, azathioprine, hydroxyurea), because of their side effects, should be reserved for severe widespread disease unresponsive to topical measures. Analgesic anti-inflammatory agents are used for the pain of the arthropathy. Sulphasalazine and methotrexate are becoming established as effective agents for the treatment of psoriatic arthropathy. Gold and penicillamine may be useful, but few controlled studies have been done. Cyclosporin may also have a place in refractory disease. Choroquine is contraindicated as it may exacerbate the skin lesions (it can even cause exfoliative dermatitis). Intra-articular steroids are useful for a single inflamed troublesome joint.

Incidence

One to 5% of Caucasians in Northwestern Europe and USA. Uncommon among Japanese, North American Indians and Afro-Americans.

See also pp. 390–392.

---

* There is no evidence of a link between the activity of the skin lesions and the arthropathy.

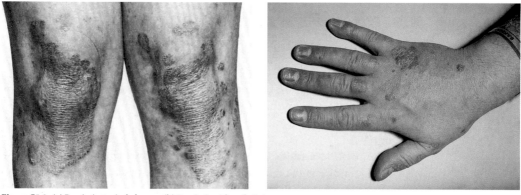

(a)

(b)

Figure C5.3 (a) Psoriasis: typical plaques. (b) Psoriasis with nail pitting.

Case 5 | **Rash of uncertain cause**

Frequency in survey: main focus of a short case in 6% of attempts at PACES station 5, skin.

It is already clear from our initial PACES survey that being faced with a rash of uncertain cause is not an uncommon situation for a candidate to arrive at in PACES, station 5. It is also clear that it is not necessarily a reason to fail. To prepare for this we suggest you study the examine *routines* 'Examine this patient's rash' (p. 54) and 'Examine this patient's skin' (p. 52). Describe the rash using appropriate terms and discuss appropriate differential diagnoses giving points in favour or against each particular diagnosis. In other words demonstrate your knowledge of the dermatological conditions that you do know about even if you are uncertain about the case before you. Mention how you might proceed to investigate, in particular by biopsy.

The following are three anecdotes from our PACES survey.

Anecdote 1: Look at this patient

This man's skin was really red. There were no plaques or scales but I said he had psoriasis. The examiners asked me how I would manage this man if it was a Friday night at 5.30 p.m. and I was in the Accident and Emergency Department and I could not get in touch with a dermatologist. I said that I would rehydrate, that I would treat any infection aggressively and that I would use simple aqueous creams. I passed the exam but on reflection I thought that I should have said that he had a drug rash and as I was walking away the examiners said, 'Did you really think it was psoriasis?' and I said, 'No!' They smiled!

Anecdote 2: Take a look at this lady's rash

She had a widespread, macular, erythematous rash and the examiners told me that the dermatologists did not know the diagnosis! I described the rash and explained that I would take a full history including a drug history and if in doubt I would do some blood tests and biopsy the lesion. They did not ask me any questions.

Anecdote 3: This patient has a rash which is congenital — what is the cause?

The patient had dysmorphic features and an old tracheostomy scar. There were also bilateral small scars over the carotids/jugular veins. There was a papular rash over the neck and shoulders. I had no idea what it was. I felt the examiners were after a specific syndrome. I expected to fail this station but got a clear pass from both examiners for station 5.

Case 6 | Dermatomyositis

Frequency in survey: main focus of a short case in 3% of attempts at PACES station 5, skin.

Record

There is a *heliotrope** *rash* over the *eyelids* and *periorbital* areas and the *backs* of the *hands,* especially around the *knuckles* (Gottron's papules) and *fingernails* (prominent nail-fold telangiectasia is characteristic). It is also present (may be) over the extensor surfaces of the elbows and knees. There is subcutaneous oedema (mainly around the eyes and due to a transient increase in capillary permeability). There is *proximal muscle weakness* and (may be) tenderness.

The diagnosis is dermatomyositis.

Male to female ratio is 2 : 1

Other features of dermatomyositis

Features and associations similar to polymyositis (p. 254)

Association with malignancy (the current recommendation is that patients over 40 years of age with dermatomyositis should be investigated for an associated malignancy particularly in the breasts, ovary, lungs and GI tract — see footnote, p. 254)

Overlap with rheumatic fever, rheumatoid arthritis, scleroderma, lupus erythematosus and other connective tissue diseases may occur (steroid responsiveness more likely)

Signs of other connective tissue diseases commoner than in pure polymyositis

Dysphagia due to upper oesophageal involvement

Raynaud's and arthralgia are frequent

Subcutaneous and intramuscular calcifications may occur

Helpful investigations include serum muscle enzymes (aldolase and CPU), urinary creatine, EMG (fibrillation, polyphasic action potentials and in some patients high frequency bizarre repetitive discharges) and muscle biopsy. The ESR is often normal despite active disease

The mainstay of treatment is steroids (initially in high doses). High dose intravenous immunoglobulin may be effective in refractory cases. Immunosuppressive agents, such as azathioprine, may be used to control the condition with a reduced steroid dose

May present with pseudohaematuria due to myoglobulinaemia

There is a juvenile form occurring in the first decade. Myopathy is severe, healing occurs with contractures and calcification in the skin and muscles, but Raynaud's is rare. There is no association with malignancy.

---

* From the shrub *heliotropium* which has fragrant purple flowers. The characteristic rash is a purple/violet/lilac colour. The skin changes may be subtle and easily overlooked. The classical heliotrope rash is diagnostic of the condition and, though it is most commonly seen in the childhood form, it also occurs in the adult form. Other skin manifestations include *local and diffuse erythema, erythema nodosum–like lesions, eczema, exfoliating dermatitis, blisters and scaling* and *maculopapular eruptions.* The skin lesions may occasionally ulcerate.

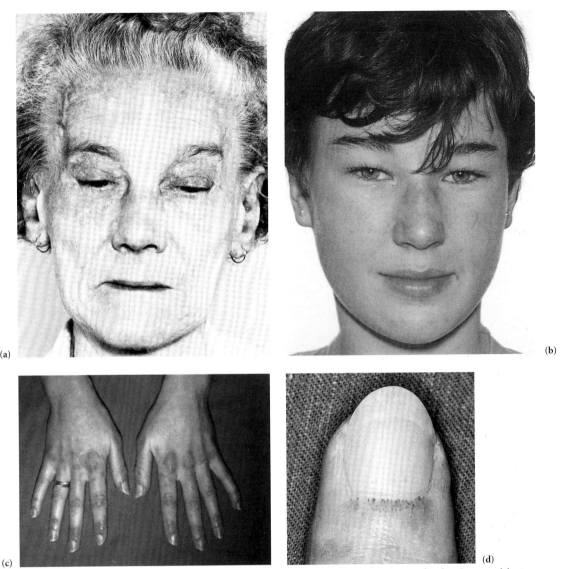

(a)

(b)

(c)

(d)

Figure C5.4 (a) Note the characteristic distribution of the rash. (b) Note the oedema and heliotrope discoloration around the eyes. (c) Gottron's papules: flat-topped, violaceous papules over the knuckles and interphalangeal joints. (d) Nail-fold telangiectasia is characteristic.

Case 7 | Xanthomata

Frequency in survey: main focus of a short case in 2% of attempts at PACES station 5, skin. Additional feature in a further 2%.

Record 1

There are *tendon xanthomata* (?corneal arcus, xanthelasma) in the *extensor tendons* on the back of the *hand*, and on the *Achilles* and *patella* tendons.

They suggest *familial hypercholesterolaemia*. (In this condition raised and nodular *tuberous xanthomata* may also occur, usually symmetrically, over the *extensor aspects of the joints* and on the *buttocks*. They may be several millimetres to several centimetres in size.)

Record 2

There are (orange or) *yellow papules* (up to 5 mm in diameter) on the *extensor surfaces* particularly over the *joints*, on the *limbs* and on the *buttocks* and *back*. They are (sometimes) surrounded by a rim of erythema (and may be tender).

This is *eruptive xanthomatosis* (?lipaemia retinalis on fundoscopy. There is often abdominal pain and there is a risk of acute pancreatitis. It suggests severe *hypertriglyceridaemia* — plasma triglycerides of the order of 20–25 mmol l^{-1} — 'milky plasma' syndrome).*

Familial hypercholesterolaemia is associated with premature development of vascular disease. Familial hypertriglyceridaemia does not appear to be an important risk factor for atherosclerosis but equivalent hypertriglyceridaemia due to familial combined hyperlipidaemia† is associated with an increased risk. Multivariate analysis suggests that the associated low levels of HDL with hypertriglyceridaemia are related to the risk of ischaemic heart disease.

Order of priorities in treating hyperlipidaemia‡

1 Secondary prevention:§

(a) patients who have had a myocardial infarction should be treated (low fat diet and statin therapy) if their total cholesterol level is 4.8 mmol l^{-1} or the LDL level is 3.2 mmol l^{-1}

(b) patients who have angina or other clinically overt atherosclerotic disease (e.g. a peripheral vascular disease, symptomatic carotid disease, or who have had a bypass graft or angioplasty) should be treated if they

---

* This level of hypertriglyceridaemia is usually due to overproduction of triglycerides occurring at the same time as hindrance of removal. For example, the coexistence of familial hypertriglyceridaemia (type IV), diabetes and/or alcohol consumption. Treatment of the secondary cause usually leads to a dramatic reduction in triglyceride levels and greatly reduces the risk of acute pancreatitis which is the main threat of this condition.

† Affected family members show either a combined rise in plasma cholesterol and triglycerides, or hypercholesterolaemia alone, or hypertriglyceridaemia alone.

‡ NB The screening and treatment of families with hypercholesterolaemia.

§ Guidelines for treatment are changed from time to time. Candidates are advised to check the current guidelines before going for the exam. In 2000 the joint recommendations of the British Cardiac Society, British Hyperlipidaemia Association, British Hypertension Society and British Diabetic Association were that, in the context of primary prevention, drug treatment for raised blood pressure or lipid concentrations should be based strongly on CHD risk. There are widely available computer programs and nomograms to measure CHD risk based on the Framingham equation. 'As a minimum, those with an absolute CHD risk of ≥30% over 10 years should be targeted and treated now and, as resources allow, individuals with a risk of ≥15% should be progressively targeted'.

have a total cholesterol of 5.5 mmol l^{-1} or more (LDL 3.7 mmol l^{-1} or more)

2 Primary prevention:§

(a) patients without clinically apparent vascular disease but who have other risk factors § (e.g. a family history of hypercholesterolaemia or ischaemic heart disease, diabetes mellitus or hypertension) should also be treated if they have a total cholesterol of 5.5 mmol l^{-1} or more (LDL 3.7 mmol l^{-1} or more)

(b) asymptomatic men and postmenopausal women should also be considered if their total cholesterol is 7.5 mmol l^{-1} or more (LDL 5.0 mmol l^{-1} or more)

3 Identify and treat any causes of secondary hyperlipidaemia such as:

(a) diabetes mellitus (?fundi)

(b) alcoholism (may be the occult underlying cause of treatment failure)

(c) nephrotic syndrome (?generalized oedema)

(d) myxoedema (?facies, pulse, ankle jerks)

(e) cholestasis (?icterus)

(f) myelomatosis

(g) oral contraceptives

4 Dietary treatment for obesity.

Treatment

Every effort should be made to reduce total cholesterol below 4.2 mmol l^{-1} and the fasting triglyceride level to 2.0 mmol l^{-1}. To begin with, all patients should be started on a low fat diet, which reduces total cholesterol and triglyceride by around 20% in patients with polygenic hyperlipidaemia and hypertriglyceridaemia. Patients with familial hypercholesterolaemia are less responsive to diet alone. Alcohol consumption should be reduced. Some patients with hypertriglyceridaemia are particularly sensitive to alcohol, and their livers produce excess VLDL particles, even from a modest alcohol intake.

Patients with combined hyperlipidaemia and hypertriglyceridaemia (without hypercholesterolaemia) respond well to fibrates. Patients with hypercholesterolaemia require a diet and a lipid-lowering agent. Treatment with statins (HMG co-A reductase inhibitors) lowers serum cholesterol substantially and has been shown to reduce myocardial infarction, coronary deaths and overall mortality in recent controlled trials.

Types of hyperlipidaemia simplified

Comparatively common

Type IIa (e.g. familial hypercholesterolaemia) — raised cholesterol only

Type IIb (e.g. familial combined hypercholesterolaemia) — raised cholesterol and triglycerides

Type IV (e.g. familial hypertriglyceridaemia) — raised triglycerides.

Rare

Type I — raised chylomicrons

Type III — an inherited defect in apolipoprotein E synthesis (mostly intermediate density remnants) and triglycerides to an equal extent. It is characteristically associated with palmar xanthomata and is very responsive to fibrates.

Type V — raised chylomicrons and triglycerides.

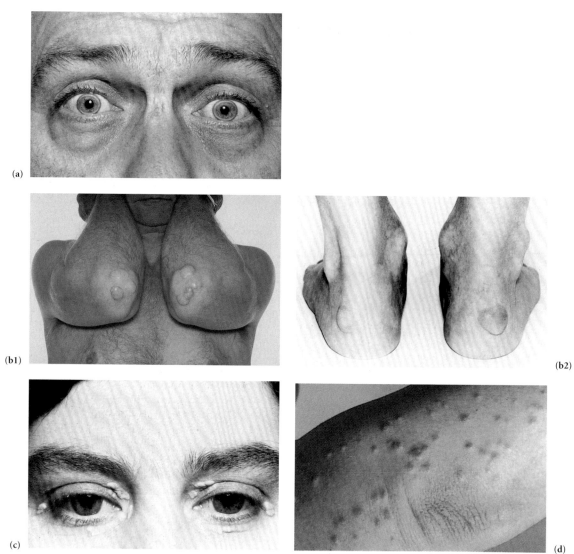

Figure C5.5 (a) Arcus senilis. (b1,2) Elbows and Achilles of the same patient. (c) Xanthelasma. (d) Eruptive xanthomata.

Case 8 | Vitiligo

Frequency in survey: main focus of a short case in 2% of attempts at PACES station 5, skin.

Record

There are *areas* of *depigmentation* around the eyes, mouth, on the knees and on the dorsum of the feet (the hands, axillae, groins and genitalia are the other commonly affected areas).

    The patient has vitiligo.

Vitiligo affects up to 1% of the population. It is equal in both sexes, although females present in dermatology clinics for cosmetic reasons. There is family history in about one-third of the patients.

    Sites subject to friction and trauma are often affected and Koebner's phenomenon (a lesion appearing at the site of skin damage) is common. Vitiligo is usually symmetrical but occasionally the depigmentation can be unilateral and follow the pattern of a dermatome. It is inherited as a dominant trait and individuals are usually otherwise healthy. Halo naevi (hypopigmented rings surrounding dark naevi), leucotrichia, premature greying of the hair and alopecia areata as well as vitiligo may all be associated with any of the **organ-specific autoimmune diseases:**

Myxoedema (?pulse, ankle jerks, facies — p. 438)

Hashimoto's disease (?goitre — p. 438)

Graves' disease (?exophthalmos, fidgety, goitre, tachycardia, etc. — p. 432)

Pernicious anaemia (?pallor, spleen, SACD — p. 518)

Atrophic gastritis associated with iron deficiency anaemia

Addison's disease (?buccal, skin crease, scar and general pigmentation, hypotension, etc. — p. 446)

Idiopathic hypoparathyroidism (Chvostek's and Trousseau's signs, tetany, paraesthesiae and cramps, cataracts, ectodermal changes, moniliasis, mental retardation, psychiatric disturbances, bradykinetic rigid syndrome, epilepsy)

Premature ovarian failure

Diabetes mellitus (?fundi)

Renal tubular acidosis

Fibrosing alveolitis (?basal crepitations — p. 72)

Chronic active hepatitis (?icterus, etc.)

Primary biliary cirrhosis (?xanthelasma, pigmentation, icterus, scratch marks, etc. — p. 121).

The organ-specific autoimmune diseases tend to occur in association with each other (*polyglandular autoimmune disease*) so that patients with one have an above normal chance of also developing another. Some patients are prone to extensive mucocutaneous candidiasis* (candidiasis-endocrinopathy syndrome) and from this two distinct syndromes emerge. The clinical features of the syndromes are compared in Table C5.1.

Vitiligo, the cutaneous marker of organ-specific autoimmune disease, may occur in the non-organ-specific autoimmune disease systemic sclerosis.† Other disorders associated with vitiligo are morphoea and malignant melanoma.

---

*The mucocutaneous candidiasis is associated with hypergammaglobulinaemia, IgA deficiency and anergy to *Candida albicans.*
†Rarely there is an overlap between the organ-specific and non-organ-specific autoimmune diseases. Sjögrens syndrome occupies an intermediate position being associated with rheumatoid arthritis on the one hand and autoimmune thyroiditis on the other. Primary biliary cirrhosis is another condition which bridges the gap. It is associated with Sjögren's syndrome, Hashimoto's thyroiditis and renal tubular acidosis on the one hand, and systemic sclerosis, CRST syndrome, rheumatoid arthritis, coeliac disease, dermatomyositis and mixed connective tissue disease, on the other.

Table C5.1 Comparison of the clinical features of the major syndromes characterized by multiple endocrine gland hypofunction (from *Cecil's Textbook of Medicine*, 19th edn, 1992, p. 1389)

	Multiple endocrine deficiency syndrome (Schmidt's syndrome)	Polyglandular deficiency with mucocutaneous candidiasis
Hypoadrenalism	Common	Common
Hypothyroidism	Common	Rare
Diabetes mellitus (type I)	Common	Rare
Gonadal failure	Less common	Less common
Hypoparathyroidism	Rare	Common
Pituitary insufficiency	Rare	Rare
Autoantibodies to endocrine tissues and gastric parietal cells	Often present	Often present
Sex distribution	Strong female predominance	Female preponderance about 4 : 1
Inheritance	Usually 'sporadic', but susceptibility related to HLA haplotype and may be inherited as autosomal dominant	Generally inherited as autosomal recessive; no apparent HLA association; siblings characteristically affected
Time of onset	Usually becomes evident during adult life	Typically becomes evident during childhood preceded by chronic mucocutaneous moniliasis
Other associated 'autoimmune' diseases and characteristics	Pernicious anaemia; hyperthyroidism; coeliac disease; alopecia; vitiligo; myasthenia gravis; isolated red-cell aplasia	Pernicious anaemia; malabsorption; alopecia; vitiligo; IgA deficiency; hypergammaglobulinaemia; chronic active hepatitis; proliferative glomerulonephritis

Treatment

There is a general misconception, even among physicians and some dermatologists, that vitiligo is untreatable. Affected subjects asking for help should be referred to those dermatologists who have a special interest in this condition, who can select the appropriate options for treatment, and who can be persistent until desirable cosmetic improvement is achieved. The available management strategies are sunscreens, camouflaging cover-up creams, topical glucocorticoids, topical and systemic photochemotherapy (sunlight or artificial UVA and oral 5-methoxypsoralen), narrow-band UVB 311 nm, mini-grafting and bleaching. The duration of vitiligo has no effect on the success of the repigmentation with PUVA photochemotherapy.

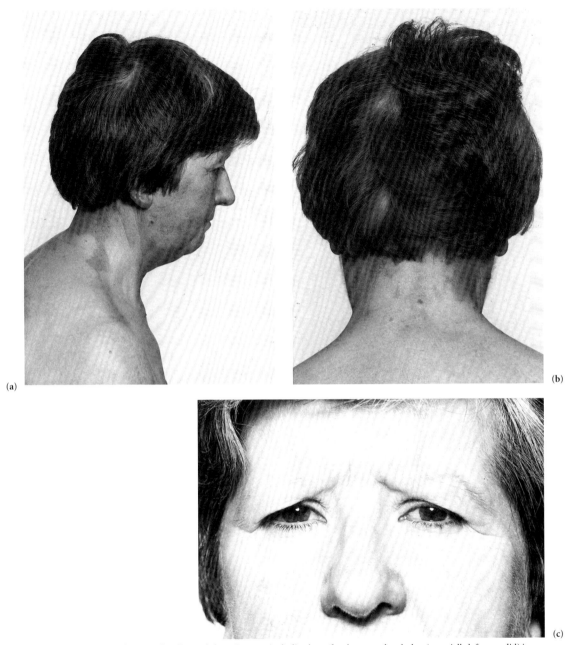

Figure C5.6 (a–c) Note the areas of vitiligo and alopecia areata including loss of eyebrows and eyelashes (especially left upper lid) in this patient with diabetes mellitus.

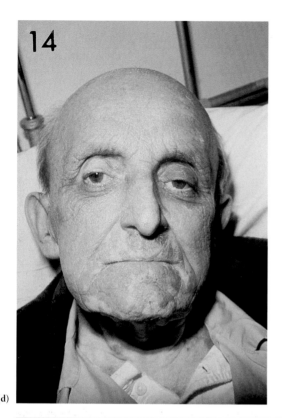

(d)

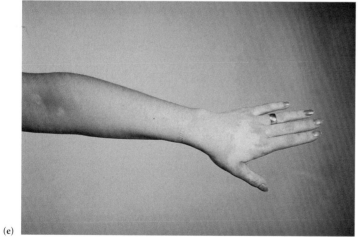

(e)

Figure C5.6 (*continued*) (d) Vitiligo. (e) Vitiligo of the hand.

Case 9 | Tuberous sclerosis/adenoma sebaceum

Frequency in survey: main focus of a short case in 2% of attempts at PACES station 5, skin.

Survey note: candidates were asked to look at the face; the clue was usually given that the patient had epilepsy or funny turns.

Record

There is a *papular, salmon-coloured* eruption on the centre of the face (over the *butterfly* area), especially in the *nasolabial* folds. These angiomatous, glistening papules and their configuration have the appearance of adenoma sebaceum (check for *periungual fibromata* and *shagreen patches*).

There may be a history of *epilepsy* and *mental deficiency** which together with *adenoma sebaceum* make up the triad associated with tuberous sclerosis (*epiloia*).

Tuberous sclerosis is a phakomatosis (see also footnote, p. 281). Autosomal dominant but 80% are sporadic due to new mutations.† The gene is on chromosomes 16p13 and 9q34.

Hamartomata

Tuberous sclerosis is characterized by the development of hamartomata of the skin, central nervous system, kidneys, retina, heart, lungs and bone. Hamartomata consist of excessive overgrowth of mature, normal cells and tissues in an organ.

Skin lesions

A number of hamartomatous lesions of the skin are seen. The term *adenoma sebaceum* is a misnomer; the lesions are actually angiofibromata. They usually appear around the age of 4 and become more prominent after puberty. The leathery *shagreen patches* (flesh-coloured lumpy plaques which resemble studded leather) over the lower back and ungual *fibromata* (firm pink periungual papules which appear at puberty) growing out from the nail beds of the fingers and toes are seen in perhaps 40% of cases. *Hypopigmented macules* (in an oval or *mountain ash leaf* configuration, rounded at one end and tapered at

the other), especially on the trunk or buttocks, are present from birth in *nearly all patients*; they are easier to see in fair-skinned patients with a Wood's lamp. Intraoral fibromata and hyperplastic gums are also seen and there may be increased pigmentation as manifest in bronzing of the skin and *café-au-lait* macules.

Other organs

Cerebral hemispheres contain multiple hamartomata or tubers (calcified lesions are well seen on CT scans but uncalcified ones may show up better on MRI). Epilepsy occurs in 80% of cases; it usually starts below the age of 5 and is often difficult to control. The diagnosis may be missed and subtle skin lesions should be sought even in adults presenting with epilepsy

Renal hamartomata (angiomyolipomata) in two-thirds of patients (may cause pain or bleeding). There may be polycystic kidneys

Retinal hamartomata‡ (phakomata), which appear yellow, in 50% (also occur in neurofibromatosis—p. 281)

Cardiac hamartomata (rhabdomyomata) in 30% (may cause dysrhythmias or congestive cardiac failure)

Cystic lung disease due to hamartomatous lesions composed of smooth muscle cells in 1% (mostly women

---

* May be mild or severe. One-third have normal, or even superior, intelligence.

† Before concluding that an affected child of apparently normal parents is the result of a new mutation, the parents should be examined with a Wood's lamp for the presence of *ash leaf*

macules, which may be the only manifestation of the disease. They should also be examined by an ophthalmologist for *retinal phakomata* and pigmentary changes, which are present in 50% of patients.

‡ See also p. 503; optic disc drusen may also occur.

over 20 years; may cause pneumothorax, breathlessness, cyanosis and cor pulmonale).

Treatment

For cosmetic reasons, adenoma sebaceum may be destroyed by electrodesiccation or laser surgery but they tend to recur.

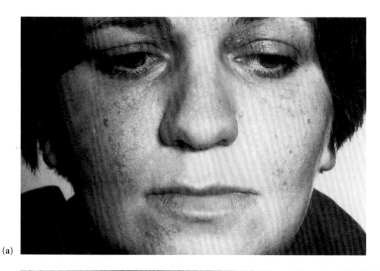

(a)

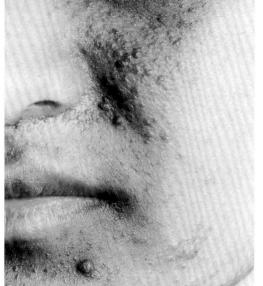

(b)

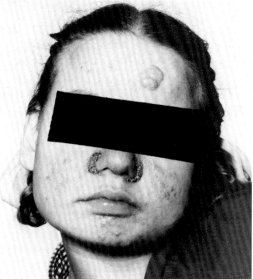

(c)

Figure C5.7 (a) Angiofibroma papules in butterfly distribution. (b) Skin-coloured papules in the nasolabial fold. (c) Clusters of angiofibromata in the nasolabial folds.

Case 10 | Pseudoxanthoma elasticum

Frequency in survey: main focus of a short case in 2% of attempts at PACES station 5, skin.

Record

There is *loose skin* mainly over the *neck, axillae, antecubital fossae* and *groins,* in which there are seen yellow, chamois-coloured papules, coalescing to form larger *yellow pseudoxanthomatous plaques* (there may be *redundant folds of lax skin*). There is a '*plucked chicken skin*' appearance because of the clear margins around the hair follicles.

This patient has pseudoxanthoma elasticum.

It is due to an inherited defect of elastin. There are four main types (two are recessive and two are dominant). An occlusive arteriopathy is the major cause of symptoms. Angina, myocardial infarction, claudication, decreased visual acuity in a young person, haematemesis and melaena are some of the presenting features. Asymptomatic skin lesions usually appear by the age of 30 years but may go undetected until old age. Steroids should be avoided and the diagnosis is confirmed by skin biopsy.

Other features which may occur

Angioid streaks* in the retina (60% have eye changes)
Blue sclerae

Macular degeneration—diminished visual acuity, blindness
Loose jointedness
Hypertension due to renovascular disease (50%)
Gastrointestinal (10%), genitourinary or respiratory haemorrhage
Coronary artery disease
Peripheral vascular disease (weak or absent pulses, claudication, often vascular calcification)
Mitral incompetence
Hypothyroidism (?due to involvement of thyroid vasculature)
Miscarriages.

---

* The triad of skin lesions, angioid streaks of the retinae and vascular abnormalities is called the *Grönblad–Strandberg syndrome.* Other causes of angioid streaks (poorly defined, greyish streaks radiating across the fundus, which represent the rupture of Bruch's membrane secondary to an elastic fibre defect) include Ehlers–Danlos syndrome, Paget's disease of the bone, sickle cell anaemia and hyperphosphataemia.

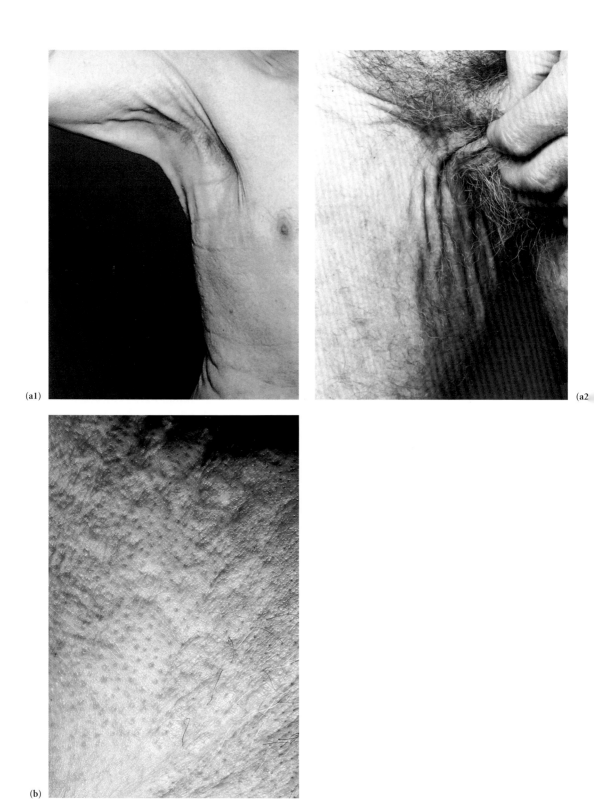

(a1)

(a2)

(b)

Figure C5.8 Pseudoxanthoma elasticum (a1,2) note the loose skin. (b) Plucked chicken skin appearance.

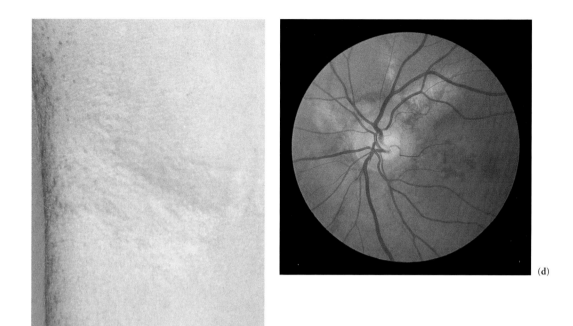

(c)

(d)

Figure C5.8 (*continued*) (c) Antecubital fossa. (d) Angioid streaks in the retina. There is a dark ring with irregular margins around the optic disc. Note a streak radiating outwards from it at 1 o'clock and another at 10 o'clock.

Case 11 | Lichen planus

Frequency in survey: main focus of a short case in 2% of attempts at PACES station 5, skin.

Record

This young (or middle-aged) patient has *flat-topped, polygonal, shiny,* reflecting light, violaceous *papules* on the wrists (and other flexor surfaces usually, though it may affect any part of the skin). Fine white streaks (*Wickham's striae*) are seen on the surface of the lesions (better seen with a hand lens). The *Koebner phenomenon* is present (i.e. lesions appear in a linear pattern along a scratch mark or on a surgical scar). There are also asymptomatic lesions in the *buccal mucosa* (in 50% of cases — white, lacy pattern).

This patient has lichen planus (itching is usual and may be quite severe, though there are seldom any excoriations because the patients tend to rub rather than scratch).

Male to female ratio is 1 : 1.

Lichen planus usually resolves in 6–24 months but it may recur. Steroids (systemic, local or intralesional) may be required if pruritus is severe and in the hypertrophic variety (see below). Certain drugs such as thiazides, methyl dopa, β-blockers, phenothiazines, gold, quinidine and antimalarials can cause lichen planus-like, generalized eruptions. Some patients with graft-versus-host disease develop a skin reaction that closely resembles lichen planus. There may be aetiological clues in this.

Other sites for lichen planus

Scalp (atrophy of the skin with patchy, permanent alopecia)
Nails (dystrophy of the nail plate with longitudinal streaking of the nail; if it is severe there may be complete loss of the nail plate)*
Palms and soles.

Other forms

Hypertrophic lichen planus (plaque-like lesions with a thick, warty surface on the front of the legs). This form is more common in Afro-Caribbean races
Erosive lichen planus (mouth). Carries an increased risk of oral squamous cell carcinoma
Bullous lichen planus.

Treatment

Intralesional triamcinolone is helpful for symptomatic cutaneous or oral mucosal lesions. Cyclosporine mouthwashes may be used in patients with erosive oral lesions. In resistant, generalized, erosive oral and hypertrophic varieties, systemic therapy with corticosteroids, cyclosporin, retinoids and PUVA photochemotherapy have all been tried with some success. Recent reports have shown successful outcomes with drugs such as mycophenolate and enoxaparin (heparin analogue) that have antiproliferative and immunomodulatory properties.

---

* A characteristic change of lichen planus of the nail is *pterygium* in which the cuticle invades the nail bed.

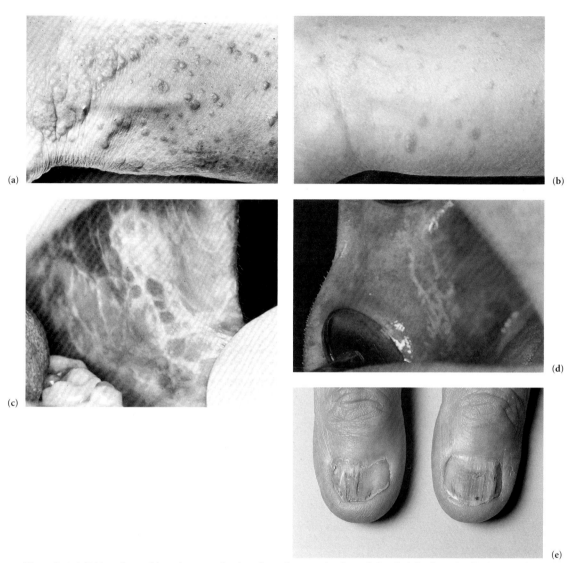

(a)

(b)

(c)

(d)

(e)

Figure C5.9 (a) Lichen planus of the wrist: grouped and confluent, flat-topped, polygonal, sharply defined papules. (b) Flat-topped violaceous, polygonal papules on the wrist. Note Wickham's striae. (c, d) The left buccal mucosa is exposed to show the characteristic lacy, white pattern. (e) Pterygium (left) and longitudinal ridging of the nails — lichen planus.

Case 12 | Yellow nail syndrome

Frequency in survey: main focus of a short case in 2% of attempts at PACES station 5, skin.

Record

The *nails* are thick, *excessively curved* from side to side and slow growing, leaving *bulbous fingertips* uncovered and pale yellow (or greenish yellow). The *cuticles* are *lost*, the lunulae are absent and there is onycholysis (though the degree is variable).

This suggests the yellow nail syndrome (check for *lymphoedema* of the extremities which may also be present).

The yellow nail syndrome is usually associated with lymphatic hypoplasia, ankle oedema and a number of *pulmonary conditions* may occur such as bronchiectasis, pleural effusion, COPD and malignant neoplasms.

Other associations include D-penicillamine therapy, nephrotic syndrome, hypothyroidism and AIDS.

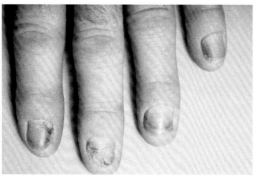 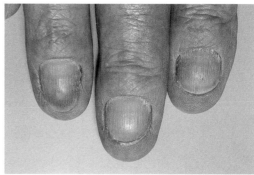

(a)

(b)

Figure C5.10 Yellow nail syndrome. (a) Thickened nails and onycholysis. (b) No cuticles or lunulae. Bulbous uncovered fingertips are suggestive of stunted nail growth.

Case 13 | **Gouty tophi**

Frequency in survey: main focus of a short case in 2% of attempts at PACES station 5, skin.

Tophaceous gout is dealt with on p. 399

Case 14 | **Alopecia**

Frequency in survey: main focus of a short case in 2% of attempts at PACES station 5, skin.

Record 1

There is a *discrete, well-circumscribed,* round (or oval) patch of *hair loss* over the back of the scalp (may involve the beard) of this patient. There is no evidence of inflammation or scarring. The empty hair follicles are easily seen and in the periphery there are tiny hairs, about 4 mm in length, with tapered ends, the so-called *exclamation mark hairs.** The eyebrows and eyelashes are preserved.

This is alopecia areata.†

Record 2

There is a complete *loss* of *hair* over the *scalp* and body. Both the *eyebrows* and *eyelashes* are *absent.*

This is alopecia universalis.

Alopecia areata may have an autoimmune cause. It is sometimes associated with Hashimoto's thyroiditis but it can also occur with other thyroid disorders, pernicious anaemia, diabetes mellitus and vitiligo (see p. 293). Most patients with alopecia areata localized to the scalp have a good prognosis. Alopecia universalis (also known as alopecia totalis) has a poor prognosis. Topical or intralesional triamcinolone leads to localized tufts of regrowth and may be used to establish eyebrows but does not affect the overall outcome. PUVA therapy may be used in patients with extensive hair loss but the results are often unsatisfactory.

Diffuse hair loss may occur during an acute febrile illness or after childbirth (telogen effluvium = hair follicles going into the resting phase), and in association with an endocrine disorder (hypopituitarism, hypo- and hyperthyroidism, hypoparathyroidism), drugs (antimitotics, anticoagulants, vitamin A excess, oral contraceptives), severe chronic illness, iron deficiency or malnutrition. Androgenetic alopecia may become diffuse, as may alopecia areata.

Sparse hair with poor development of nails and teeth, with or without defective sweat glands, is characteristic of a group of rare inherited disorders, the ectodermal dysplasias (p. 364).

Some causes of localized alopecia

Non-scarring alopecia

Alopecia areata
Androgenetic (male-pattern baldness)
Self-induced (hair pulling habit and traction alopecia caused by rollers)
Scalp ringworm from human source.

Scarring alopecia

Burns, radiodermatitis
Tinea capitis (from animal source)
Aplasia cutis
Cicatricial basal cell carcinoma
Carbuncle
Lichen planus
Lupus erythematosus
Necrobiosis lipoidica diabeticorum
Sarcoidosis.

---

* These are broken off hairs about 4 mm from the scalp, and are narrower and less pigmented proximally. They may be seen around the edges of enlarging areas of alopecia and are pathognomonic of alopecia areata.

† The hair loss of the entire scalp is called alopecia totalis.

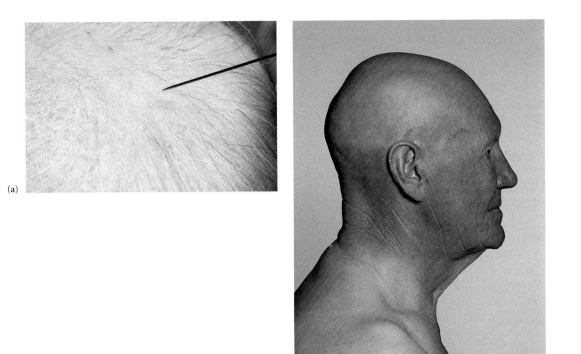

(a)

(b)

Figure C5.11 (a) Alopecia areata. Note the empty hair follicles and the short, tapering, exclamation mark hairs. (b) Alopecia universalis in a patient with diabetes mellitus.

Case 15 | **Eczema**

Frequency in survey: main focus of a short case in 2% of attempts at PACES station 5, skin.

Record 1

There is a *papulovesicular* eruption on the *face* (may be on the trunk, hands or legs) with *excoriation, scratch marks* and *lichenification*.* The *skin* is *dry*.

This is chronic atopic eczema.

Record 2

There is an area of *lichenification** on the *arm* (usually in the flexural areas) with *dryness, scratch marks* and some *vesicular lesions*.

This is chronic atopic eczema.

Record 3

There is a bilateral, *darkish, erythematous eruption* over the *face* with some *vesicular* and *crusted lesions* and *fine scales*. There is *lichenification** with *prominent skin markings* secondary to repeated scratching and rubbing.

This is contact dermatitis probably secondary to the use of some cosmetic agent.

Some common forms of eczema

Atopic dermatitis

Atopic dermatitis is a chronic, eczematous condition often associated with a personal or family history of asthma, allergic rhinitis and/or atopic eczema. It often begins before the age of 6 months but the onset may be delayed to childhood or adult life. About 40% of affected babies will 'outgrow' their eczema but the others will manifest some features of atopic dermatitis as adults. In most cases, the condition starts as an acute or subacute, red, vesicular eruption affecting the face, upper chest and the antecubital and popliteal fossae (flexural dermatitis). Pruritus is a major symptom and the consequent rubbing and scratching leads to lichenification, most typically in the flexural areas of the arms and legs. Patients with chronic atopic dermatitis have a characteristic facies with diffuse erythema, perioral pallor, and loose folds below the lower eyelids. The palms tend to be dry with an increased number of skin lines.

The incidence of atopic dermatitis is increasing in industrialized countries but the cause remains unknown.

Atopic patients demonstrate excessive T-cell activation, specifically with increased helper T-cell cytokines such as IL-4 and IL-10, usually with elevated serum IgE levels. These patients have depressed cell-mediated immunity, which probably accounts for their increased susceptibility to cutaneous infections by herpesvirus, vaccinia and molluscum contagiosum virus, and human papillomavirus. Abnormal neutrophil and monocyte chemotaxis may explain frequent staphylococcal infections, which often flare or complicate atopic dermatitis.

The treatment consists of topical steroids and emollients and systemic antihistamines. Refractory cases may require immune modulators such as methotrexate, cyclosporin or tacrolimus.

Contact dermatitis

Contact dermatitis may be due to a direct toxic or irritant effect of a substance (e.g. acids, solvents, detergents, etc.) or through an allergic, delayed (type IV) type of hypersensitivity. The original site of the eruption suggests a clue to the likely irritant or allergen, since both irritant

---

* Lichenification is dry, leathery thickening of the skin with exaggerated skin markings. It is testimony to patients' bitter complaint of itching and is a characteristic sign of atopic eczema and other irritative dermatoses such as lichen planus.

and allergic contact eczemas are initially confined to sites of contact. In chronic cases, the eczema and the maculopapular or papulovesicular rash spread to other parts of the skin, as the skin reacts as an organ.

The most common allergens causing allergic contact dermatitis are pentadecylcatechol in poison oak, ivy, cashews and mangos, paraphenylenediamine (a substance in hair dyes that cross-reacts with benzocaine and hydrochlorthiazide), nickel, mercaptobenzothiazole and thiuram (components in rubber), and ethylenediamine (a preservative found in many medications and also found in industrial dyes and insecticides).

Photodermatitis

Areas of skin exposed to too much ultraviolet become red and painful. Repeated exposure leads to pigmentation and desquamation. Photodermatitis has an immunological basis. A specific wavelength of ultraviolet light is absorbed by a topical substance or systemic drug, which is deposited in the skin from the circulation (amiodarone, chlorpropamide, nalidixic acid, oral contraceptives, phenothiazines, sulphonamides, tetracyclines and thiazides). The offending rays cause chemical conversion of the substance or drug to a hapten, that binds cutaneous proteins to become a complete antigen, capable of inducing a type IV delayed hypersensitivity reaction similar to that of allergic contact dermatitis.

Stasis dermatitis

A chronic, patchy, ill-defined eczematous eruption occurs on the lower legs secondary to peripheral venous insufficiency, with a consequent increased hydrostatic pressure and extravasation of red blood cells and serum. These blood substances set up an inflammatory, brawny, oedematous, red, scaling or weeping reaction on the distal one-third of the lower legs, which in due course becomes hyperpigmented due to haemosiderin deposition.

Nummular eczematous dermatitis

Nummular eczematous dermatitis often affects the legs and arms of middle-aged males with groups of papules and vesicles on an erythematous base. These lesions may coalesce into rounded or coin-shaped (Latin *nummularis*—like a coin) plaques, 4–6 cm in diameter, and have an erythematous base with an indistinct border.

Seborrhoeic dermatitis

Seborrhoeic dermatitis often affects those with a tendency to dandruff. It manifests as a red, exudative eruption with yellow, greasy scales localized to hairy regions of the skin with a high population of sebaceous glands (i.e. middle of the face, nasolabial folds, eyebrows, retroauricular folds, presternal and interscapular areas). Some lesions develop follicular papules or pustules (seborrhoeic folliculitis) and some manifest as intertriginous lesions of the armpits, groins and umbilicus or under spectacles or hearing aids.

It is sometimes difficult to distinguish seborrhoea from psoriasis when the latter is confined to the scalp, ears and face. The cause of seborrhoea is unknown but it is sometimes associated with emotional stress and neurological disease. Patients with Parkinson's disease or stroke may have a dramatic flare of their seborrhoea. Extensive, intractable seborrhoea may also signal infection with HIV regardless of CD4 counts or viral load and may be one of the first cutaneous clues to the diagnosis.

Antiseborrhoeic shampoos containing tar, sulphur, salicylic acid, selenium sulphide, pyrithione zinc or ketoconazole provide the most effective treatment. Continual use of shampoo and topical steroids are sometimes required for control.

Lichen simplex chronicus

This occurs as a single, lichenified plaque on the nape of the neck in women, legs in men, and orogenital areas in both sexes.

Erythroderma / exfoliative dermatitis

The whole skin may become red and scaly (exfoliative dermatitis) or red with little or no scaling (erythroderma) in patients with a previous skin disease (psoriasis, pityriasis, pemphigus, contact dermatitis, Reiter's syndrome and lymphoma). Most patients have lymphadenopathy and hepatomegaly with improper temperature regulation.

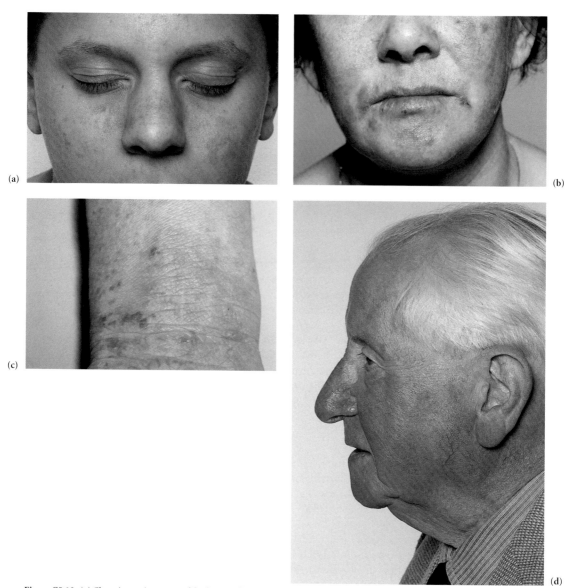

Figure C5.12 (a) Chronic atopic eczema of the face: erythematous patches and papulovesicular lesions. (b) Chronic atopic eczema. Note perioral pallor, erythematous patches and papulovesicular lesions. (c) Chronic atopic eczema of the arm with marked lichenification. (d) Photodermatitis (amiodarone face).

Case 16 | **Pretibial myxoedema**

Frequency in survey: main focus of a short case in 2% of attempts at PACES station 5, skin.

Pretibial myxoedema is dealt with on p. 451.

Case 17 | Clubbing

Frequency in survey: main focus of a short case in 2% of attempts at PACES station 5, skin. Additional feature in many cases in all stations.

Record

There is finger clubbing* (*thickening of the nail bed†* with *loss of the obtuse angle* between the nail and the dorsum of the finger—becomes >180° ‡; *increased curvature* of the nail bed—both side-to-side and lengthwise; increased *sponginess or fluctuation* of the nail bed; and sometimes, when there is marked swelling of the nail bed, the fingers may have a *drumstick appearance*).

Causes of clubbing

1 Carcinoma of the bronchus (the commonest cause—?nicotine staining, obvious weight loss with temporal dimples, lymph nodes, chest signs, evidence of secondaries, etc.—p. 81)

2 Fibrosing alveolitis (?basal crackles—p. 72)

3 Cyanotic congenital heart disease (?cyanosis, thoracotomy scars, Fallot's—p. 163, Eisenmenger's—p. 157)

4 Bronchiectasis (?productive cough, crepitations, etc.—p. 75)

5 Cirrhosis (?icterus, spider naevi, palmar erythema, Dupuytren's xanthelasma—especially in primary biliary cirrhosis, hepatosplenomegaly, etc.—p. 108).

Other causes

Subacute bacterial endocarditis (heart murmur, fever, splenomegaly, petechiae, splinter haemorrhages, Osler's nodes, Janeway's lesions, Roth's spots, etc.)

Empyema

Lung abscess

Crohn's disease

Ulcerative colitis

Asbestosis (especially with mesothelioma)

Thyroid acropachy (?exophthalmos, pretibial myx-oedema, goitre, thyroid status, etc.—p. 432)

Hereditary (rare; dominant).

---

* Indisputable clubbing is one of the important fundamental clinical signs which, when present, has clear implications. Less clear-cut changes in the finger nails are susceptible to assessment which (even if dogmatic) may be very subjective. Such finger nails are best described as showing 'debatable clubbing' (in that physicians will disagree as to whether there are significant changes or not). Genuine 'debatable clubbing' occurring in the examination may cause trouble if you recognize it as such, but you are not sure what your examiners' opinion is. The safest course in a case of doubt is to use nail bed thickening as your guide and quote the nail angle rule in a way that cannot be argued with. For example: 'The appearance of the nails (e.g. increased curvature) is initially suggestive of clubbing, but the obtuse angle between the nail and the dorsum of the finger is preserved, and therefore by definition (loss of the angle being the "official" first sign) the diagnosis of definite clubbing cannot be accepted in this case.'

† Before palpating always inspect the fingers in profile for a slightly bulbous appearance due to thickening of the nail bed.

‡ *Shamroth's sign:* if you put the fingernails of the same fingers of each of your hands together, against each other, you will see a gap at their base between them. This gap may be lost when the angle is lost in finger clubbing.

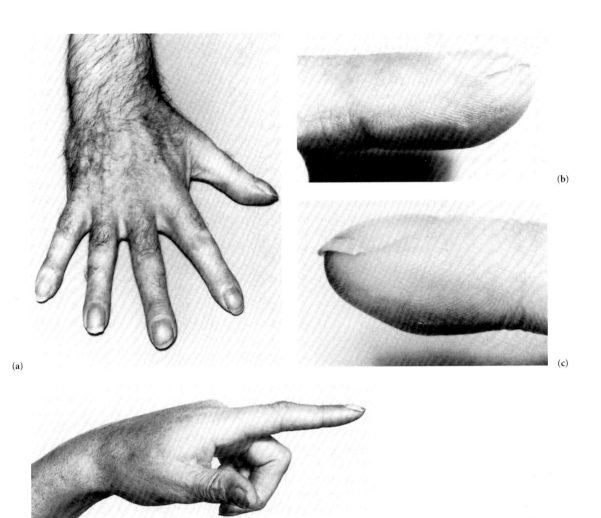

Figure C5.13 (a) Clubbing (carcinoma of the bronchus). (b) Loss of the angle. (c) Thickening of the nail bed (early drumstick appearance—same patient as in (a)). (d) Clubbing and leuconychia (cirrhosis of the liver).

Case 18 | Necrobiosis lipoidica diabeticorum

Frequency in survey: main focus of a short case in 2% of attempts at PACES station 5, skin.

Record

There are *sharply demarcated*, coalescing *oval plaques* on the *shins* (occasionally arms and elsewhere) of this lady (usually a female aged <40). The lesions have a *shiny atrophic surface,* with characteristic *waxy yellow centres* and *brownish-red edges.* There is (usually) telangiectasia over the surface.

The diagnosis is necrobiosis lipoidica diabeticorum.

It is rare, usually associated with diabetes, but can occur in the prediabetic and on its own. It may have to be differentiated from granuloma annulare, from nodular vasculitis when small, and from localized scleroderma or sarcoidosis when larger.

The lesions may ulcerate. Opinions vary as to whether good diabetic control can improve healing, but this should be tried. Gradual healing, with scarring, occurs over a period of years. Steroids (topical or local injection) administered cautiously (to avoid local atrophy) may help. Severe cases can be treated by excision and skin grafting. The histology varies, some containing large amounts of lipid, some not. There is necrosis of collagen, surrounded by pallisades of granulomatous epithelioid cells, and the aetiology is obscure.

Granuloma annulare (did not occur in original survey): pale or flesh-coloured, non-scaly (distinguishable from tinea/ringworm which has fine scales over the surface) papules coalescing in rings of usually 1–3 cm diameter, especially on the backs of the hands and fingers. Blanching by pressure reveals a characteristic beaded ring of white dermal patches. It is sometimes associated with diabetes especially when the lesions are generalized and atypical. The histology is almost identical to necrobiosis lipoidica diabeticorum. The lesions regress spontaneously.

Diabetic dermopathy (did not occur in original survey): atrophic pigmented patches (start as dull red oval papules; sometimes with a small blister) occurring mostly on the shins of diabetics. It has been suggested that they are precipitated by trauma in association with neuropathy.

Other skin lesions in diabetics

Infective (bacterial—boils, etc.; fungal—candidiasis)

Foot/leg ulcers (ischaemic and neuropathic)

Vitiligo (?other associated organ-specific autoimmune disease—p. 293)

Fat atrophy (very rare with highly purified insulins)

Fat hypertrophy (recurrent injection of insulin into the same site)

Xanthomata (associated hyperlipidaemia—may disappear with control of diabetes as this causes improvement in the hyperlipidaemia—p. 290)

Insulin allergy (immediate and delayed; though less likely this can even occur in patients on human insulin given subcutaneously)

Sulphonylurea allergy (erythema multiforme, phototoxic and other eruptions)

Acanthosis nigricans (see p. 374)

Peripheral anhidrosis (due to autonomic neuropathy)

Chlorpropamide alcohol flush.

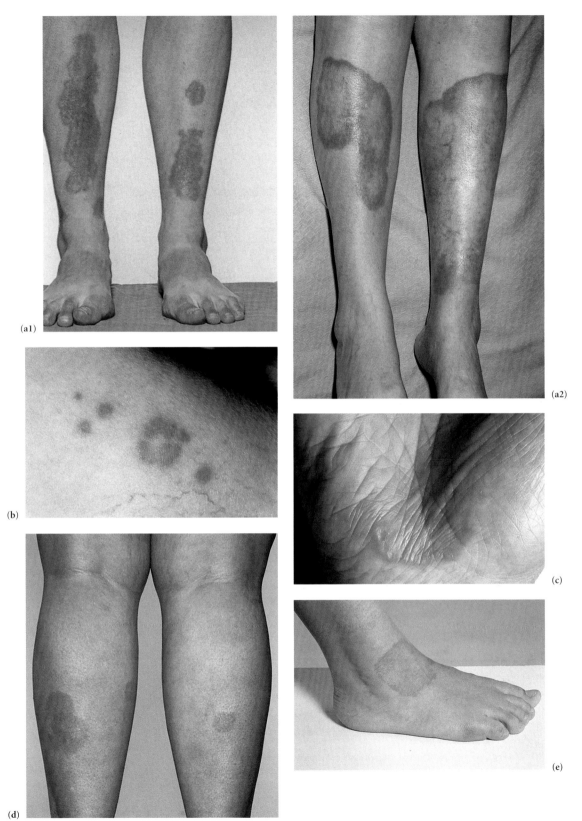

Figure C5.14 (a1, 2) Necrobiosis lipoidica diabeticorum: bilateral, well-demarcated plaques. (b–e) Granuloma annulare: circular, well-demarcated plaques with central regression.

Case 19 | Lupus pernio

Frequency in survey: main focus of a short case in 2% of attempts at PACES station 5, skin.

Survey note: candidates often gave differential diagnoses such as SLE and rosacea before being led to the correct diagnosis. We suggest that candidates try to see real life cases of all three conditions affecting the face before the examination so that they can recognize the differences.

Record

There is (in this female patient) a *diffuse*, livid, *purple–red infiltration* of the *nose* (and/or cheeks, ears, hands and feet).*

The diagnosis is lupus pernio (usually associated with *chronic pulmonary sarcoidosis* which progresses to *fibrosis; chronic uveitis* and *bone cysts* in the phalanges are often present).

Other complications which may occur in chronic sarcoidosis

Facial palsy (may be bilateral; parotid enlargement not always present)

Peripheral neuropathy

Meningeal infiltrations and tumour-like deposits

Hypopituitarism and diabetes insipidus (granulomata extending from the meninges into the hypothalmus)

Hypercalcaemia and its nephropathy (probably hypersensitivity to vitamin D)

Mikulicz's syndrome (diffuse swelling of lachrymal and salivary glands with conditions such as sarcoidosis, lymphoma or leukaemia — p. 510)

Cardiomyopathy (clinical evidence rare; there may be arrythmias or heart block; cor pulmonale is more likely to be the cardiac consequence)

Chronic arthritis

Hypersplenism if sufficient splenomegaly

Infiltration of old scars by sarcoid tissue

Polymyositis (progressive muscle wasting).

Hepatic granulomata can be found in two-thirds of patients with sarcoidosis (symptoms rare). Sarcoidosis may affect most tissues.

---

* *Other skin lesions*: multiple scattered maculopapular or papular lesions, 0.5–1 cm, yellowish brown or purple, that occur mainly on the face and extremities. Larger, brownish–purple plaques with annular, polycyclic or serpiginous margins, and central atrophy, also occur mainly on the extremities, buttocks and trunk. Sarcoid granulomata tend to infiltrate old scars, as translucent, purple or yellowish papules and nodules. On the scalp, sarcoidosis may cause scarring alopecia with brownish infiltration of the scarred tissue.

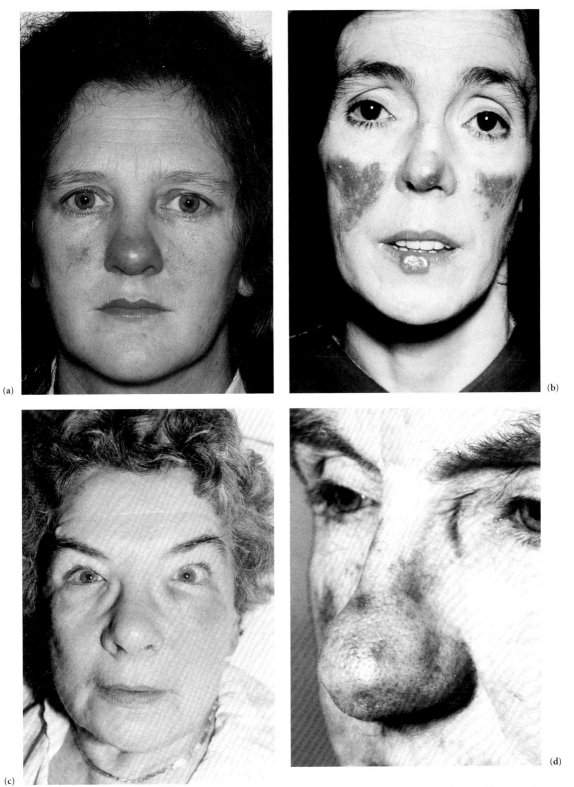

Figure C5.15 (a,b) Lupus pernio on cheeks, nose and lip. (c) Lesions under the eyes especially on the left. (d) A close-up of lupus pernio on the nose. The treated case may just show a faint purplish discoloration on the end of the nose or cheeks.

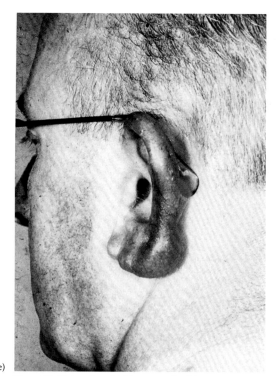

(e)

Figure C5.15 (*continued*) (e) Lupus pernio of the ear.

Case 20 | **Tinea**

Frequency in survey: main focus of a short case in 2% of attempts at PACES station 5, skin.

Record 1

There is a well-defined, *annular, erythematous plaque* with *central clearing* on the *face* and *scalp* (can be on the trunk or limbs). The *erythema* and papular lesions with *fine scaling* are more *pronounced* in the *periphery of the plaque.**

    This is tinea capitis caused by a fungal (dermatophyte) infection of the keratin.

Record 2

The *palms* of this patient are *erythematous* with *exaggerated creases* and *hyperkeratosis.* There is characteristic *powdery, dry scaling* in the creases. There may be similar changes on the soles (ask to examine the feet).

    The appearance is characteristic of chronic dermatophyte infection (tinea) of the hands.

Record 3

There are widespread but *well-demarcated, erythematous plaques* in both *groins* spreading over the thighs (look over the abdomen for contiguous spread) with *scaling in the periphery.* There is some *clearing* in the *centre.*

    This is tinea of the groins (cruris).

Record 4

The skin between the fourth and fifth toes (commonest site of infection) is *soggy* and *macerated* with *fine scaling.*

    This is tinea pedis, also known as athlete's foot.†

Dermatophyte infections (ringworm) are either transmitted to humans by animals (zoophilic) or from person to person (anthrophilic fungi). Dermatophytes invade keratin only, live on dead tissue and cause inflammation by their metabolic products and/or by delayed hypersensitivity. The sites of predilection are the trunk (tinea corporis), scalp (tinea capitis), groins (tinea cruris), hands, feet, fingernails and toenails.

Diagnosis

The appearances are sufficiently characteristic for a clinical diagnosis to be made, though the lesion may have to be distinguished from eczema, psoriasis, erythrasma, interdigital intertrigo and granuloma annulare. Microscopic examination of a skin scraping, nail clipping or a plucked hair can provide confirmatory evidence.

Treatment

Local application of one of the imidazole preparations such as miconazole may be all that is necessary for tinea of the trunk, hands and feet. Systemic treatment with griseofulvin or terbinafine is often needed for tinea of the scalp and of the nails, and for widespread or chronic infection of the skin that has not responded to local measures.

* The lesions expand slowly outwards and healing in the centre leaves a ring-like pattern, hence the name ringworm.

† This is the commonest type of fungal infection in humans. The sharing of wash places and swimming pools predisposes to infection, which is often aggravated by occlusive footwear.

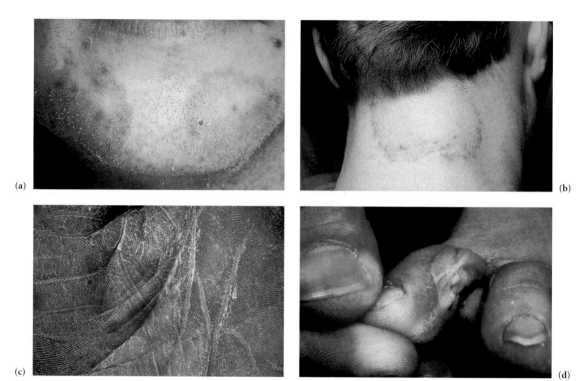

Figure C5.16 (a) Tinea of the face: annular, erythematous border. (b) Tinea of the neck: note central clearing. (c) Tinea of the hand: prominent creases with powdery scales. (d) Tinea of the toes.

Case 21 | **Koilonychia**

Frequency in survey: main focus of a short case in 2% of attempts at PACES station 5, skin.

Record
The nails are *thin*, *concave* and *spoon-shaped* with *everted edges* in this patient who also has *pallor* of the *skin* and *conjunctiva* (check for this).

This is koilonychia associated with iron deficiency anaemia.

Koilonychia is common in infancy as a benign feature. In adults it has a familial pattern and is most commonly associated with iron deficiency anaemia and haemochromatosis. All fingers and toes may be affected; most prominently the thumb or the great toe, which are sometimes the only nails that show the characteristic appearance.

Causes of koilonychia
Hereditary and congenital forms
Ectodermal dysplasia
Adenoma sebaceum
Osteo-onychodysplasia (the nail–patella syndrome).

Acquired forms
Iron deficiency states (e.g. Plummer–Vinson syndrome, polycythaemia rubra vera)
Some haematological conditions (e.g. haemoglobinopathy, haemochromatosis)
Infections (e.g. fungal diseases)
Endocrine disorders (e.g. acromegaly, hypothyroidism)
Traumatic
Malnutrition
Dermatoses (e.g. lichen planus, psoriasis, acanthosis nigricans)
Connective tissue diseases
Carpal tunnel syndrome.

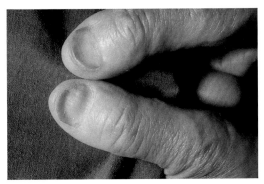

Figure C5.17 Koilonychia.

Case 22 | Raynaud's phenomenon

Frequency in survey: main focus of a short case in 0.5% of attempts at PACES station 5, skin. Additional feature in a further 2% of station 5, locomotor.

Record

The *fingers* are *cold* and *cyanosed** with (maybe) *atrophy* of the *finger pulps* (and in severe cases gangrene of the fingertips).

The patient is likely to have Raynaud's phenomenon (now look for features of underlying connective tissue diseases, especially systemic sclerosis).

Causes of Raynaud's phenomenon

1 Idiopathic Raynaud's disease* (common, especially in young females, thumbs often spared, starts in childhood, usually benign)
2 Vibrating tools (e.g. pneumatic drills, polishing tools)
3 Systemic sclerosis (Raynaud's may be the first symptom; ?smooth, tight, shiny skin on the hands and face, typical mask-like facies, telangiectasia, etc. — p. 393)
4 Other connective tissue disorders (especially mixed connective tissue disease but also SLE, polymyositis, Sjögren's syndrome and rheumatoid arthritis)
5 Cervical rib (?supraclavicular bruit, ipsilateral diminished radial pulse especially during a Raynaud's attack, wasting of the small muscles of the hand and C8/T1 sensory impairment though neurological signs of cervical rib are often minimal if vascular signs are prominent).

Other causes

Cold agglutinins
Cryoglobulinaemia
Hypothyroidism
Heavy metal poisoning.

Women who develop toxaemia of pregnancy are more likely to have a history of Raynaud's disease (suggesting an abnormal vascular reactivity or unidentified humoral agent underlying both conditions).

Treatment

Hand warmers, vasodilators both oral (calcium-channel blockers, ACE inhibitors) and, if necessary, parenteral (prostacyclin analogues and calcitonin gene-related peptide). In severe cases, lumbar (feet) and digital sympathectomy may help.

---

* In idiopathic Raynaud's disease the arteries show an exaggerated physiological response to cold and go into intense spasm to produce numb, dead-white fingers. With rewarming the classic colour sequence is white to blue (cyanosis) then blue to red (rebound hyperaemia which is painful). If taking a history from the patient ask about precipitating events, frequency, severity, progression, ulcers and for features of associated connective tissue diseases. The patient (usually with systemic sclerosis) in whom Raynaud's is discussed in the MRCP examination may have chronically impaired arterial circulation leading to cyanosis even in the warm hospital environment.

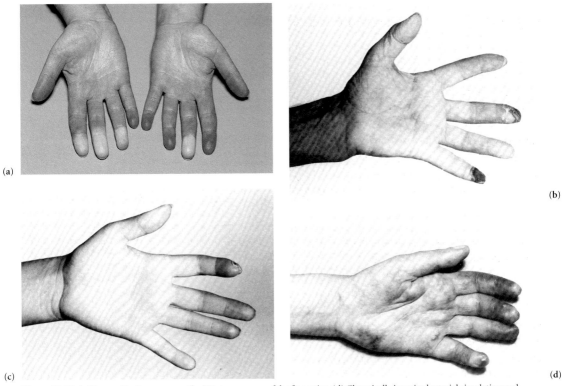

Figure C5.18 (a)Raynaud's phenomenon. (b,c) Note gangrene of the fingertips. (d) Chronically impaired arterial circulation and atrophy of the finger pulps.

Case 23 | Erythema nodosum

Frequency in survey: did not occur in the initial small survey of PACES station 5, skin.

Predicted frequency from older, more extensive MRCP short case surveys: main focus of a short case in 5% of attempts at PACES station 5, skin.

Survey note: in the original, pre PACES, survey this usually occurred as a spot diagnosis followed by questions about the possible causes. Histology was asked for on one occasion.

Record

There are in this (usually) female patient *raised* (become flat with healing) *red* (pass through the changes of a *bruise* with healing), *tender* lesions 2–6 cm in diameter on the *shins* (and occasionally thighs and upper limbs).

The diagnosis is erythema nodosum (?fever, arthralgia).

Possible causes

1 Acute sarcoidosis (bilateral hilar lymphadenopathy; fever, arthralgia, palpable cervical and axillary lymph nodes, mild iridocyclitis)
2 Streptococcal infection (e.g. throat)
3 Rheumatic fever (tachycardia, murmur, nodules, etc.)
4 Primary tuberculosis (?ethnic origin, chest signs, etc.)
5 Drugs (sulphonamides, penicillin, oral contraceptives, codeine, salicylates, barbiturates).

Other causes

Pregnancy
Ulcerative colitis
Crohn's disease
Yersinia enterocolitis
Malignancies (lymphoma and leukaemia)
Syphilis
Leprosy (important cause on a worldwide basis)
Coccidioidomycosis
Toxoplasmosis
Lymphogranuloma venereum
Behçet's disease (orogenital ulceration, iridocyclitis, etc.)
Idiopathic.

Histology

This is a classic example of septal penniculitis where the inflammation is mostly in the septa of fat, with little or no vasculitis.* These septa are thickened and infiltrated with inflammatory cells that extend to the periseptal areas of the fat lobules. The composition of the infiltrate varies with age of the lesion. In early stages, oedema, haemorrhage and neutrophils cause septal thickening, whereas fibrosis, periseptal granulation tissues, lymphocytes and giant cells are found in late-stage erythema nodosum.

---

* The idea that erythema nodosum is vasculitic in origin is a misleading one which has been passed from book to book far too long!

Treatment

The ideal treatment, though not always possible, is to identify and eliminate the cause (e.g. penicillin if a streptococcal infection is confirmed). NSAIDs are helpful. Systemic steroids are seldom necessary. Empirically, a short course of potassium iodide in a dose of 400–900 mg day^{-1} may be helpful.

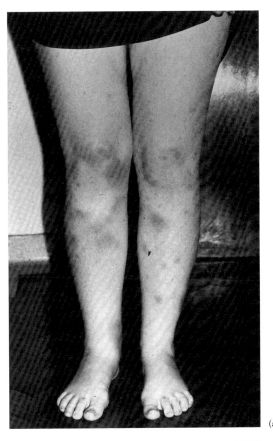

(a)

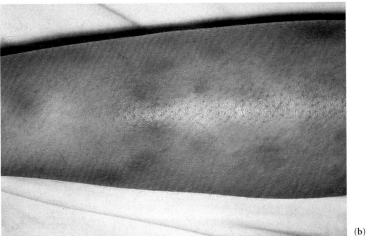

(b)

Figure C5.19 Erythema nodosum: subcutaneous swellings with erythematous overlying skin.

Case 24 | Sturge–Weber syndrome

Frequency in survey: did not occur in the initial small survey of PACES station 5, skin.

Predicted frequency from older, more extensive MRCP short case surveys: main focus of a short case in 5% of attempts at PACES station 5, skin.

Survey note: patients with unilateral and bilateral lesions were seen. One case had buphthalmos. These was discussion on the skull X-ray appearance including the site of calcification and, on one occasion, on temporal lobe epilepsy.

Record

There is a *port-wine stain* (capillary haemangioma) involving the area supplied by the first (and/or second) division of the trigeminal nerve on the R/L side (it does not cross the midline although the skin supplied by the opposite nerve may also be involved). There may be an associated ipsilateral intracranial capillary haemangioma* of the pia arachnoid with *tramline calcification* (which outlines the cortical mantle in an undulating manner) on skull X-ray and a history of *epilepsy*, in which case the diagnosis would be Sturge–Weber syndrome.†

There may be a genetic predisposition.

Congenital abnormalities may be found in the eye on the affected side:
Glaucoma (blindness frequent)
Strabismus
Buphthalmos or ox eye
Angiomata of the choroid
Optic atrophy.

If the port-wine stain is in the area supplied by the first division of the trigeminal nerve the intracranial lesion is often in the occipital lobe. A facial naevus is more commonly associated with involvement of parietal and frontal lobes. The calcification seen on skull X-ray is in the cortical capillaries. The capillary haemangioma does not contain large vessels and does not fill on arteriography. The underlying brain damage is a rare cause of infantile hemiplegia (?hemismallness) and mental retardation as well as epilepsy. Most lesions occur on the face or trunk in a dermatomal distribution. The lesion is present at birth and persists throughout life. In middle age it may darken and become studded with angiomatous nodules. Treatment is unsatisfactory but encouraging results have been obtained with careful, and time-consuming, laser therapy.

---

* Rare association with port-wine stain in real life but common in the examination!

† A phakomatosis, see footnote, p. 281.

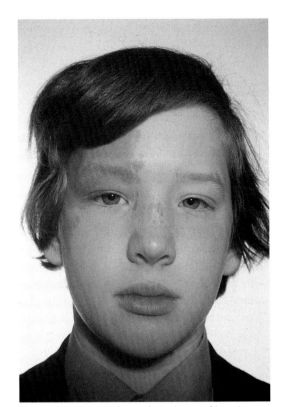

Figure C5.20 Sturge–Weber syndrome (note strabismus).

Case 25 | **Purpura**

Frequency in survey: did not occur in the initial small survey of PACES station 5, skin.

Predicted frequency from older, more extensive MRCP short case surveys: main focus of a short case in 4% of attempts at PACES station 5, skin. Additional feature in some others in all stations (Cushingoid).

Record
There is purpura.*
  Now look at the patient and note:
?Age ('senile purpura')
?Cushingoid features with thin skin (if present observe for features of underlying steroid-treated disease, e.g. asthma, rheumatoid arthritis, cryptogenic fibrosing alveolitis)
?Rheumatoid arthritis (phenylbutazone and gold as well as steroids)
?Anaemia (leukaemia, bone marrow aplasia or infiltration)
—as well as the distribution and type of purpura.

Causes of purpura
Can be divided into:
Thrombocytopenic purpura such as:
Idiopathic thrombocytopenic purpura (purpuric rash in a young female, ?spleen—may respond to steroids and/or splenectomy)
Marrow replacement by leukaemia (acute and chronic; ?spleen, nodes, liver, anaemia, oral and pharyngeal infection)
Marrow replacement by secondary malignancy (?cachexia, evidence of primary)
Marrow aplasia (idiopathic, secondary to drugs, hepatitis A or B)

Capillary defect (vascular; platelet count normal) such as:
Senile and steroid-induced purpura (purpura over loose skin areas); skin atrophy/fragility
Henoch–Schönlein purpura (children > adults; purpuric rash (a leucocytoclastic vasculitis, with appearance ranging from papular to vesiculopustular) over the extensor surfaces of the limbs particularly at the ankles and on the buttocks; associated with arthritis of medium-sized joints, colicky abdominal pains, occasionally gastrointestinal bleeding and acute nephritis; see p. 344)
Coagulation deficiency such as:†
Haemophilia
Christmas disease
Anticoagulant therapy.

---

* Purpura refers to a spontaneous extravasation of blood from the capillaries into the skin; petechiae = pin-head size, ecchymoses = large lesions. The lesions are non blanching.

† These conditions may cause ecchymoses rather than purpura.

Other causes of purpura

Other drugs (e.g. sulphonamides, chloramphenicol, thiazides)

Hypersplenism (large spleen)

Von Willebrand's disease

Infective endocarditis (?heart murmur, splenomegaly, splinters, clubbing, Osler's nodes, etc.)

Systemic lupus erythematosus (?typical rash)

Polyarteritis nodosa (?arteritic lesions)

Osler–Weber–Rendu syndrome (p. 283)

Venous stasis (ankle and lower legs; obesity or varicose veins; accompanied by progressive pigmentation due to deposition of haemosiderin)

Scurvy (NB the neglected elderly patient with ecchymoses on the legs)

Paroxysmal nocturnal haemoglobinuria

Amyloidosis (periorbital purpura)

Uraemia (pale, brownish-yellow tinge to skin)

Disseminated intravascular coagulation

Thrombotic thrombocytopenic purpura

Haemolytic–uraemic syndrome

Paraproteinaemia

Meningitis (especially meningococcal)

Septicaemia (especially meningococcal)

Viral haemorrhagic fevers

Kaposi's sarcoma

Factitious purpura

Ehlers–Danlos syndrome (p. 334)

Scarlet fever

Measles

Rubella

Glandular fever

Typhoid

Cyanotic congenital heart disease.

Investigations

These will be dictated by the clinical circumstances. For example, it may be immediately clear that the patient is on steroids and that this is the cause and no further investigation is required. If it is not clear, in addition to a full blood count and biochemical screen, protein electrophoresis (to exclude paraproteinaemia and hyper-gammaglobulinaemia) and a full coagulation screen, including measurement of fibrin degradation products, should be carried out. A bone marrow biopsy will establish the diagnosis of idiopathic thrombocytopenic purpura. A trephine biopsy of the iliac crest may be necessary if marrow aplasia is suspected. Skin biopsy will confirm a small vessel vasculitis.

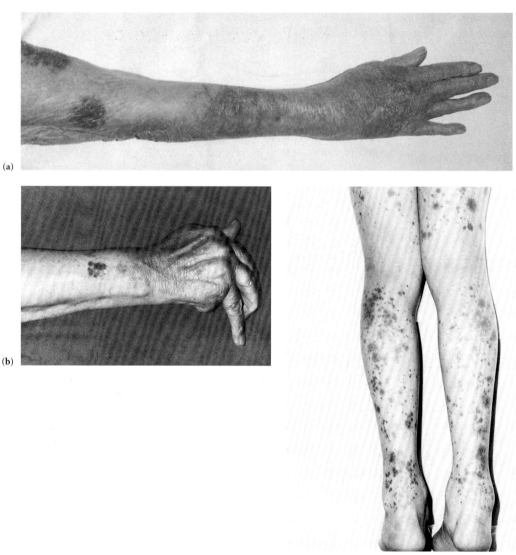

Figure C5.21 (a) Purpura from steroid therapy for rheumatoid arthritis. (b) Purpura on forearm (note rheumatoid arthritis). (c) Henoch–Schönlein purpura.

Case 26 | Peutz–Jeghers syndrome

Frequency in survey: did not occur in the initial small survey of PACES station 5, skin.

Predicted frequency from older, more extensive MRCP short case surveys: main focus of a short case in 4% of attempts at PACES station 5, skin.

Record

There are (sparse or profuse) small brownish-black *pigmented macules* (2–5 mm) (lentigines) on the lips, around the *mouth* (and/or eyes or nose) and *buccal mucosa* (but never on the tongue). They are also (may be) seen on the hands and fingers.

This pigmentation (which tends to reduce in adult life*) may be associated with *intestinal polyposis* (single or multiple polyps, which are *hamartomasta*, may occur in the small and large bowel) in which case the diagnosis would be Peutz–Jeghers syndrome.

Autosomal dominant.

Complications
Recurrent colicky abdominal pain
Intestinal obstruction or intussusception
Iron deficiency anaemia
Frank gastrointestinal haemorrhage

Malignant transformation (rare)†
Increased incidence of breast, ovarian (approximately 10% of affected women) and pancreatic cancer.

Multiple polypectomy may be required for disabling symptoms but excision of bowel is to be avoided, if possible, as polyps may recur.

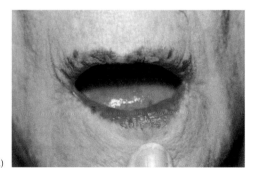
(a)

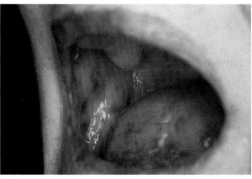
(b)

Figure C5.22 (a) Peutz–Jeghers syndrome. (b) Pigmentation of the buccal mucosa.

* Macules on the lips may disappear over time but mouth pigmentation persists, and is the *sine qua non* for the diagnosis.
† Cf. familial polyposis coli—adenomatous tumours in which malignant transformation is inevitable and for which premalignant treatment is colectomy, ileorectal anastomosis and fulgarization of remaining rectal polyps. This is followed by careful life-long 6-monthly follow-up with sigmoidoscopy and polyp fulgarization.

Case 27 | Vasculitis

Frequency in survey: did not occur in the initial small survey of PACES station 5, skin.

Predicted frequency from older, more extensive MRCP short case surveys: main focus of a short case in 4% of attempts at PACES station 5, skin. Additional feature in some others in station 5, locomotor.

Record

There are (may be) small *nail-fold* and nail-edge *infarcts* (due to small vessel vasculitis affecting the terminal digital arteries—in severe cases there may be *digital gangrene*). There is (may be) a purpuric rash (macules, papules, nodules or pustules). There are (may be) chronic leg ulcers. There is (may be) a peripheral neuropathy (due to involvement of the vasa nervorum).

This patient has vasculitis (look for obvious signs of a cause, e.g. rheumatoid arthritis, SLE).

The term vasculitis refers to a broad grouping of disorders involving the small vessels and larger arteries of the skin, either alone or in association with other organs (there is chronic inflammation in and around the vessel wall). This is usually caused by deposition of immunoglobulin and is sustained by complement activation. The clinical hallmark is *palpable purpura*.

Conditions associated with vasculitis

Rheumatoid arthritis (?hands, nodules, etc.—p. 384)
SLE (?rash, etc.—p. 416)
Polyarteritis nodosa* (medium and small arteries and adjacent veins—fever, hypertension, abdominal pain, mononeuritis multiplex, peripheral neuropathy, proteinuria, haematuria, renal failure, myocardial infarction)
Churg–Strauss syndrome (eosinophilic granulomatous vasculitis—similar to polyarteritis nodosa but asthma, eosinophilia, IgE elevation and pulmonary infiltrates are prominent; it may present as asthma)
Australia antigenaemia and vasculitis (a variant of polyarteritis nodosa)

Infectious diseases—hepatitis B and C viruses, group A haemolytic streptococci, *Staphylococcus aureus*, *Mycobacterium leprae*
Wegener's granulomatosis* (granulomatous ulceration of the upper and lower respiratory tract associated with generalized arteritis and glomerulitis)
Antiphospholipid antibody syndrome (?livedo reticularis, history of recurrent DVT, recurrent spontaneous abortion—p. 336)
Other connective tissue diseases (systemic sclerosis, etc.)
Drug reactions—sulphonamides, penicillin, serum, etc.
Infective endocarditis
Mixed cryoglobulinaemia
Hypergammaglobulinaemia
Lymphoproliferative disorders
Henoch–Schönlein syndrome (leucocytoclastic vasculitis; children > adults; purpuric rash over the extensor surface of the limbs, particularly at the ankles and often on the buttocks; associated with arthritis of medium-sized joints, colicky abdominal pains, occasionally GI bleeding and acute nephritis—p. 344)

---

* Antineutrophil cytoplasmic antibodies (ANCA) occur in two staining patterns—cytoplasmic (cANCA) and perinuclear (pANCA). High titre cANCA strongly suggests necrotizing vasculitis of the Wegener's granulomatosis type. pANCA is particularly associated with microscopic polyarteritis nodosa.

Persistent (>24 hours) urticaria (urticarial vasculitis)

Giant cell arteritis (large and medium-sized vessels; elderly patients — headache, temporal artery tenderness, polymyalgia rheumatica — danger of blindness)

Behçet's disease (oral ulcers, uveitis, phlebitis, photosensitivity, spontaneous pustules)

Thromboangiitis obliterans — Buerger's disease (young man, nicotine staining, peripheral ischaemia, gangrene, migratory superficial thrombophlebitis; see also p. 514).

Rheumatoid patients with vasculitis often have

Nodules

Circulating immune complexes

Cryoglobulins

Low complement levels

Rheumatoid factor

Antinuclear factor

Immunoglobulins and complement in the cutaneous lesions.

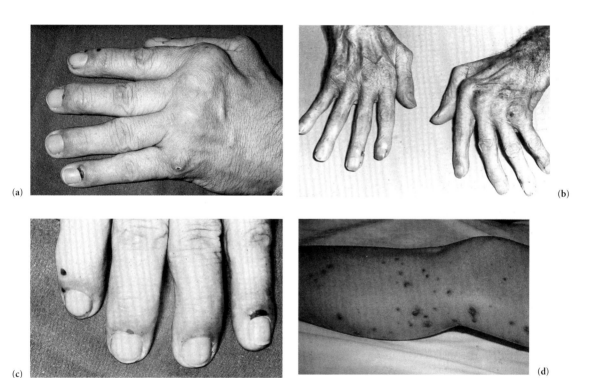

(a)

(b)

(c)

(d)

Figure C5.23 (a) Vasculitis (rheumatoid arthritis). (b) Rheumatoid arthritis. (c) Nail-fold infarcts (rheumatoid arthritis). (d) Vasculitis with 'palpable purpura' (bright red, well-demarcated petechiae with a central, dot-like haemorrhage) on the lower limb.

Case 28 | Ehlers–Danlos syndrome

Frequency in survey: did not occur in the initial small survey of PACES station 5, skin.

Predicted frequency from older, more extensive MRCP short case surveys: main focus of a short case in 2% of attempts at PACES station 5, skin.

Record

The patient (may be wearing glasses; myopia common) has *epicanthal folds*, a *flat nasal bridge* and prominent ears which point downwards. There is *hyperextensibility* of the skin which is *elastic* and *very thin*. There is evidence of *poor healing* with *thin, 'cigarette-paper' scars* (the skin tears with minor injury, usually over the knees and elbows, producing *fish-mouth* wounds). *Purpura* is present and there are (commonly) *pseudotumours* over the knees and elbows (trauma→haematoma which organizes→ fatty degeneration→calcification). The joints are (remarkably) *hyperextensible* and the patient has kyphoscoliosis, genu recurvatum and flat feet.

The diagnosis is Ehlers–Danlos syndrome.

There are at least seven distinct types which vary from mild to severe and show different patterns of inheritance (dominant, recessive, X-linked).

Complications

Bleeding (mostly from the gut)
Poor healing which makes surgery difficult
Recurrent dislocations of patellae, shoulders, hips, etc.
Recurrent hydrarthrosis
Repeated falls (poor control due to hypermobile joints), frequent skin lacerations and prominent scars — may suggest child abuse before the diagnosis is made
Diaphragmatic herniae
Diverticula of the GI and respiratory tracts
Spontaneous pneumothorax
Dissecting aneurysms
Spontaneous rupture of large arteries
Mitral valve prolapse (p. 159).

Other causes of hypermobile joints

Osteogenesis imperfecta* (p. 516)
Marfan's syndrome (tall, long bones, dislocated lens, etc. — p. 156)
Turner's syndrome (p. 456)
Noonan's syndrome (males and females; short stature, webbed neck etc. — p. 456)
Down's syndrome (p. 517)
Pseudoxanthoma elasticum (p. 299)
Familial tendency in otherwise normal patients.

Cutis laxa: in this condition the skin may also be hyperextensible, but in contrast to Ehlers–Danlos syndrome it has decreased elasticity, and hangs in loose folds. Late in Ehlers–Danlos, the skin in localized areas may resemble that seen in cutis laxa.

* Blue sclerae often occur in Ehlers–Danlos also.

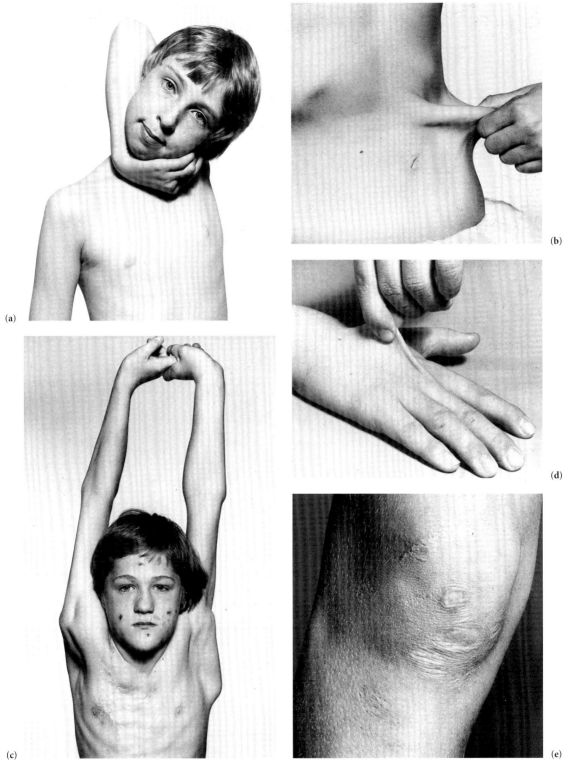

Figure C5.24 Ehlers–Danlos syndrome: (a,c) markedly hyperextensible joints; (b,d) loose hyperelastic skin; (e) thin, 'cigarette-paper' scars.

Case 29 | Livedo reticularis

Frequency in survey: did not occur in any of our MRCP surveys. Nevertheless we suspect it has occurred in MRCP, and will occur in PACES since a skin case is mandatory and it is a skin marker of a systemic problem.

(Erythema ab igne did not occur in the initial small survey of PACES station 5, skin. However it did occur in our older, more extensive, MRCP short case surveys and from this the frequency in PACES is predicted to be 2%.)

Record 1

There is (say where) an *arborescent pattern* of *reddish-blue* erythema (or pigmentary change).

The changes are suggestive of livedo reticularis. (Now if allowed ask for any history of deep venous thrombosis, transient cerebral ischaemic attacks or cerebrovascular accidents, migraine, epilepsy or recurrent abortions).

Livedo reticularis may be associated with antiphospholipid antibody syndrome (APAS), collagen vascular disease—especially polyarteritis nodosa, cryoglobulinaemia or a hyperviscosity syndrome. APAS is a hypercoagulable condition leading to both venous and arterial occlusions. Lupus anticoagulant and *anticardiolipin antibodies* are the serological markers. DVT, transient ischaemic attack, cerebrovascular accident, migraine, epilepsy and recurrent abortions may all be manifestations. Other arterial and venous thromboses may occur, as may heart valve disease. Sudden widespread organ failure may occur (catastrophic APAS). Sometimes, but not always, it may occur in the context of a connective tissue disease, particularly SLE (see p. 416). APAS (or APS) is also recognized as occurring as a primary condition (PAPS). APAS now tends to be referred to as *Hughes' syndrome*.

Other conditions which show a reticuloid pattern in the skin are erythema ab igne (see below) and cutis marmorata (a physiological reaction to cold seen in 50% of normal children and many adults).

Record 2

There is a *reticular pigmented* rash on the . . . (describe the site—usually lateral aspect of one *leg*).

It is characteristic of erythema ab igne.* (As it is due to long-term exposure to local heat, the patient obviously feels the cold. Look at the face and feel the pulse— ?hypothyroidism.)

---

* Erythema ab igne is due to repeated infrared heat injury. It can occur anywhere where heat is applied, e.g. on the back or abdomen where a hot water bottle is used over a prolonged period in an attempt to alleviate pain. The condition is common in Northern Europe ('tinker's tartan'), but rare in the USA where central heating is almost universal. In long-standing cases, premalignant keratosis and squamous cell carcinoma can develop.

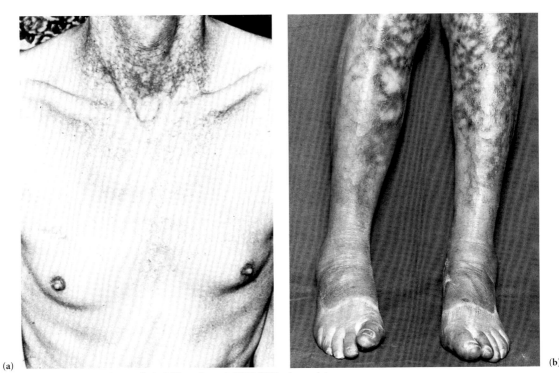

(a)

(b)

Figure C5.25 (a) Livedo reticularis visible on the neck (SLE). (b) Erythema ab igne.

Case 30 | Pemphigus/pemphigoid

Frequency in survey: did not occur in the initial small survey of PACES station 5, skin.

Predicted frequency from older, more extensive MRCP short case surveys: main focus of a short case in 2% of attempts at PACES station 5, skin.

Record 1

This middle-aged (or elderly) patient has flaccid, *thin-roofed blisters* containing serous fluid, and arising on normal skin (usually over the axillae and trunk), which vary in size (usually 1–2 cm in diameter). Most of the blisters have *burst* leaving *red* and *exuding areas* (which are extremely tender). There are also (not always) red denuded patches in the *mouth* (the first site involved in up to 50% and may precede by months the appearance of skin lesions), *pharynx* and *eyes*.

  The patient has pemphigus.

Record 2

This elderly patient has *tense blisters* (containing serous/haemorrhagic fluid, arising on normal/erythematous skin) varying in size from a few millimetres to a few centimetres in diameter involving . . . (describe where—usually it is the limbs but it can be widespread). There are also *reddened* and *urticarial* (sometimes eczematous) *patches* surrounding and separate from the blisters. There are no lesions in the mouth (they do occur but are uncommon).

  The diagnosis is pemphigoid.

Pemphigus vulgaris

This condition occurs most commonly in Jewish people. The site of the blister is in the epidermis. Occasionally lesions may occur without initial blister formation. The mucous membranes never have blisters, only denuded, painful patches. It is a progressive and fatal condition if not treated with corticosteroids in very high doses (initially 100–200 mg daily of prednisolone). Azathioprine may reduce the maintenance dose of steroid. It can be caused by penicillamine, captopril, phenylbutazone and rifampicin. In most cases the eruption resolves after withdrawal of the offending drug. There is an increased incidence in patients with thymoma and myasthenia gravis. *Acantholysis* (rounded keratinocytes floating free within the blister) is a characteristic histological feature.

Nikolsky's sign* is invariably present. Immuno-fluorescence of biopsy shows intercellular epidermal deposits of immunoglobulins (usually IgG) and/or complement factor C3.

Pemphigoid

The site of the blisters is at the basement membrane between the epidermis and the dermis; therefore the blister is thicker and less likely to rupture than in pemphigus. Mucosal lesions are less common in pemphigoid. Though it is self-limiting (2 years) systemic steroids are usually given (initially 60–80 mg day^{-1}) and azathioprine may reduce the maintenance dose. It does not have a high mortality like pemphigus. It has been alleged that it is sometimes a manifestation of underlying malignancy

---

* Firm pressure on apparently normal skin causes it to slide off. Nikolsky's sign may also occur in other severe bullous eruptions, such as toxic epidermal necrolysis.

but this point is not proven. Biopsy shows a band of IgG and complement at the basement membrane zone.

Other bullous disorders

Dermatitis herpetiformis (groups of blisters on the elbows, knees and buttocks; associated with coeliac disease—p. 356)

Epidermolysis bullosa congenita (congenital blistering disorders usually of the hands and feet; genetically determined; range from simple blisters to severe scarring with contractures; teeth and nails abnormal in some forms)

Epidermolysis bullosa acquisita (associated with inflammatory bowel disease, amyloidosis and internal malignancy)

Pemphigoid gestationis—previously called herpes gestationis (pregnancy or early puerperium, erythematous/urticarial lesions with blistering; no relation to herpes virus; resolves a few weeks after the birth; may require steroids; recurs with increased severity in subsequent pregnancies)

Hailey–Hailey disease (benign familial pemphigus, onset age 10–30 years; unrelated to pemphigus).

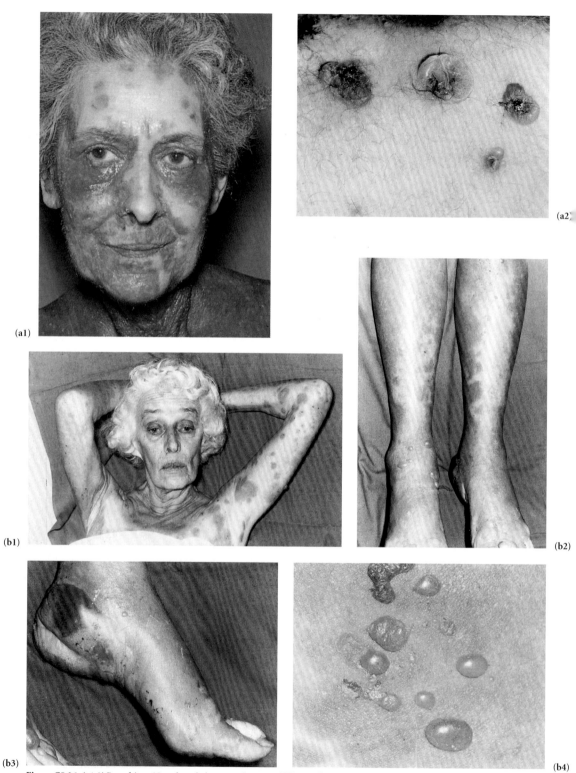

Figure C5.26 (a1,2) Pemphigus. Note denuded areas and ruptured blisters. (b1–4) Pemphigoid. Note the tense blisters.

Case 31 | Radiation burn on the chest

Frequency in survey: did not occur in the initial small survey of PACES station 5, skin.

Predicted frequency from older, more extensive MRCP short case surveys: main focus of a short case in 1% of attempts at PACES station 5, skin. Additional feature in some others in station 1, respiratory.

Survey note: usually one of many physical signs in a patient with carcinoma of the bronchus (see experience 1, vol. 2, p. 325), sometimes causing superior vena cava obstruction. Rarely other intrathoracic malignancy. Occasionally the main focus of a short case.

Record

There is an area of *erythema* on the *chest* wall. The chest has been marked (radiotherapy *field markings* or 'Red Indian' marks) for deep X-ray therapy and this (or the signs of *intrathoracic malignancy*) suggests that it is due to a radiotherapy burn (see p. 81).

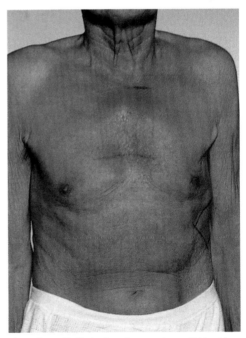

Figure C5.27 Radiation burn between the two field marks over the chest, and marks over the left lower chest wall (carcinoma of the lung).

Case 32 | Herpes zoster

Frequency in survey: did not occur in the initial small survey of PACES station 5, skin.

Predicted frequency from older, more extensive MRCP short case surveys: main focus of a short case in 1% of attempts at PACES station 5, skin.

Record

This elderly (or middle-aged) patient has *grouped and confluent papules, vesicles* and *crusted erosions* in the *area supplied by the . . . nerve* (say which/where).* The lesions are in *clusters* at different stages of development—the stages each cluster goes through is papule → vesicle → (pustule, sometimes haemorrhagic) → crusting → scar. The regional lymph nodes are enlarged.

The diagnosis is herpes zoster.

About two-thirds of patients are older than 50 years of age. Risk factors include diminishing immunity to varicella-zoster virus with advancing age, malignancy and immunosuppression from lymphoproliferative disorders, chemotherapy, radiotherapy and HIV infection (eight times more susceptible than normal subjects).

Complications

Cranial nerve palsy—especially facial nerve palsy which may occur not only with lesions of the external auditory meatus (Ramsay Hunt syndrome), but also with trigeminal zoster and zoster of the head, neck and mouth†

Peripheral motor palsy (lower motor neurone deficit from involvement of the motor root—sometimes permanent)

Post-herpetic neuralgia (10%; commoner in the elderly, approaching 40% in patients older than 60 years of age; can be very severe and difficult to treat)

Eye damage (ophthalmic zoster)

Zoster sine herpete (typical pain, etc., but no rash—serological evidence confirms).

Other complications

include visceral nerve involvement (pain or dysfunction in an organ), myelitis (transverse or ascending—rare), disseminated encephalitis (rare), cerebellar ataxia (rare) and diffuse polyneuritis (rare).

Generalized herpes zoster

is usually associated with an underlying reticulosis (especially Hodgkin's), leukaemia, HIV or carcinoma (especially bronchogenic).

---

* The commonest is a thoracic dermatome (>50%). Cranial nerve involvement is next in frequency (10–20%). The ophthalmic division of the trigeminal nerve is the commonest cranial nerve. With cranial nerve involvement there are often signs of meningeal irritation and sometimes mucous membranes are affected.

† In true Ramsay Hunt (see p. 211) the zoster is probably of the geniculate ganglion. In other cases there may be multiple cranial ganglia involvement (see anecdote 31, vol. 2, p. 364) and an associated localized encephalitis and neuronitis. Eighth nerve involvement (vertigo and deafness) is a particularly common association with facial palsy due to herpes zoster. Aciclovir given as soon as possible after the start of the infection is the treatment of choice.

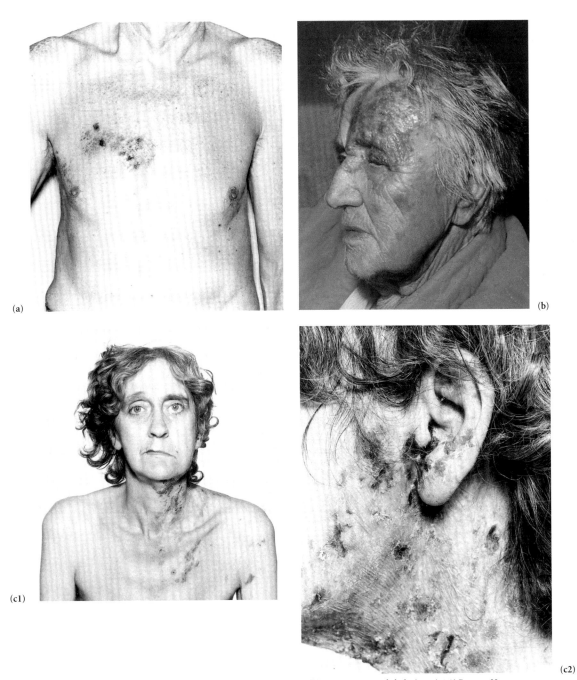

(a)

(b)

(c1)

(c2)

Figure C5.28 (a) Involvement of a thoracic dermatome (probably T3). (b) Herpes zoster ophthalmicus. (c1,2) Ramsay Hunt syndrome.

Case 33 | Henoch–Schönlein purpura

Frequency in survey: did not occur in the initial small survey of PACES station 5, skin.

Predicted frequency from older, more extensive MRCP short case surveys: main focus of a short case in 1% of attempts at PACES station 5, skin.

Record

This patient (usually a male child or a young adult) has a *palpable purpuric rash* (initially macules which rapidly urticate and become purpuric and may go on to develop central necrosis with overlying crusts) over the *extensor* surfaces of his *limbs* (usually forearms and the back of the legs) and *buttocks*.

The rash is typical of Henoch–Schönlein purpura. The patient may have other features of the Henoch–Schönlein syndrome—*polyarthralgia* (70%—large joints, usually knees and ankles), *bowel involvement* (25%—colic and haemorrhage) and *renal involvement* (30%—usually focal necrotizing glomerulonephritis).

The Henoch–Schönlein syndrome is also called *anaphylactoid purpura* or leucocytoclastic vasculitis.

Other features of Henoch–Schönlein syndrome

There may be a history of *recent infectious illness* (most commonly viral). Usually remits after 1 week but the cutaneous lesions may take several weeks to regress and the course is often punctuated by recurrent flare ups of the symptoms and/or signs

There may be self-limiting hypertension

Polyarthralgia is common but frank arthritis is rare

Colicky abdominal pain may mimic an acute surgical abdomen

Patients may experience nausea, vomiting, diarrhoea, constipation and occasionally the passage of blood and mucus per rectum. *Intussusception* may occur rarely

Renal disease typically develops within 3 months of the onset of the other systemic manifestations of the Henoch–Schönlein syndrome. It is usually only a glomerulitis with microscopic haematuria and without any significant impairment of renal function. Renal failure is rare in children. Up to 25% of adults develop a severe crescentic lesion with rapidly progressive glomerulonephritis; nephrotie syndrome occurs in 50%

Patients usually recover spontaneously and completely. Corticosteroids may lead to symptomatic improvement and should be considered in patients with renal involvement. In difficult cases colchicine or dapsone may be worth a trial, but such patients will require careful monitoring for side effects

Involved tissues, including the skin, demonstrate vasculitis with IgA and complement deposition

IgA nephropathy (*Berger's disease*) is now regarded as a monosymptomatic form of the Henoch–Schönlein syndrome with manifestations usually confined to the kidney

Histology of the biopsy shows leucocytoclastic vasculitis.

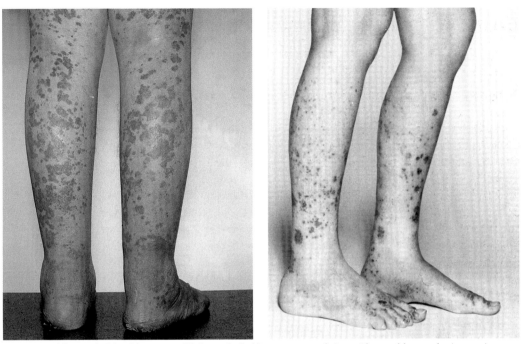

(a)
(b)

Figure C5.29 (a) Henoch–Schönlein purpura. (b) Crops of palpable purpura, some lesions with central, haemorrhagic necrosis.

Case 34 | Mycosis fungoides

Frequency in survey: did not occur in the initial small survey of PACES station 5, skin.

Predicted frequency from older, more extensive MRCP short case surveys: main focus of a short case in 0.9% of attempts at PACES station 5, skin.

Record

There are (in this middle-aged or elderly patient) erythematous, *well-defined thickened, indurated, scaly plaques* (which itch) over . . . (describe the site; can be on any part of the body though in the early stages exposed areas are often spared). There are also (may be) raised ulcerated nodules.

The appearances are suggestive of mycosis fungoides (cutaneous lymphoma*).

Males > females.

Mycosis fungoides is a T-cell (CD4+) tumour of the skin* which usually shows no evidence of visceral involvement for several years. The initial lesions may be confused with psoriasis or eczema.† They usually progress very slowly to nodules which may ulcerate. Diffuse exfoliative erythroderma may develop. Extensive nodular infiltration of the face can cause characteristic *leonine facies*. Extracutaneous involvement (especially lung, liver and spleen) does not usually become manifest for many years (though it can be found in two-thirds of patients at autopsy). Lymph node involvement suggests the likelihood of further extracutaneous spread.

Other reticuloses, for example Hodgkin's disease and leukaemia, may present as infiltrative papules or plaques in the skin diagnosed by skin biopsy.

Treatment

Treatment includes steroids, cytotoxic agents, PUVA and radiotherapy. In early stages, PUVA photochemotherapy is the most effective treatment. Topical chemotherapy in the form of nitrogen mustard in an ointment base, with or without total body electron-beam therapy, is also used with good effect. Isolated tumours should be treated with local X-ray or electron-beam therapy. For the extensive plaque stage with multiple tumours, electron-beam with chemotherapy is the recommended combination at present.

---

* Cutaneous T-cell lymphomata are lymphoproliferative disorders of helper T lymphocytes with an affinity for the skin in which atypical lymphocytes accumulate in clusters in the epidermis. They represent at least three types of lymphoma: mycosis fungoides, Sézary's syndrome and adult T-cell lymphoma (HTLV-ɪ

antibodies, hepatosplenomegaly, osteolytic bone lesions, *hypercalcaemia*).
† In fact, a high index of suspicion should be maintained in patients with atypical or refractory 'eczema' or 'psoriasis'.

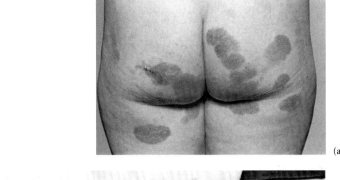

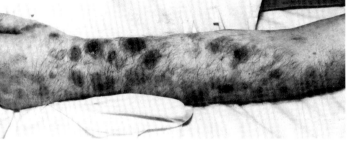

Figure C5.30 (a) Early lesions of mycosis fungoides showing well-demarcated, scaly, atrophic, erythematous patches. (b) Mycosis fungoides showing early ulceration of plaques.

Case 35 | **Morphoea**

Frequency in survey: did not occur in the initial small survey of PACES station 5, skin.

Predicted frequency from older, more extensive MRCP short case surveys: main focus of a short case in 0.9% of attempts at PACES station 5, skin.

Record 1

There is an *indurated, poorly defined plaque* under the breast (may be anywhere on the trunk, face, axillae or perineum). The lesion is multicoloured (initially violaceous, later ivory-coloured) with a central yellowish area, 2–5 cm in diameter (say how big), the surface is (may be) *smooth* and *shiny* with *no hair follicles* and *no sweat ducts*. There is (may be) a *lilac border* (diagnostic, if present). There is *hypoaesthesia* over the plaque which is adherent to deeper tissues. The plaque looks like a depressed area due to *atrophy* of the *underlying tissue.**

The appearances are suggestive of localized scleroderma.

Record 2

There is a solitary indistinct induration over the trunk (say where). The area looks *discoloured* and *depressed* and there is (may be) telangiectasis.

This is probably a small patch of solitary, localized scleroderma.

Morphoea is also known as *localized* or *circumscribed scleroderma*. The aetiology is unknown but some patients (predominantly in Europe) with classic morphoea have sclerotic skin changes due to *Borrelia burgdorferi* infection. Occasionally, morphoea develops after X-ray irradiation for breast cancer.

Lichen sclerosus is a chronic atrophic disorder characterized by a *white*, angular, *well-defined indurated* plaque or plaques, which can usually be distinguished from morphoea by its characteristic clinical and histological features.

Treatment

There is no effective treatment for morphoea. Morphoea-like lesions associated with borreliosis may be treated successfully in the early stages with parenteral penicillin or cefotaxime. The course is slowly progressive, but spontaneous remission may occur in some cases.

---

* Deep involvement may be associated with *atrophy* of *muscles* and *bone*. There may be *scarring alopecia* on the scalp. A variant of morphoea, involving the frontoparietal scalp and face usually in a linear distribution, with or without hemiatrophy of the face, is rarely seen (*en coup de sabre*).

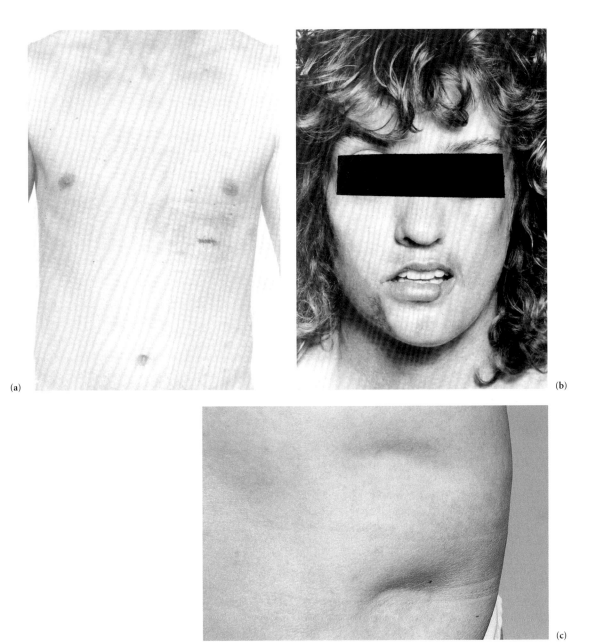

Figure C5.31 (a) Morphoea — central pale area from which a biopsy has been taken. (b) Localized scleroderma of the lower lip. (c) Depression caused by the atrophy of underlying tissues.

Case 36 | Kaposi's sarcoma (AIDS)

Frequency in survey: did not occur in the initial small survey of PACES station 5, skin.

Predicted frequency from older, more extensive MRCP short case surveys: main focus of a short case in 0.9% of attempts at PACES station 5, skin.

Record

There are (may be numerous or solitary; may be firm; are palpable even at the macular stage) reddy-purple and bluish-brown macules, plaques and nodules (may appear initially as a dusky stain, especially about the toes).

The lesions are suggestive of Kaposi's sarcoma.

Kaposi's sarcoma classically occurs in four major clinical settings:

1 African—endemic Kaposi's (extremities; 9–12.8% of all malignancies in Zaïre)

2 Elderly Jewish or Mediterranean males (purplish on distal extremities; indolent course)

3 Immunodeficiency conditions (widespread, reddish-purple papules; rapidly progressive; may regress if immunosuppression discontinued)

4 AIDS* (reddy-brown; wide distribution).

Features of Kaposi's sarcoma

Herpesvirus type 8 is thought to be involved in the pathogenesis of all variants of Kaposi's sarcoma

May also occur in the viscera

May infiltrate the lymphatics of the leg leading to chronic oedema

Associated with cytomegalovirus on electron microscopy

May complicate treatment with immunosuppression for SLE or renal transplant

Especially affects homosexual men (most commonly fourth decade): smaller lesions than non-AIDS Kaposi's. May affect viscera first.

Natural history of HIV infection

Primary infection

Leads to transient fall in CD4+ cells and may lead to opportunistic infection (usually oesophageal candidiasis) and an increase in cytotoxic CD8+ T lymphocytes

Self-limiting (2–4 weeks), febrile myalgic illness often associated with oral and oesophageal ulceration, a maculopapular rash on the trunk and elsewhere, generalized lymphadenopathy (CD8+ lymphocytes), 'aseptic meningitis-like' picture; conventional HIV antibody tests positive 2–6 weeks after onset of illness

Seroconversion at a median of 2 months after exposure, 6 months in over 95%

At least 50% progress to severe immunodeficiency over a variable period—on average 10 years

After infection, despite immune response which results in an approximately 1000-fold decrease in the amount of HIV, a slow but relentless destruction of CD4+ T lymphocytes occurs rendering the patient susceptible to opportunistic infections.

Early HIV disease (asymptomatic phase)

Attacks usually mild: generalized lymphadenopathy (B lymphocytes), irregular and unpredictable fevers, hypersensitivity reactions, reactivation or worsening of eczema, psoriasis or folliculitis. Polyclonal hypergammopathy (IgG, IgA) is usual. CD8+ titre elevated; CD4+ normal. Less common features: thrombocytopaenia; vasculitis.

Intermediate stage (AIDS-related complex)

Number of CD4+ lymphocytes starts to fall;*

---

*In HIV-infected individuals, the risk for Kaposi's sarcoma is 20 000 times that of the general population.

delayed-type hypersensitivity to common antigens (*Trichophyton*, mumps, *Candida*, tetanus, tuberculin) lost

Increased susceptibility to pathogens not usually considered opportunistic (e.g. *Pneumococcus, Shigella, Salmonella, Haemophilus*) with more serious illness

Increased vaginal thrush, pelvic inflammatory disease and cervical intraepithelial neoplasia (due to human papillomavirus infection)

Shingles more common

Kaposi's sarcoma at this stage or later.

Late phase HIV infection

Fall in CD4+ lymphocytes,* sometimes to zero, leads to profound immunodeficiency. CD8+ lymphocytes start to fall. Oral thrush common. Significant opportunistic infections depending on level of CD4+ count:

CD4+ level <300 cells μl^{-1} — reactivation of tuberculosis and syphilis

CD4+ level <200 cells μl^{-1} — *Pneumocystis carinii* pneumonia, cerebral toxoplasmosis, fungal infections (including cryptococcal meningitis)

CD4+ level <100 cells μl^{-1} — *Mycobacterium avium*

CD4+ level <50 cells μl^{-1} — cytomegalovirus retinitis, GI disease.

In late phase HIV infection, direct HIV CNS involvement may occur (dementia, myelopathy); Kaposi's may be extensive and aggressive; high grade B-cell lymphomata are more likely to occur.

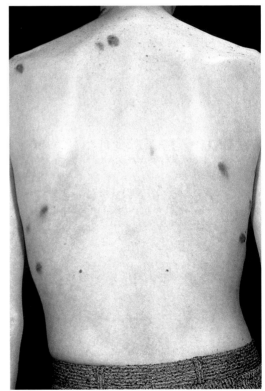

Figure C5.32 Kaposi's sarcoma: multiple, well-demarcated, purplish macules, papules and plaques.

---

* CD4+ count gives the most consistent predictive measure of the risk of progression. CD4+ <250 cells μl^{-1} or CD4+ to CD8+ ratio < 0.3 indicates 2:3 chance of progression to AIDS in the next 2 years. Oral thrush and serum HIV p24 antigen are also predictors of progression.

Case 37 | **Porphyria**

Frequency in survey: did not occur in the initial small survey of PACES station 5, skin.

Predicted frequency from older, more extensive MRCP short case surveys: main focus of a short case in 0.9% of attempts at PACES station 5, skin.

Survey note: only variegate porphyria and porphyria cutanea tarda were reported as short cases in the original, pre PACES surveys.

Record 1

There is *muscular weakness* in the upper and lower limbs particularly in the *proximal* groups. The *tendon reflexes* are *absent* (or diminished) and the plantars are flexor (or unresponsive). There are no sensory changes. The backs of the hands show *crusts, scarring*, areas of *fragility of the skin* and *blisters*.

These features suggest a diagnosis of variegate porphyria.*

Record 2

The skin on the backs of the hands shows *thin* and *traumatized areas, vesicles* and *bullae, crusts* and *scarring* and a few (say how many) *pearly white* to *yellow, subepidermal papules* or *milia*, 1–5 mm in diameter, particularly over the knuckles. There are areas of hyperpigmentation with some patches of hypopigmentation, periorbital suffusion and *hypertrichosis* over the temples and cheeks. There is one crusted lesion on the pinna of the ear, presumably a remnant of a bulla.

The features of *cutaneous fragility, photosensitivity* and *bullous lesions* suggest a diagnosis of porphyria (possibly porphyria cutanea tarda†), though one has also to consider the possibility of a pseudoporphyria.‡ A complete clinical assessment and laboratory investigations are necessary for a more specific diagnosis.

---

* *Variegate porphyria* has both the cutaneous changes of porphyria cutanea tarda and the systemic features of acute intermittent porphyria. The latter does not show photosensitivity or have any cutaneous changes.

† Patients with porphyria cutanea tarda excrete increased amounts of porphyrin into the urine, which can be demonstrated with a Wood's lamp as pinkish-red fluorescence. Freshly voided urine may look orange–red. A quick way to demonstrate orange–red fluorescence is by adding a few drops of 10% hydrochloric acid or acetic acid to the urine sample. A rapid screening test demonstrating excess porphobilinogen (PBG) in the urine can be done to diagnose acute intermittent porphyria. Freshly voided urine should be *exposed to sunlight* for several hours and a *deep red colour develops* which suggests that there is some excess

PBG. Alternatively, a *few drops* of freshly voided *urine* are added to *2 ml* of *Ehrlich's reagent* and the urine forms a *cherry-red* colour suggesting the presence of PBG. A markedly elevated faecal protoporphyrin level is diagnostic of variegate porphyria.

‡ The term *pseudoporphyria* is applied when patients clinically exhibit cutaneous manifestations of porphyria cutanea tarda without the characteristic abnormal porphyrin profile. The disorder may develop in association with certain drugs (frusemide (furosemide), tetracycline, naproxen and pyridoxine), diabetes mellitus, and chronic renal failure on maintenance haemodialysis. In the initial stages the porphyrin levels in the urine, faeces and plasma may be normal in the last condition, but some studies have reported true porphyria cutanea tarda with excess porphyrins in dialysed patients.

Acute intermittent porphyria (the skin is not affected), *variegate porphyria** and *hereditary coproporphyria* (very rare) all exhibit acute episodes, the clinical features of which may be abdominal pain, vomiting and constipation; peripheral neuropathy with weakness or paralysis; confusion and psychosis; tachycardia and hypertension.

Drugs and chemicals associated with the clinical expression of acute hepatic porphyria are ethyl alcohol, oestrogen hormones, hexachlorobenzene, chlorinated phenols, iron, etc. There is a long list of potentially hazardous drugs including barbiturates, carbamazepine, amphetamines, chloroquine, danazol, ethosuximide, frusemide (furosemide), methyldopa, sulphonamides, rifampicin, hydralazine and valproic acid.

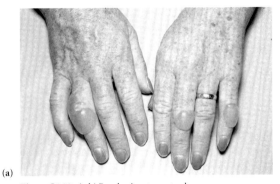 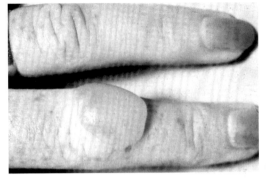

(a)

(b)

Figure C5.33 (a,b) Porphyria cutanea tarda.

Case 38 | Lupus vulgaris

Frequency in survey: did not occur in the initial small survey of PACES station 5, skin.

Predicted frequency from older, more extensive MRCP short case surveys: main focus of a short case in 0.9% of attempts at PACES station 5, skin.

Record

There is a *reddish-brown flat plaque* with irregular edges of about 5×7 cm on the R/L side of the face.* The appearance is smooth (may be hyperkeratotic in later stages) and glistening but there is *fine scaling* over the middle (look for this). The *consistency* is *soft*† and there is some *scarring* (say where).

The characteristic appearance of this plaque with scarring and its soft consistency support the diagnosis of lupus vulgaris.‡

Lupus vulgaris is a progressive form of cutaneous tuberculosis occurring in a person with a moderate or high degree of immunity. A cool, moist dull climate (as in Northern Europe) seems to favour its development, but nowadays it is rare in Europe and the USA. Lupus vulgaris is disproportionately uncommon in Eastern countries where other forms of TB are frequently seen. Its clinical presentation falls into five general patterns:

Plaque form—starts as a tiny reddish-brown, flat plaque and extends gradually with little or no scarring. There may be excessive scaling which gives it a psoriasiform appearance. The edges often become thickened and hyperkeratotic

Ulcerative form—scarring and ulceration with crusts over the areas of necrosis are the major features of this type. The lesion erodes into deep tissues and cartilages producing deformities and contractures

Vegetating forms—ulcerates, sometimes quite rapidly, producing necrosis, but there is minimal scarring. Mucous membranes may be invaded. Response to chemotherapy is excellent

Tumour-like forms—these lesions are deeply infiltrating and stand out over the surface of the skin as a group of soft, smooth nodules. Scaling and scarring are absent. In the 'myxomatous' form, large soft tumours occur, mostly on the ear lobes which become enlarged. The response to treatment may be poor

Papular and nodular forms—this is often the disseminated variety and multiple papular and nodular lesions may occur on the body ('miliary lupus'). The papulonodular lesions may be confined to the face and resemble acne.

Treatment

Standard antituberculous therapy should be given. Despite long periods of indolence, the natural course of an untreated lesion is inexorably progressive. The older the patient, the more rapid is the spread of the lesion. Spontaneous resolution may occur but leaves contractures, scars and mutilation.

---

* The lesion commonly appears on normal skin of the head and neck in about 80% of the cases in Europe. The face, particularly around the nose, is the area of predilection. The arms and legs are sometimes involved but the trunk is often spared. In India the face is affected less frequently than the buttocks and trunk.

† The lesions of lupus vulgaris are soft and this, together with the associated scarring, is the main feature that distinguishes it from the lupus pernio of sarcoidosis. If the lesion is probed, the instrument breaks through the overlying epidermis. Diascopy (i.e. looking at a glass slide pressed against the lesion) reveals an 'apple-jelly' (yellowish-brown) colour of the infiltrate.

‡ In the early stage (i.e. a small plaque/nodule on the face), lupus vulgaris may be confused with lymphocytoma, lupus pernio,† juvenile melanoma, lupus erythematosus and a 'port-wine' stain. Of these lupus pernio, and lymphocytoma are the two conditions which may have solitary lesions on the face without any other manifestations and may present a diagnostic problem. Lymphocytoma cutis is often a red, even violaceous, nodule with an indurated centre. Lupus pernio (p. 316) is usually a purple–red induration of the skin. On diascopy these lesions look a pale, brownish-red colour.

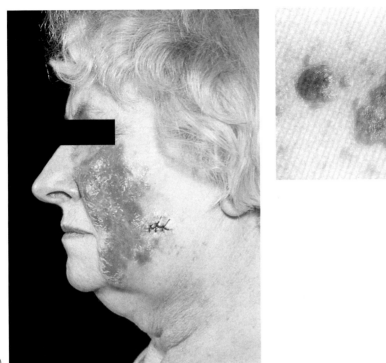
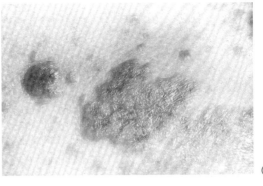

(b)

(a)

Figure C5.34 (a) Lupus vulgaris: note the glistening, transparent surface of the lesion. (b) Plaques with scaling and irregular edges.

Case 39 | Dermatitis herpetiformis

Frequency in survey: did not occur in the initial small survey of PACES station 5, skin.

Predicted frequency from older, more extensive MRCP short case surveys: main focus of a short case in 0.5% of attempts at PACES station 5, skin.

Record

This middle-aged (or elderly) patient has *groups* of *erythematous papules* and *excoriations* on the *elbows, knees, buttocks, scalp, upper back* and at *pressure points* (very occasionally it is generalized). There are (may be) *vesicles* which have (usually) a raised, reddened background (vesicles may be present but have usually been ruptured by scratching — the lesions are intensely *pruritic*).

The diagnosis is dermatitis herpetiformis and this is nearly always associated with a gluten-sensitive enteropathy* (*coeliac disease*).

Male to female ratio is 2 : 1.
About 85% of patients are HAL-B8/DRw3.

Ingestion of iodides and gluten overload may bring on an attack.

Dermatitis herpetiformis can occur at any stage of adult life (rare in childhood). Once developed it is persistent. It is treated with a gluten-free diet and/or dapsone (has a dramatic response, often within hours of starting dapsone, but side effects include rashes, haemolysis and agranulocytosis). The G6PD level should be checked before starting sulfones; methaemoglobin levels should be determined during the initial 10 weeks; and blood counts should be monitored for the first few months. The differential diagnosis is from pemphigus, pemphigoid and other bullous disorders (see p. 338) and from scabies. Involvement of the oral mucosa is uncommon. There may be a higher incidence of developing malignancies than in the general population.

Histology — subepidermal blister with microabscesses at dermal papillae.

Direct immunofluorescence (diagnostic) — IgA deposit at basement membrane (dermal papillae).

---

* There may not be overt symptoms of malabsorption, which occurs in 10–20% of patients, though an abnormal D-xylose absorption may be found in up to 70% of patients.

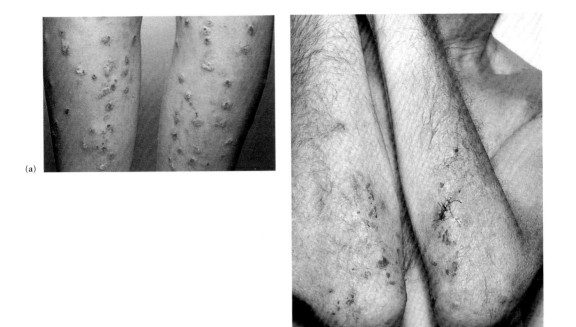

(a)

(b)

Figure C5.35 (a) Dermatitis herpetiformis. (b) Grouped lesions.

Case 40 | Urticaria pigmentosa (mastocytosis)

Frequency in survey: did not occur in the initial small survey of PACES station 5, skin.

Predicted frequency from older, more extensive MRCP short case surveys: main focus of a short case in 0.5% of attempts at PACES station 5, skin.

Record

There are *multiple*, small, discrete, round (or oval), reddish-brown (or yellowish-brown) *pigmented macules* (and/or papules). After *friction*, *rubbing* or *stroking*, *itching*, *urticarial weals* develop (due to histamine release from the mast cells — *Darier's sign*).

The diagnosis is urticaria pigmentosa.

Urticaria pigmentosa, the commonest skin manifestation, is seen in more than 90% of patients with indolent mastocytosis, and in less than 50% of patients with mastocytosis and an associated haematological disorder or those with aggressive mastocytosis.

If involvement is extensive, a hot bath followed by vigorous drying and certain drugs (alcohol, dextran, polymyxin B, morphine, codeine and NSAIDs) may lead to flushing, hypotension, bronchospasm and diarrhoea. In a minority, systemic involvement may occur with in-volvement of the liver, spleen and bone marrow. Bowel involvement may lead to malabsorption. A small percentage of patients develop leukaemia which can be, but is not usually, mast cell leukaemia.

Treatment

Drugs that may cause mast cell degranulation should be avoided (see above). Both H_1 and H_2 antihistamines and disodium cromoglycate can ameliorate itching, flushing, diarrhoea and abdominal pains.

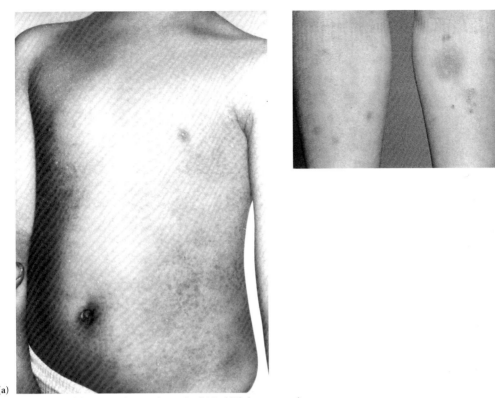

Figure C5.36 (a) Discrete pigmented macules. (b) Reddish-brown macules.

Case 41 | Tylosis

Frequency in survey: did not occur in the initial small survey of PACES station 5, skin.

Predicted frequency from older, more extensive MRCP short case surveys: main focus of a short case in 0.5% of attempts at PACES station 5, skin.

Record

There is *diffuse, thick, yellowish hyperkeratosis* of the *palms* and (ask to see the feet) of the *soles* with painful fissuring. The margins are delineated by a reddish line at the lateral border of the feet and at the wrist, beyond which there is no hyperkeratosis (does not involve the extensor surfaces). The areas are *moist* (*hyperhidrosis*) and there is (may be) evidence of dermatophyte infection.

The diagnosis is of diffuse palmoplantar keratoderma or tylosis.

Tylosis is transmitted through an autosomal dominant gene with high penetrance and occurs in all races. The condition is usually obvious by the age of 4. This is the commonest variety of hereditary palmoplantar keratoderma. Many associated disorders including *internal malignancy* (particularly of the oesophagus) have been reported, but sporadic cases occur commonly without any coexisting disorder.

A distinctive pattern, *keratoderma climactericum*, is sometimes seen in middle-aged women at the menopause. Regular chiropody attention with paring and keratolytic ointments are often helpful.

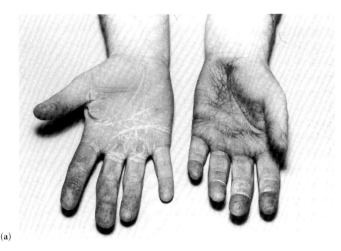

(a)

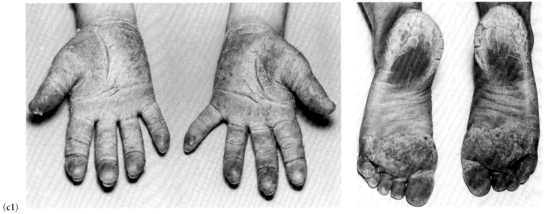

(b)

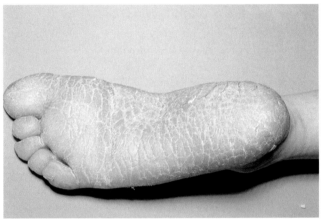

(c1)

(c2)

Figure C5.37 (a) Tylosis. (b) Tylosis—note the diffuse hyperkeratotic areas. (c) Hyperkeratosis with secondary fungal infection on (1) the palms and (2) the soles.

Case 42 | Secondary syphilis

Frequency in survey: did not occur in the initial small survey of PACES station 5, skin.

Predicted frequency from older, more extensive MRCP short case surveys: main focus of a short case in 0.5% of attempts at PACES station 5, skin.

Record

There are firm, well-demarcated round to oval papules, 0.5–1 mm in diameter, on the palms and (ask to see the feet) the soles of this patient. There are (maybe) similar lesions on the trunk, face and the legs. Scattered among the papules are some macules. Both of these lesions are pinkish-brown, and many of the papules have some fine scaling in the centre.

The differential diagnosis lies between secondary syphilis, pityriasis rosea, a drug eruption (especially captopril), tinea versicolor, lichen planus and infectious mononucleosis.*

The characteristic maculopapular (sometimes pustular, papulosquamous or acneform) lesions with scaling and their predilection for the palms and soles favour the diagnosis of secondary syphilis.

Mucosal and other associated findings

Small, asymptomatic, flat-topped, round or oval, somewhat elevated macules and papules covered with a hyperkeratotic greyish membrane, occur on the oral or genital mucosa. There may be mucocutaneous papules (*split papules*) at the angles of the mouth. About 80% of patients with secondary syphilis have cutaneous or mucocutaneous lesions. The patient may have lymphadenopathy (cervical, suboccipital, epitrochlear and axillary), splenomegaly or hepatosplenomegaly, periostitis of the long bones, diffuse pharyngitis and acute iritis. The diagnosis can be confirmed by dark-field examination and serology.

---

* In *pityriasis rosea* there is often (about 80%) a bright red, oval, 2–5 cm, *herald plaque*, with *delicate scaling, adherent peripherally* (a collarette), and a fine scaling maculopapular rash is usually scattered on the trunk in a 'Christmas tree' distribution. A *drug eruption* will mimic any rash but generally tends to be distributed symmetrically over the trunk. *Tinea versicolor* is a chronic, asymptomatic fungal infection of the *trunk* characterized by sharply marginated scaly macules which often take on a colour in contrast with the normal colour of the patient's skin. The flat-topped maculopapules of *lichen planus* (see p. 302) may be mistaken for secondary syphilis but their predilection for the wrist and the presence of characteristic mucosal lesions should help make the diagnosis.

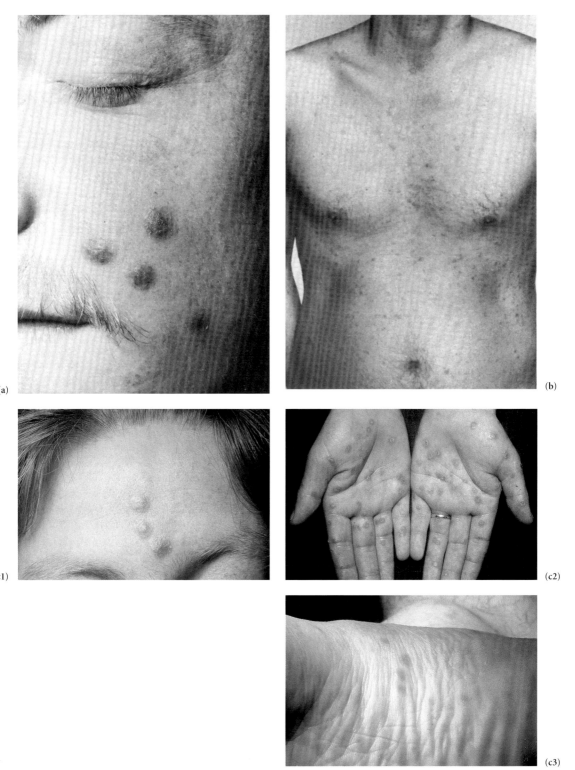

Figure C5.38 (a) Round papules with a keratotic top of secondary syphilis. (b) Scattered papules and macules (c) on the forehead (1), palms (2) and sole (3).

Case 43 | **Ectodermal dysplasia**

Frequency in survey: did not occur in the initial small survey of PACES station 5, skin.

Predicted frequency from older, more extensive MRCP short case surveys: main focus of a short case in 0.5% of attempts at PACES station 5, skin.

Record 1

The striking feature in this patient is *alopecia* with *sparse, dry, thin, spindly,* short hair. The *skin is dry* and finely wrinkled around the eyes. The nails are short, thin, ridged and brittle (ask the patient to show *his* teeth). The *incisors* and *canine teeth* are *under-developed, conical* and are *pointed.*

These features suggest that this patient has hypohidrotic ectodermal dysplasia.

Record 2

The *scalp hair* is *sparse, fine* and *brittle.* The eyebrows are (may be) absent. The *teeth* are *normal.* The *palms* and *soles* show diffuse *hyperkeratosis.* The *nails* are *short, thickened* and *discoloured.* The *skin feels moist.*

The nail dystrophy and sparse hair with normal teeth and facial appearance suggest that this patient has hidrotic ectodermal dysplasia.

Ectodermal dysplasia is a congenital condition with one or more defects of hair, teeth, nails and sweating. Two main groups are identified. Hypohidrotic (or anhidrotic) ectodermal dysplasia is X-linked (over 90% of patients are males, but female carriers may show dental defects, sparse hair and reduced sweating) and characterized by partial or complete *absence of sweat glands, hypotrichosis* and *hypodontia.* In the complete form, the facial features are distinctive with prominent frontal ridges and chin, saddle-nose, sunken cheeks, thick lips, large ears and sparse hair. Absent or reduced sweating causes heat intolerance and affected individuals may present with unexplained fevers.

The *sweat glands* are *normal* in the other main group (hidrotic ectodermal dysplasia) which is transmitted as an autosomal dominant trait. This variety is characterized by *nail dystrophy, defects of the hair* and *keratoderma of the palms and soles.*

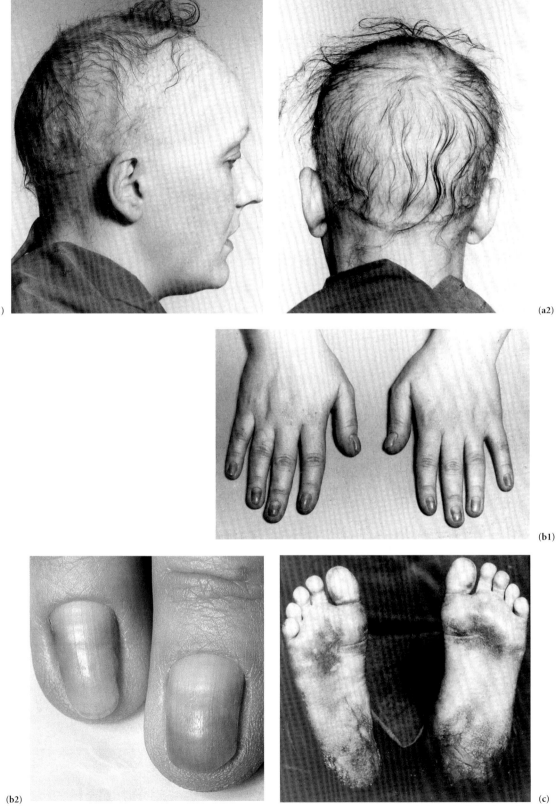

Figure C5.39 (a1,2) Hydrotic ectodermal dysplasia showing alopecia with sparse, thin, spindly hair. (b1,2) Thin, ridged, discoloured and excessively curved nails. (c) Diffuse hyperkeratosis.

Case 44 | **Partial lipodystrophy**

Frequency in survey: did not occur in the initial small survey of PACES station 5, skin.

Predicted frequency from older, more extensive MRCP short case surveys: main focus of a short case in 0.5% of attempts at PACES station 5, skin.

Record

There is *loss of fat* in the *face* and *upper half* of the body.* The prominent muscles and inframaxillary dimples give the face a characteristic masculine appearance. There is (may be) hypertrophy of fat† on the lower half of the body.

This suggests the diagnosis of partial lipodystrophy, a condition which may be associated with *renal disease.*

Male to female ratio is 1 : 5.

Usually begins in children or young adults. A history of infection, frequently measles, has often been noted prior to onset.

Retinitis pigmentosa has been reported to occur in patients with partial lipodystrophy.

Association with renal disease

Patients with partial lipodystrophy often develop progressive mesangiocapillary glomerulonephritis and hypocomplementaemia. The prognosis depends on the severity of the renal disease.

HIV-associated lipodystrophy syndrome

A curious combination of *lipohypertrophy* (buffalo hump and axial adiposity involving the neck, breast and abdomen) and *lipoatrophy* (face and proximal extremities) occurs in HIV-infected patients treated with a protease inhibitor. The pathogenesis is not clear though it is thought that it is not a drug toxicity effect and probably results from the substantial suppression of HIV in advanced patients. Carbohydrate tolerance is impaired in 16% and type 2 diabetes mellitus develops in 7% of these patients.

Total lipoatrophy

Complete loss of subcutaneous fat* may occur in children or young adults with associated diabetes, which may be difficult to treat because of extreme insulin resistance. Severe hepatic dysfunction may occur, sometimes with terminal liver failure.

---

* The lack of fat may give the appearance of emaciation, but closer inspection reveals that the muscles are not wasted, being well developed with clearly visible outlines beneath the skin. The whole appearance may give a false suggestion of virilization in females.

† The legs may be grossly fat and may give chronic discomfort.

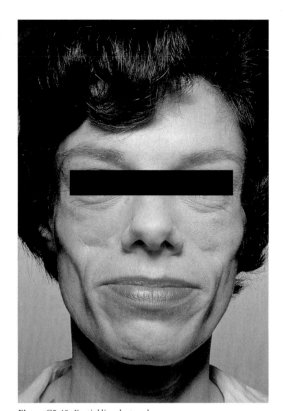

Figure C5.40 Partial lipodystrophy.

Case 45 | Fabry's disease

Frequency in survey: did not occur in the initial small survey of PACES station 5, skin.

Predicted frequency from older, more extensive MRCP short case surveys: main focus of a short case in 0.5% of attempts at PACES station 5, skin.

Record

The *skin* is *dry* and *lax*, and there is (may be) *arthropathy* of the *terminal interphalangeal joints*. There is conjunctival injection with dilated and tortuous vessels. There are groups of *darkish-red* and *black telangiectatic macules* and *papules* (*angiokeratomata*), about 2–4 mm in diameter, over the thigh (see p. 330) and around the umbilicus in this young man. The skin is somewhat roughened because of *hyperkeratosis*, and the *papules do not fade on pressure*.

These lesions are characteristic of Anderson–Fabry disease. The patient also has *superficial corneal dystrophy* (cornea verticillata) which is almost specific to this condition*

Most cases of Fabry's disease occur in males and the female carriers are mostly symptomless. The cutaneous eruption first appears at, or soon after, puberty. The prognosis is usually grave with death occurring in the third or fourth decade from a *vascular accident* or *uraemia*. Patients are often mildly *hypertensive*, and there may be *varicose veins* and *stasis oedema*. *Albuminuria*, *haematuria* and *specific lipophages* may be seen in the urine resulting from lipid infiltration of the glomerular vessels. The homozygous males have attacks of excruciating unexplained pain in their hands, TIAs and myocardial infarction.

Fabry's disease is also called *Anderson–Fabry disease* and *angiokeratoma corporis diffusum*. It is a rare hereditary disorder (X-linked recessive) characterized by a *deficiency* of the *lysomal hydrolase α-galactosidase A*, resulting in the progressive deposition of uncleaved, neutral glycosphingolipids in the small blood vessels of the skin and viscera. The characteristic cutaneous eruption (*angiokeratomata*) may be seen on the limbs, buttocks, around the umbilicus (periumbilical rosette), lower trunk and on the shaft of the penis.

---

*Superficial corneal dystrophy is frequently present both in the affected patients as well as in female carriers. It is asymptomatic but of great diagnostic importance since the only other condition resembling it is *chloroquine keratopathy*.

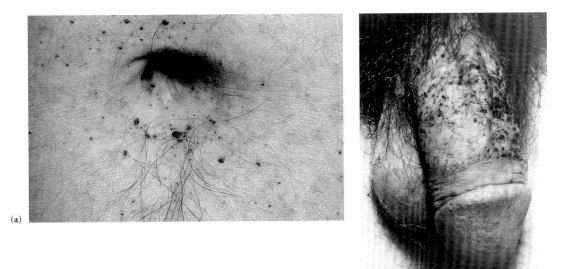

(a)

(b)

Figure C5.41 (a) Fabry's disease. Groups of fleshy macules and papules (angiokeratomata) around the umbilicus (periumbilical rosette). (b) Macules and papules with fine, keratotic crusts.

Case 46 | Reiter's syndrome/ keratoderma blenorrhagica

Frequency in survey: did not occur in the initial small survey of PACES station 5, skin.

Predicted frequency from older, more extensive MRCP short case surveys: main focus of a short case in 0.5% of attempts at PACES station 5, skin.

Record

On the *soles* of this patient's feet* and on the *palms* of his hands* there are *brownish-red macules* (early lesions), some *vesicopustules* (further developed lesions) and some crusted limpet-like masses of yellowish-brown scales (late lesions).

The appearances are those of keratoderma blenorrhagica.* If the patient has a history of *urethritis, conjunctivitis, arthritis, buccal ulceration* or *balanitis*, the combination would suggest the diagnosis of Reiter's syndrome.

The classic triad of Reiter's syndrome is urethritis, conjunctivitis and arthritis. However, it may manifest as a tetrad with the addition of buccal ulceration or balanitis to the triad; alternatively, only two of the cardinal features may be present. Classically arthropathy develops within 1 month of urethritis or *cervicitis*. However, it may follow either a dysenteric (e.g. *Shigella*) or venereal infection.

Other features which may occur

Uveitis

Balanitis may progress to *balanitis circinata* (scaling red patches evolve encircling the glans penis and within the groin)

Plantar fasciitis

Sausage-shaped digit is a typical manifestation of the arthropathy

Sacroiliitis†

Ascending spinal disease†

Nail involvement with subungual pustules that progress to onycholysis and extensive subungual hyperkeratosis with erythema surrounding the nail

Plantar spurs on X-ray

Periosteal new bone formation on X-ray

Cardiac complications similar to ankylosing spondylitis as a late manifestation

HLA-B27 may predispose

Sex distribution is difficult to define as the syndrome is diagnosed in women with difficulty because the urethritis and cervicitis are often clinically unapparent

Formes frustes of the syndrome (e.g. a woman with an inflammatory arthropathy of the knee, in association with HLA-B27, with or without uveitis, may have Reiter's syndrome)

High level of complement in synovial fluid (low level in rheumatoid arthritis)‡

About 80% of patients still have evidence of disease activity after 5 years.

---

* At times Reiter's syndrome may be confused with psoriasis as pustular psoriasis on the palms and soles looks like keratodermic blenorrhagica. Psoriatic arthropathy is also a seronegative arthropathy with an HLA-B27 association. In severely affected Reiter's patients, the skin lesions may occur anywhere on the body. The toes and fingernails in Reiter's may be affected with thickening, ridging and opacity of the nails. The skin lesions of psoriasis and Reiter's are often indistinguishable clinically or histologically. In Reiter's the lesions are typically confined to the palms and soles and the presence of urethritis, iritis or conjunctivitis, balanitis,

asymptomatic lesions on the tongue and buccal mucosa, and occasionally diarrhoea should suggest the diagnosis.

† Occasionally the diagnosis of ankylosing spondylitis and Reiter's syndrome may be difficult to disentangle. The original urethritis of Reiter's may be forgotten or the patient with ankylosing spondylitis may happen to have an unrelated episode of urethritis.

‡ The high level in Reiter's reflects a non-specific inflammatory reaction whereas the low level in rheumatoid reflects immune-complex disease.

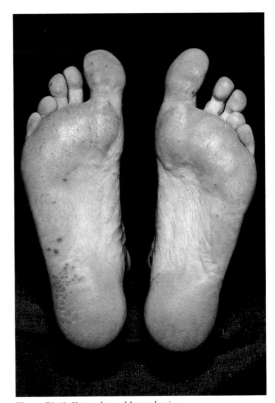

Figure C5.42 Keratoderma blenorrhagica.

Case 47 | Malignant melanoma

Frequency in survey: did not occur in the initial small survey of PACES station 5, skin.

Predicted frequency from older, more extensive MRCP short case surveys: main focus of a short case in 0.5% of attempts at PACES station 5, skin.

Record

There is a *violaceous* (or darkish-brown, reddish-brown or black)* nodule with *variegated* appearance and *irregular edges* on this patient's leg (it may also be present on the trunk or face). It is about 8 mm in diameter (measure). The shape is asymmetrical (i.e. *one half is unlike the other half*), it is unevenly pigmented* and it is elevated above the level of the skin.†

These features suggest the diagnosis of a malignant melanoma.

Diagnosis

The North American approach to the diagnosis is to use the ABCDE mnemonic: A = *asymmetry*; B = *irregular border*, C = *colour variation*, mottled, haphazard shades of brown, black, grey and white; D = *diameter > 6 mm*; E = *elevated* above the skin. A seven-point check list is used in the UK consisting of three major (the first three) and four minor criteria: (i) change in size; (ii) change in shape; (iii) change in colour; (iv) diameter more than 7 mm; (v) the presence of inflammation; (vi) oozing or bleeding; and (vii) mild itch.

Cutaneous malignant melanomata

Superficial spreading melanoma: this variety appears mostly in the fourth or fifth decade on the trunk (mostly males) or legs (mostly females). Starts as a brown macule with well-defined but irregular margins. It may be present for years before it becomes invasive. The majority of invasive melanomata are preceded by a superficial and radial growth phase, seen as an expanding, irregularly pigmented macule. It is then followed by a horizontal growth phase. As it expands and becomes palpable, it is entering a vertical growth phase. Partial regression may cause central pigment loss while extension continues peripherally

Nodular melanoma: this usually occurs in the fifth or sixth decade and the male : female ratio is 2 : 1. It presents as an elevated, dome-shaped or pedunculated nodule with reddish-brown colour. There may be a varied red central area, with only a faint brown ring of melanin peripherally. Ulceration and bleeding occur frequently. This variety of malignant melanoma is frequently confused with a vascular lesion because of its rapid growth and paucity of melanin pigment. It is a tumour in the vertical growth phase and carries a poor prognosis

Lentigo maligna melanoma: this occurs equally in males and females on sun-exposed areas, and tends to occur in the elderly. Most lesions occur on the face, commonly on the upper cheek or forehead. Initially, it is a flat, brown, stain-like lesion. This flatness with loss of skin markings is useful in distinguishing it from such lesions as actinic keratoses or seborrhoeic keratoses

Acral lentiginous melanoma (palmoplantar malignant melanoma): this represents 10% of all melanomata on white skin but almost 50% of all melanomata in Japan. The lesions are found mainly on the sole of the foot or the palm of the hand, and are characterized by a large, macular, lentiginous pigmented area around an invasive raised tumour

---

* There is usually an array of colours in a gradation of red, grey or blue and mixed with brown or black. The colour may vary from one part to the other, and from the centre to the periphery, of the tumour.

† The prognosis of malignant melanoma depends on the thickness of the tumour.

Desmoplastic melanoma: a rare variant of melanoma which may complicate any of the above, but is most commonly seen in lentigo maligna.

A pigmented naevus without any inflammation or granulation is unlikely to be mistaken for a malignant melanoma. The commonest errors occur with *benign pigmented lesions, seborrhoeic keratosis, pigmented angiomata* and *basal cell carcinoma.* In general *any change* in a *pigmented lesion* in an adult between 20 and 40 years of age should be regarded with suspicion, and any *unusual pigmented lesion* on the lower leg of a female should be examined carefully. The correct diagnosis can be made on excision biopsy.

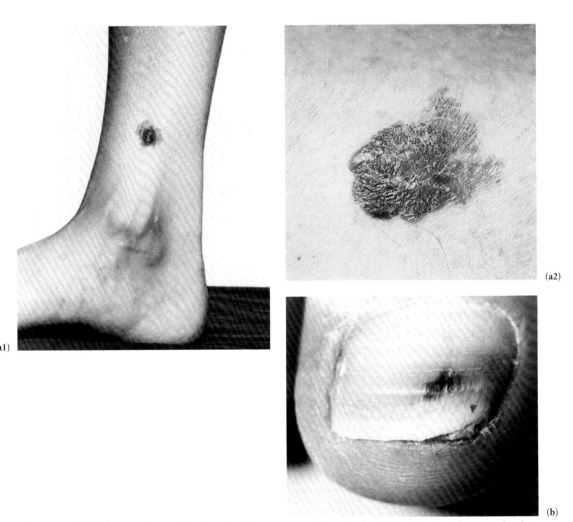

(a1)

(a2)

(b)

Figure C5.43 (a1) Malignant melanoma. Note the variegated appearance and irregular edge. (2) Irregular edge with variegated surface. (b) Subungual melanoma.

Case 48 | Acanthosis nigricans

Frequency in survey: did not occur in the initial small survey of PACES station 5, skin.

Predicted frequency from older, more extensive MRCP short case surveys: main focus of a short case in 0.5% of attempts at PACES station 5, skin.

Record

There is a soft, *velvety*, verrucous, *brown* hyperpigmentation of the body folds, especially those of the *neck, axillae* and groin.

The diagnosis is acanthosis nigricans.

Patient age under 40 years (most common)

Associated with:

*Obesity** and *insulin resistance* (high insulin levels; there may be glucose intolerance or frank diabetes, though glucose tolerance may be normal, depending on the severity of the insulin resistance; rarely insulin receptor antibodies are found)

Endocrinopathies (it is said that it may also be associated with a variety of endocrinopathies such as Cushing's disease, acromegaly, polycystic ovaries, hypothyroidism and hyperthyroidism)

May be familial.

Patient age over 40 years

May indicate:

Underlying malignancy (usually adenocarcinoma especially of the *stomach*, gastrointestinal tract and uterus; less commonly, ovary, prostate, breast and lung; rarely lymphomata. Involvement of the tongue and oral mucosa highly suggestive of malignancy. Acanthosis nigricans may appear before the malignant neoplasm becomes manifest in 20% of cases. May regress with response to therapy for the tumour and worsen again with reactivation of the tumour, raising the possibility of a humoral secretion from the tumour as the cause of the skin lesion).

Other cutaneous manifestations of malignancy
Non-genetic

Paget's disease of the breast (underlying intraductal mammary carcinoma)

Stewart–Treves syndrome (angiomatous, livid or dusky-red blebs and nodules exuding fluid indicating lymphangiosarcoma as a complication of chronic lymphoedema, especially after radical mastectomy)

Dermatomyositis (heliotrope rash around eyes and backs of hands, proximal muscle weakness — but see footnote, p. 254). Neoplasm should be suspected if the dermatomyositis is unresponsive to conventional treatment, or if there are atypical symptoms, or the patient has a history of previous malignant disease.

---

* Particular concern should be exercised over the appearance of acanthosis nigricans in non-obese adults.

The Leser–Trélat sign (sudden appearance and growth of multiple seborrhoeic keratoses in the elderly may be a sign of underlying malignancy; however there is increasing doubt about this nowadays. Multiple seborrhoeic keratoses are very common in the elderly and one needs to exercise caution in chasing internal malignancy in everyone with multiple seborrhoeic keratoses)

Necrolytic migratory erythema (associated with glucagonomata of the pancreas; gradually enlarging erythematous patches with central superficial blister formation, progressing to central crusting and healing; annular and figurate lesions result, with exudative, erosive and crusting areas especially in the perineum, groin and perioral areas; similar lesions are seen in severe zinc deficiency)

Bazex's syndrome or *acrokeratosis paraneoplasia* (red to violaceous scaling, psoriatic-like patches confined to the bridge of the nose, fingers, toes and margins of the ear helices; nail folds may be red, scaling and tender with nail grooving and onycholysis; associated with asymptomatic squamous cell carcinomata of the oral, pharyngeal, laryngeal and bronchial areas primarily in men; as the tumour progresses the rash may spread and develop, and can become very widespread)

Clubbing of the fingers (p. 312)

Hypertrophic pulmonary osteoarthropathy (clubbing in association with subperiosteal new bone formation, shafts of long bones of extremities and digits; ankles, knees, wrists and hands may be painful and swollen*)

Carcinoid erythema (eventually the flush becomes permanent and telangiectasis and tortuous veins evolve in the flushed areas — p. 125)

Urticaria pigmentosa (multiple reddish-brown or yellowish-brown macules showing Darier's sign — p. 358; may rarely be associated with myeloproliferative disorders — mast cell leukaemia, myelofibrosis, myeloid metaplasia, polycythaemia, granulocytic leukaemia)

Bowen's disease of the skin (multiple, discrete, red, scaling, flat to slightly raised patches that mimic eczematous or psoriatic patches, occurring in non-sun-exposed areas; each represents a squamous cell cancer (*in situ*); may progress to invasive squamous carcinoma if not excised; relationship to internal malignancy controversial; particularly associated with

long-term exposure to arsenicals — well water, insecticides, industrial chemicals).

Genetic

Gardener's syndrome (multiple epidermoid and sebaceous cysts of the face and scalp, fibrous tissue tumours of the skin, osteomata of the membranous bones of the face and head, and polyps of the colon and rectum; all patients develop adenocarcinoma of the bowel before the seventh decade)

Cowden's disease (numerous hamartomata of the skin, mucous membranes and internal organs; present as keratotic, warty papules and nodules on the hands, arms and central face; may be papular, cobblestone lesions on the gingiva, palate, tongue and larynx; associated with malignant neoplasms of the breast and thyroid in a high percentage of cases)

Torre's syndrome (dominant; multiple sebaceous gland tumours, sebaceous adenomata, sebaceous hyperplasia, and basal cell cancers with sebaceous differentiation; present as yellowish or red papules and nodules; associated with cancers of the colon, duodenum, ampulla of Vater, uterus and genitourinary tract)

MEN type IIb (multiple whitish to pink papular mucosal neuromata studding the lips, tip of tongue and, less often, the buccal mucosa, gingivae, palate and pharynx; neuromata on the conjunctivae and corneas; associated with medullary carcinoma of the thyroid and phaeochromocytoma — see footnote, p. 435)

Ataxia telangiectasia (recessive; telangiectasiae over the ears, eyelids, nose, butterfly facial area, and conjunctivae in association with progressive cerebellar ataxia, profound immunological deficiency and sinopulmonary infections; lymphoma develops in 10%; other malignancies may occur less frequently)

Wiscot–Aldrich syndrome (skin changes similar to atopic dermatitis; there may be petechiae due to thrombocytopaenia; widespread humoral and cell mediated immunological abnormalities; 80% have lymphoma and 15% leukaemia by the age of 10 years)

Neurofibromatosis (dominant; *café-au-lait* spots, axillary freckles, multiple neurofibromata; 10% develop phaeochromocytoma by the age of 60; acoustic neuromata and neurofibrosarcomata are also associated — p. 281)

---

* Occasionally in hypertrophic pulmonary osteoarthropathy, cutaneous thickening of the forearms and legs leads to cylindrical enlargement of the limbs. Facial features may become coarse with deep facial furrows reminiscent of acromegaly. Deep confluent skin wrinkles may evolve over the forehead and scalp, these latter features with the acromegalic features being termed *pachydermoperiostosis*.

Peutz–Jeghers syndrome (dominant; numerous brown–black macules on the lips, perioral regions and hands and feet; associated with hamartomatous polyps of the small bowel, stomach and, less commonly, colon — p. 331).

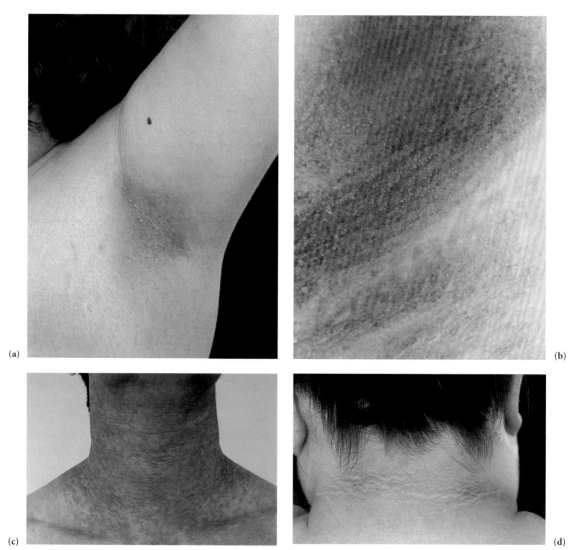

(a)

(b)

(c)

(d)

Figure C5.44 (a) Hyperpigmented, thickened fold in the axilla. (b) Note multiple verrucous lesions. (c) Marked acanthosis nigricans of the neck, and (d) less marked acanthosis nigricans at the back of the neck in an overweight female.

Case 49 | **Keratoacanthoma**

Frequency in survey: did not occur in the initial small survey of PACES station 5, skin.

Predicted frequency from older, more extensive MRCP short case surveys: main focus of a short case in 0.5% of attempts at PACES station 5, skin.

Record

There is (say where — usually *sun-exposed areas*, face, backs of hands and forearms) a *round*, firm, cherry-sized, *flesh-coloured*, shell-like *tumour* with a *central crater containing horny material*. It is well demarcated and seems to be stuck on the skin.

The likely diagnosis is keratoacanthoma.

Commoner in males (3:1); also called *molluscum sebaceum*.

Microscopic appearance is so like a low grade squamous cell carcinoma that differentiation is often impossible. In keratoacanthoma (self-healing epithelioma), however, the edge is regular, the surrounding skin is undamaged and the age of onset is younger (middle age) than in squamous cell carcinoma.

They begin as flesh-coloured papules that *rapidly grow* (unlike squamous cell carcinoma) to full size (1–2.5 cm in diameter) over a period of about 6 weeks, evolving a central keratin-filled crater. The lesions remain for about 6 or 8 weeks and then undergo spontaneous involution leaving a depressed scar.

Although spontaneous regression occurs within a few months, lesions are best excised because the scars are unsightly and because of the difficulty of differentiation from squamous cell carcinoma.

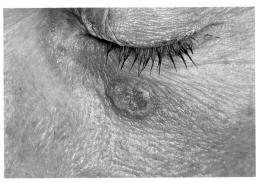
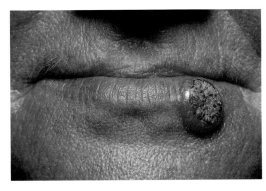

(a) (b)

Figure C5.45 (a,b) Keratoacanthoma.

Case 50 | Pyoderma gangrenosum

Frequency in survey: did not occur in the initial small survey of PACES station 5, skin.

Predicted frequency from older, more extensive MRCP short case surveys: main focus of a short case in 0.2% of attempts at PACES station 5, skin.

Record

There are large *necrotic ulcers* with *ragged* bluish-red *overhanging edges* together with areas containing erythematous plaques with pustules. They are situated . . . (describe site — usually legs but can occur anywhere on the body).*

The appearances are suggestive of pyoderma gangrenosum. The patient may have *ulcerative colitis* or Crohn's disease.

It may also be associated with *rheumatoid arthritis* and myeloproliferative disorders. Fifty per cent of patients with pyoderma gangrenosum have ulcerative colitis.† It is frequently an indicator of the severity of the disease. Healing often parallels that of the colitis and colectomy may allow this to be rapid. Systemic corticosteroids often help. The adjunctive use of minocycline may reduce corticosteroid requirements. The histopathological findings are non-specific.

Other skin manifestations of ulcerative colitis

Aphthous ulcers
Erythema nodosum
Erythema multiforme
Perianal fistulae and abscess formation
Purpura.

Other causes of leg ulcers

Venous ulceration (only 50% have superficial varices)
Ischaemic arterial ulceration (usually anterior or lateral lower leg, pain, cold pulseless cyanotic feet, shiny hairless lower legs — p. 514)
Diabetes mellitus (p. 396)
Vasculitis (rheumatoid arthritis or other connective tissue disorder)
Infection (acute pyogenic, tuberculous, syphilitic, cutaneous leishmaniasis)
Tumour (squamous cell, basal cell, melanoma)
Haematological (sickle cell, thalassaemia, acholuric jaundice, paroxysmal nocturnal haemoglobinuria)
Neurological (diabetes, tabes dorsalis, leprosy, syringomyelia).

---

* Pyoderma gangrenosum may occur as an example of *Koebner's phenomenon* in which skin diseases occur in scars or sites of trauma. It may rarely complicate surgical wounds and needs to be recognized and distinguished from infection as it responds to corticosteroids.

† Pyoderma gangrenosum can precede the onset of chronic inflammatory bowel disease.

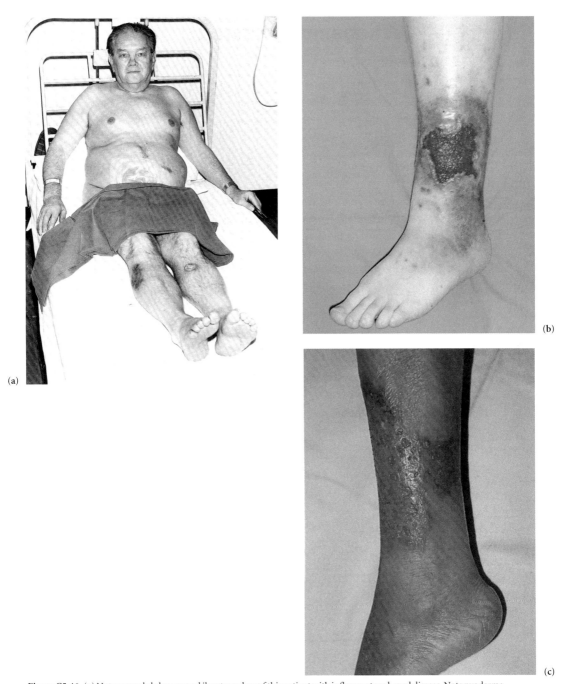

(a)

(b)

(c)

Figure C5.46 (a) Note scarred abdomen and ileostomy bag of this patient with inflammatory bowel disease. Note pyoderma gangrenosum on the legs. (b,c) Pyoderma gangrenosum. Note ragged, bluish-red edge to the ulcer.

Case 51 | **Psychogenic/factitious**

Psychogenic and factitious illnesses occur in everyday clinical practice and it would seem from the following anecdote and from those on p. 275, from our original, pre PACES surveys, that it is possible that they have also occasionally appeared in the Membership!

Anecdote

A candidate was shown a rash on a female patient. The rash was only in accessible areas and there were some bullae. He asked the patient a few question and then gave a differential diagnosis of bullous lesions. The examiners asked if there were any other causes. There was a period of silence. One examiner said 'Yes, it seems to be in accessible areas'. The candidate asked the invigilating registrar later about the case and was told that 'Apparently no one yet knows the cause!' In retrospect the candidate feels it may have been a case of dermatitis artefacta.

For discussion see p. 275.

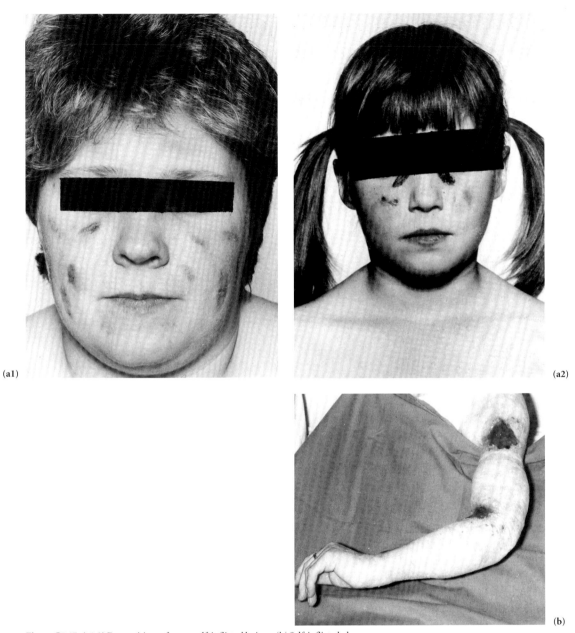

Figure C5.47 (a1,2) Dermatitis artefacta—self-inflicted lesions. (b) Self-inflicted ulcers.

Station 5
Locomotor

1 Rheumatoid arthritis
2 Psoriatic arthropathy
3 Systemic sclerosis/CRST syndrome
4 Diabetic foot/Charcot's joint
5 Tophaceous gout
6 Ankylosing spondylitis
7 Paget's disease
8 Osteoarthritis
9 Marfan's syndrome
10 Vasculitis

11 Proximal myopathy
12 One leg shorter and smaller than the other
13 Radial nerve palsy
14 Arthropathy associated with inflammatory bowel disease
15 Polymyositis
16 Systemic lupus erythematosus
17 Old rickets
18 Juvenile chronic arthritis
19 Swollen knee

Case 1 | Rheumatoid arthritis

Frequency in survey: main focus of a short case in 31% of attempts at PACES station 5, locomotor. Additional feature in some others, especially station 1, respiratory.

Record

There is a *symmetrical deforming arthropathy*. There is *spindling* of the fingers due to soft tissue swelling at the *proximal interphalangeal joints* and *metacarpophalangeal joints*. The *terminal interphalangeal joints* are *spared*. There is generalized *wasting* of the *small muscles* of the hand and use is restricted by weakness, deformity and pain. There are *nodules* at the elbow, over the extensor tendons, and in the palm. There is *ulnar deviation* of the fingers (consequent upon subluxation and dislocation at the metacarpophalangeal joints). There are arteritic lesions* in the nail folds. (The presence of erythema, warmth, pain and swelling suggests that there is active inflammation at present.)

The patient has rheumatoid arthritis.

The ratio of males to females is 1 : 3.

Other features which may occur

'Swan neck' deformity (*hyperextension of proximal interphalangeal* joint with fixed flexion of MCP and terminal interphalangeal joints)

Boutonnière's deformity (flexion deformity of proximal interphalangeal joint with *extension contracture of terminal interphalangeal* and MCP joints)

Z deformity of the thumb

Triggering of the finger (flexor tendon nodule)

Palmar erythema

Iatrogenic Cushing's (?facies, thin atrophic skin, purpura)

Swollen or deformed knees (see p. 422)

Elbow and shoulder disease

Cervical spine disease (upper cervical spine, especially atlantoaxial joint—subluxation can occur with *spinal cord compression*; a lateral X-ray centred on the odontoid peg with the neck in full flexion, shows the distance from the odontoid to the anterior arch of the atlas as abnormal at more than 3 mm—general anaesthesia is dangerous and requires extreme care in neck handling)

Anaemia (five causes†)

Chest signs (?pleural effusions; fibrosing alveolitis‡)

Neurological signs (?peripheral neuropathy, mononeuritis multiplex, carpal tunnel syndrome, cervical myelopathy)

Eye signs (episcleritis, painful scleritis, scleromalacia perforans, cataracts due to chloroquine or steroids)

Sjögren's syndrome (?dry eyes, dry mouth)

Felty's syndrome (?spleen—p. 134)

---

* As well as causing nail-fold infarcts and chronic leg ulceration, the vasculitis (p. 332), which is immune complex induced and may affect small, medium or large vessels, may also lead to digital gangrene. A purpuric rash may occur due to capillaritis. Raynaud's phenomenon (p. 322) may occur. Pyoderma gangrenosum (p. 378) is a rare cause of ulceration.

† Five causes of anaemia in rheumatoid arthritis are:

1 Anaemia of chronic disease (normochromic normocytic)

2 Gastrointestinal bleeding related to NSAIDs

3 Bone marrow suppression (gold, indomethacin, methotrexate, sulphasalazine, penicillamine)

4 Megaloblastic anaemia (folic acid deficiency or associated pernicious anaemia; see organ-specific autoimmune disease, p. 293 and footnote)

5 Felty's syndrome (p. 134)

‡ The lungs may also be affected in other ways. Rheumatoid nodules may occur in the lung fields on chest X-ray and in patients exposed to certain dusts—especially coal miners—nodules may be accompanied by massive fibrotic reactions (Caplan's syndrome). Obliterative bronchiolitis is a severe but rare complication which may be associated with penicillamine therapy.

Leg ulceration (vasculitic)*

Cardiac signs (pericarditis is present in up to 40% of patients at autopsy but is rarely apparent clinically; myocarditis, conduction defects and valvular incompetence are rare consequences of granulomatous infiltration)

Secondary amyloidosis (?proteinuria, hepatosplenomegaly, etc.—see footnote, p. 108)

Other autoimmune disorders (see pp. 438, 242 and 293).

Management
General measures
Education (patient, carer)

Exercise (affected joints, general)

Physiotherapy (electrical therapy (ultrasound or interferential); heat, cold or specific exercise techniques; joint protection in the form of splinting to prevent deformity during episodes of acute pain; advice regarding transference of load or alternative ways of performing)

Dietary advice (weight reduction, fish oil, fish supplements or evening primrose oil†).

NSAIDs
These have no effect on long-term disability but provide symptom relief. Pure analgesic agents such as paracetamol can provide pain relief and reduce the dose requirements for NSAIDs. NSAIDs reduce prostaglandin synthesis. Prostaglandins have a major role in maintaining normal body function, particularly in the gastric and renal tracts and interference with these processes leads to a variety of adverse reactions (see below).‡ Patients need to try these drugs for up to 10 days before it can be decided whether they are likely to respond.

Disease-modifying antirheumatic drugs (DMARDS)
Features include:
Adverse events (require monitoring—Table 5.2) are relatively common, though the incidence of toxicity is probably similar to that with NSAIDs

Onset of effect is usually delayed (4 weeks to 3 months)

Various mechanisms of action

Can alter laboratory markers of inflammation such as C-reactive protein and ESR

Meta-analyses of randomized controlled trials of DMARDs show a favourable benefit to toxicity ratio

with low-dose methotrexate and antimalarial drugs. Hydroxychloroquine is significantly less effective than other DMARDs but is still better than placebo

Despite this efficacy, most patients commenced on a DMARD will not be taking that particular drug 3–4 years later because of adverse drug reactions or lack of efficacy. Some patients respond initially to these drugs but their disease subsequently reactivates

Most patients are given combinations of DMARDs.

DMARDs include:
Methotrexate (the most widely used and effective; given weekly—oral or intramuscular; associated with pulmonary disease in up to 10% of patients, including opportunistic infections and pneumonitis)

Sulphasalazine (has been shown to slow joint erosions)

Gold complexes (suppresses disease activity in many patients; intramuscular gold is more effective than oral; can be used over long periods of time)

Penicillamine (now seldom used but effective in some patients; has multiple mechanisms of action)

Chloroquine and hydroxychloroquine (3–4 months before steady-state concentrations and maximal efficacy are achieved)

Other DMARDs (such as azathioprine, cyclophosphamide, chlorambucil and cyclosporin can be tried in refractory patients)

Combinations of DMARDs (may prove beneficial in some patients; cyclosporin and methotrexate or methotrexate and sulphasalazine have been shown to be superior to methotrexate alone).

Corticosteroids
Features of corticosteroid therapy in rheumatoid arthritis include:
Still commonly used

Dose of 7.5 mg/day^{-1} effective in slowing the rate of erosion

May be used as:

Continuous oral background therapy (up to 7.5 mg daily)

Short courses of a rapidly decreasing dose for disease flares

Large oral pulse doses (100 mg to 1 g)

Intra-articular injections into inflamed joints

---

† Fish oil substitutes have enabled reduction or discontinuation of NSAIDs in some patients with rheumatoid arthritis.

‡ The cyclo-oxygenase (COX) enzyme system involved in producing prostaglandins comprises two enzymes—(i) COX-1, which produces prostaglandins for normal body functions; and (ii) an

inducible enzyme, COX-2, which produces prostaglandins found at sites of tissue inflammation. NSAIDs selective for COX-2 seem to be associated with a lower incidence of gastric and renal side-effects.

Table C5.2 Major adverse effects of antirheumatic drugs

Drug	Recommended monitoring*
Antimalarials Visual disturbances, retinopathy (occasionally) Rash	Regular fundoscopy, visual field evaluation or use of an AMSLER grid (4–6 monthly)
Sulphasalazine Hepatic reactions, nausea, dizziness, rash, discoloration of urine and sweat, oligospermia	Full blood count and liver function tests fortnightly for 3 months, then 3 monthly
Gold Rash, eosinophilia, cytopenia, proteinuria, diarrhoea (oral gold)	Intramuscular — full blood count and urinalysis before and after each injection initially; urinalysis monitored by patient Beware co-administration of ACE inhibitors Oral — full blood count and urinalysis every 2 weeks to monthly
D-penicillamine Rash, proteinuria, thrombocytopenia Taste disturbances	Full blood count and urinalysis every 2 weeks on initiating or changing dose, then monthly full blood count and urinalysis
Corticosteroids Weight gain, bruising, fluid retention, susceptibility to infection, diabetes Osteoporosis	Consider annual bone density measurements
Methotrexate Hepatic fibrosis, nausea, cytopenia, pneumonitis	Full blood count and liver function tests every 2 weeks, then 1–3 monthly; liver biopsy in at-risk patients
Azathioprine Oncogenicity Cytopenia	Full blood count every 1–2 weeks initially, then 3 monthly; full blood count and urinalysis after initial weekly tests
Cyclosporin Renal impairment Hypertension	Full blood count, serum creatinine level and blood pressure measurement weekly, then every 2–4 weeks with maintenance dose
Cyclophosphamide Interstitial nephritis and haemorrhagic cystitis Oncogenicity	Full blood count and urinalysis monthly after initial weekly tests

* None of these monitoring strategies have been tested for cost-effectiveness.

Intravenous pulse therapy during a flare-up or as induction treatment at the time of commencement of DMARDs

Intramuscular injection during a flare-up

High doses should be given only to patients who demonstrate severe systemic features and/or vasculitis

Low-dose background therapy may be beneficial in maintaining mobility in patients with active disease on other DMARDs

Variety of long-term side effects (see pp. 441–45)

Antiosteoporotic therapies (calcium supplements, 1,25-dihydrocholecalciferol or bisphosphonates) should be considered in all patients on long-term (>3 months) therapy

A slow dose reduction (1 mg every month) should be tried in patients in whom disease is relatively quiescent or in whom the side effects are becoming a problem.

Biological agents
Include molecules targeted at:
The major histocompatibility complex/T-cell receptors

Cells involved in inflammation (e.g. T cells)

Cytokines (e.g. IL-1, IL-1 receptor antiagonist, TNFα, TNF receptor fusion proteins, interferon-α, IL-6, IL-10, IL-4).

Clinical trials of these agents show a variety of responses but some (e.g. with TNFα) show a dramatic improvement in symptoms and apparent halting of disease progression.

Nevertheless there is caution because of the potential for long-term side effects, possibly associated with immunosuppression, and the cost of therapy.

Potential adverse effects of NSAIDs

Gastrointestinal (common; indigestion, ulceration, haemorrhage, perforation; small bowel ulceration; stomatitis)

Renal (common; increased serum creatinine; renal failure; oedema, worsening of heart failure; interstitial nephritis; papillary necrosis)

Neurological (uncommon; headache; dizziness; nausea)

Pulmonary (rare; asthma)

Dermatological (rare; erythema multiforme or variants (Stevens–Johnson syndrome, toxic epidermal necrolysis); bullous eruptions; fixed drug eruption; urticaria)

Haematological (rare; aplastic anaemia; haemolytic anaemia (mefenamic acid only))

Hepatic (rare; hepatitis)

Systemic (rare; anaphylactoid reactions).

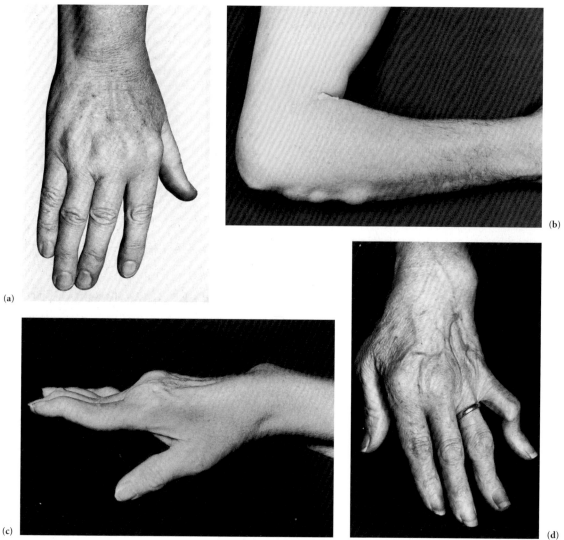

Figure C5.48 (a) Early changes—swelling of the MCP joints, slight ulnar deviation. (b) Rheumatoid nodules. (c) 'Swan neck' deformity. (d)Boutonnière deformity.

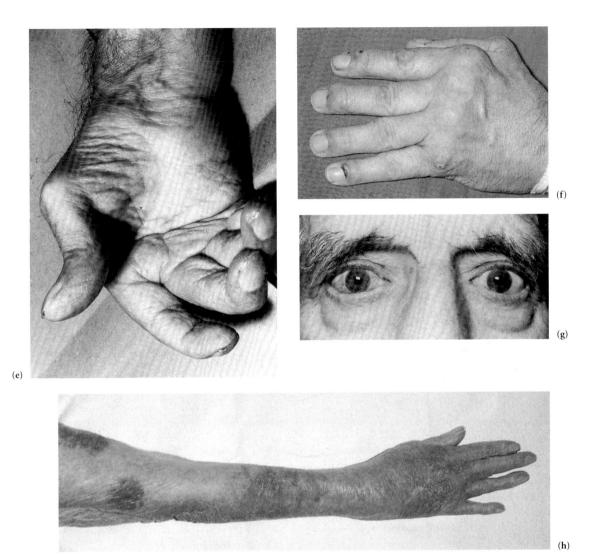

(e)

(f)

(g)

(h)

Figure C5.48 (*continued*) (e) Z-shaped thumb. (f) Vasculitis. (g) Episcleritis. (h) Purpura: steroid therapy for rheumatoid arthritis.

Case 2 | **Psoriatic arthropathy**

Frequency in survey: main focus of a short case in 12% of attempts at PACES station 5, locomotor. Additional feature in a further 1%.

Survey note: patients had arthropathy and/or skin lesions. Questions such as treatment were only occasionally asked.

Record

There is an *asymmetrical arthropathy* involving mainly the *terminal interphalangeal joints*. There is *pitting* of the fingernails and *onycholysis*. Some of the nail plates (say which) are thickened and there is a thick scale (*hyperkeratosis*) under them. There are patches of psoriasis at the *elbows*. The plaques are circular with well-defined edges and they are *red* with a *silvery scaly* surface.

The patient has psoriatic arthropathy.

Psoriatic arthropathy (even if severe) can occur with minimal skin involvement.* If there is no obvious psoriasis at the elbows the following areas should particularly be checked for skin lesions:

1 Extensor aspects
2 Scalp
3 Behind the ears
4 In the navel.

Other forms of psoriatic arthropathy

Arthritis mutilans
Arthritis clinically indistinguishable from rheumatoid arthritis but consistently seronegative
Asymmetrical oligo- or monoarthropathy
Ankylosing spondylitis occurring alone or in conjunction with any of the other forms.

Treatment

Treatments of the skin lesions include sunlight, UV light, coal tar, dithranol, local steroids, calipotriol and PUVA.

Systemic treatment with acitretin (a retinoid) or antimetabolites (methotrexate, azathioprine, hydroxyurea), because of their side effects, should be reserved for severe widespread disease unresponsive to topical measures. Analgesic anti-inflammatory agents are used for the pain of the arthropathy. Sulphasalazine and methotrexate are becoming established as effective agents for the treatment of psoriatic arthropathy. Gold and penicillamine may be useful, but few controlled studies have been done. Cyclosporin may also have a place in refractory disease. Choroquine is contraindicated as it may exacerbate the skin lesions (exfoliative dermatitis). Intra-articular steroids are useful for a single inflamed troublesome joint.

Incidence

One to 5% of Caucasians in Northwestern Europe and USA. Uncommon among Japanese, North American Indians and Afro-Americans.

---

* There is no evidence of a link between the activity of the skin lesions and the arthropathy.

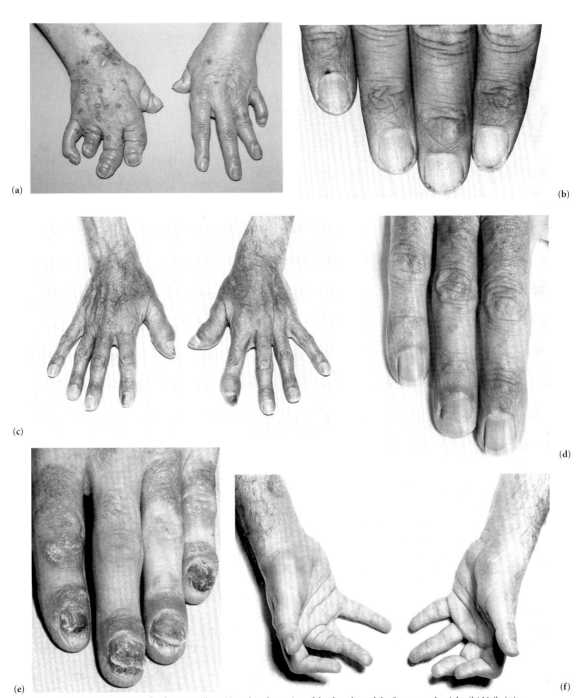

(a)

(b)

(c)

(d)

(e)

(f)

Figure C5.49 (a) Psoriasis and arthritis mutilans. Note the telescoping of the thumbs and the fingers on the right. (b) Nail pitting. (c) Terminal interphalangeal arthropathy and nail changes. (d) Onycholysis. (e) Advanced nail changes (note the psoriatic plaques and hyperkeratosis of the nail beds). (f) Note the typical plaque on the forearm and telescopic middle finger.

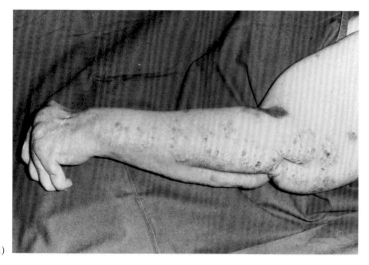

(g1)

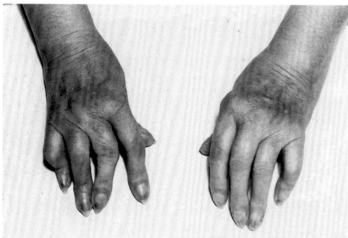

(g2)

Fig. C5.49 (*continued*) (g1,2) Indistinguishable from rheumatoid arthritis. Note plaques in (1) and nails in (2).

Case 3 | Systemic sclerosis/CRST syndrome

Frequency in survey: main focus of a short case in 12% of attempts at PACES station 5, locomotor. Additional feature in a further 1%.

Record

The *skin* over the *fingers* and *face* (of this middle-aged female) is *smooth, shiny* and *tight*. There is *sclerodactyly*, the *nails* are *atrophic* and there is evidence of *Raynaud's phenomenon* (see p. 322). There is atrophy of the soft tissues at the ends of the fingers. There is *telangiectasia* of the face and pigmentation. There are nodules of *calcinosis** palpable in some of the fingers.

The diagnosis is systemic sclerosis or CRST† syndrome.

Other signs which may be present

Skin ulcers
Vitiligo (p. 293)
Dry eyes and dry mouth (Sjögren's syndrome—p. 510)
Dyspnoea or inspiratory crackles (diffuse interstitial fibrosis‡—decreased pulmonary diffusion capacity is the first sign; overspill pneumonitis may also occur).

Other systems which may be involved

Oesophagus (dysphagia or other oesophageal symptoms are present in 45–60%; oesophageal manometry is abnormal and shows diminished peristalsis in 90%)
Kidney (renal failure occurs in 20%—it is late but often fatal; it may be associated with malignant hypertension which tends to be responsive to ACE inhibitors but is otherwise resistant to therapy)
Heart (pericardial effusion is not an uncommon finding if careful echocardiography is performed; cardiomyopathy may occur but is rare)
Musculoskeletal (inflammatory arthritis or myositis—their presence raises the possibility of mixed connective tissue disease§ and therefore increased likelihood of improvement with steroid therapy)
Intestine (rarely hypomotility with a dilated second part of the duodenum leads to bacterial overgrowth, which in turn leads to steatorrhoea and malabsorption; widemouthed colonic diverticuli, and the rare pneumatosis cystoides are other abnormalities which may occur)
Liver (may be associated with primary biliary cirrhosis—p. 121).

Management

No drug or treatment has proved safe and effective in altering the underlying disease process in scleroderma. Management includes:

General—education, counselling and family support
Contractures—exercises and lubricants may limit
Raynaud's—hand warmers, vasodilators both oral (calcium-channel blockers, ACE inhibitors) and parenteral (prostacyclin analogues and calcitonin gene-related peptide). In severe cases lumbar and digital sympathectomy may help

---

* If there is diffuse deposition of calcium in subcutaneous tissue in the presence of acrosclerosis this is termed the Thibierge–Weissenbach syndrome.
† CRST or CREST is the association of calcinosis, Raynaud's, oesophageal involvement, sclerodactyly and telangiectasia. It may be a variant of systemic sclerosis associated with a more benign prognosis.
‡ Pulmonary hypertension may develop independent of parenchymal changes, suggesting primary pulmonary vessel disease. Renal failure has now been replaced by pulmonary complications as the major cause of death in systemic sclerosis. Pleural effusions, pulmonary hypertension, interstitial lung disease, progressive pulmonary fibrosis and obstructive airways disease, all contribute to respiratory failure. Pulmonary hypertension can develop suddenly; all patients should be followed closely for the changes in P_2. The appearance of tricuspid regurgitation is evidence of established pulmonary hypertension. Aggressive vasodilatation therapy should be used to treat pulmonary hypertension.
§ Mixed connective tissue disease is a clinical overlap between systemic sclerosis, SLE and polymyositis. The serum has a high titre of antiribonuclear protein antibody. The fluorescent antinuclear antibodies are typically distributed in a speckled pattern.

Oesophageal symptoms—proton-pump inhibitors and prokinetic drugs (cisapride)

Malabsorption—low-residue diets, nutritional supplements, rotational antibiotics

Renal—intensive hypertensive control (with either ACE inhibitors or calcium antagonists). High-dose corticosteroids should be avoided and may precipitate renal crisis

Pulmonary vascular disease—vasodilators

Fibrotic process—D-penicillamine and interferon-γ are suggested therapies. The treatment of lung fibrosis has paralleled that of cryptogenic fibrosing alveolitis and has been a mixture of corticosteroids, and cyclophosphamide or azathioprine.

The efficacy of these treatments remains to be proven in placebo-controlled trials.

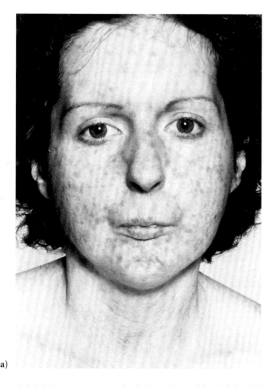
(a)

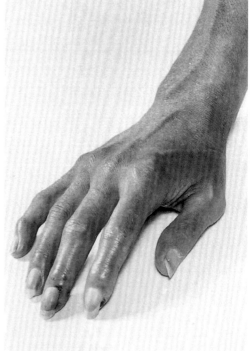
(b)

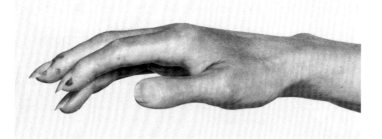
(c)

Figure C5.50 (a) Perioral tethering with pseudorhagades. (b) Tight, shiny, adherent skin and vasculitis. (c) Atrophy of the finger pulps.

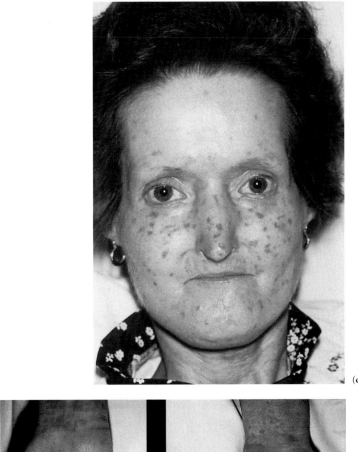

(d1)

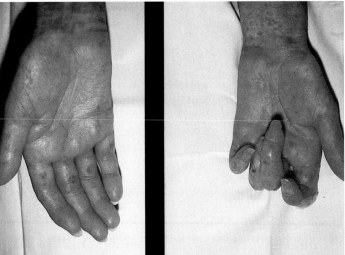

(d2)

Fig. C5.50 (*continued*) (d1,2) The face and hands of the same patient, note the tight shiny skin, pinched nose and telangiectasia.

Case 4 | Diabetic foot/Charcot's joint

Frequency in survey: main focus of a short case in 7% of attempts at PACES station 5, locomotor. Additional feature in a further 2%, especially station 3, CNS.

Record 1

There is an *ulcer* on the sole of the R/L foot (most commonly at the site of the pressure point under the head of the first metatarsal) and two of the toes have previously been amputated. There is thick *callous* formation over the pressure points of the feet, and the normal concavity of the transverse arch at the head of the metatarsals is lost. There is *loss* of *sensation* to light touch, vibration and pinprick in a *stocking distribution*. The feet are *cold*, the foot pulses are not palpable* and there is *loss of hair* on the lower legs which are *shiny*.

This patient has *peripheral neuropathy*, a *neuropathic ulcer* on the sole of his foot and evidence of *peripheral vascular disease*. It is likely that he has underlying diabetes mellitus (?fundi).

Record 2

As relevant from *record* 1, plus: the ankle joint is greatly *deformed* and *swollen*, and there is loud *crepitus* accompanying *movement* which is of an *abnormal range*.

This is a Charcot's joint (neuropathic arthropathy—gross osteoarthrosis and new bone formation from repeated minor trauma without the normal protective responses which accompany pain sensation; the joint is painlessly destroyed).

Factors which may contribute to the production of diabetic foot lesions

Injury—always a provocative factor

Neuropathy—trivial injury is not noticed

Consequent formation of callosities at repeatedly traumatized pressure points

Small vessel disease

Large vessel disease producing ischaemia and gangrene of the foot

Increased susceptibility to infection

Maldistributed pressure and foot deformity leading to increased likelihood of friction and trauma.

From the list of the other causes of peripheral neuropathy (see p. 180) **neuropathic ulcers** are particularly associated with:

1 Tabes dorsalis (?facies, pupils, etc.—p. 265)
2 Leprosy
3 Porphyria (?vesicles, crusts—p. 352)
4 Amyloidosis
5 Progressive sensory neuropathy (both familial and cryptogenic) and rarely as a late manifestation of
6 Charcot–Marie–Tooth disease (distal muscle wasting, pes cavus, etc.—p. 188).

Main causes of a Charcot's joint

Diabetes mellitus (toes—common; ankles—rare)

---

* NB In the predominantly neuropathic foot the pulses may be present or even bounding, and the veins may be prominent (Ward's sign)—autonomic denervation opens up arteriovenous shunts; as a consequence blood passes down the arteries, through the shunts and back up the veins, missing out the nutrient capillaries on the way—this contributes to the poor healing.

Tabes dorsalis (especially hip and knee; ?facies, pupils, etc.)

Syringomyelia (elbow and shoulder; ?Horner's, wasted hand muscles, dissociated sensory loss, etc. — p. 303)

Leprosy (important on a worldwide basis).

Other rare causes include yaws, progressive sensory neuropathy (familial and cryptogenic), other hereditary neuropathies (e.g. Charcot–Marie–Tooth), and neurofibromatosis (pressure on sensory nerve roots), though any cause of loss of sensation in a joint may render it liable to the development of a neuropathic arthropathy.

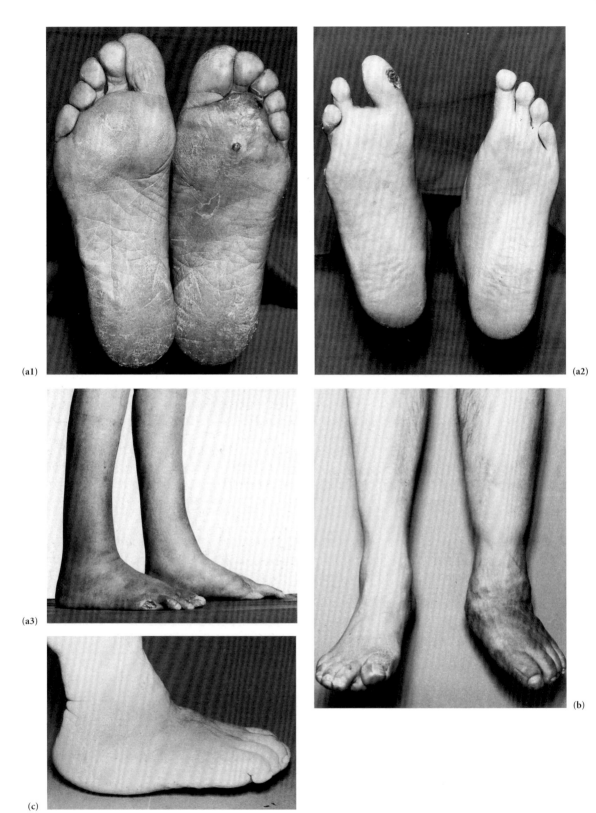

Figure C5.51 (a1–3) Note ulcers, missing digits, hyperkeratinization over pressure areas and loss of arches. (b,c) Charcot's ankle.

Case 5 | Tophaceous gout

Frequency in survey: main focus of a short case in 6% of attempts at PACES station 5, locomotor.

Record

There is *asymmetrical swelling* affecting the *small joints* of the *hands* and feet with *tophi* formation (in the periarticular tissues). These joints are (occasionally) severely *deformed*. There are tophi on the *helix* of the *ear* and in some of the tendon sheaths (especially the ulnar surface of the forearm, olecranon bursa, Achilles tendon and other pressure points).

This patient has chronic tophaceous gout.

Chronic tophaceous gout results from recurrent acute attacks. Tophus formation is proportional to the severity and duration of the disease. However, patients with severe tophaceous disease appear to have milder and less frequent acute attacks than non-tophaceous patients. Large tophi may have areas of necrotic skin overlying them and may exude chalky or pasty material containing monosodium urate crystals. Sinuses may form. Tophi may resolve slowly with effective treatment of hyperuricaemia. Effective antihyperuricaemic therapy has reduced the incidence and severity of the tophaceous disease. A major complication is renal disease (urolithiasis, urate nephropathy). Carpal tunnel syndrome may occur.

Associations include obesity, type IV hyperlipidaemia and hypertension. These associations may be the cause of an association which has also been recognized between gout and two other conditions—diabetes mellitus and ischaemic heart disease.

Secondary hyperuricaemia may occur in many situations including:

Drugs—diuretics (especially thiazides), ethambutol, nicotinic acid, cyclosporin
Myeloproliferative and lymphoproliferative disorders (and other conditions with increased turnover of pre-formed purines)
Chronic renal failure
Alcoholism
Obesity.

Treatment of gout

Acute attack

NSAIDs* (oral or suppository) or oral colchicine (effective but can cause nausea, diarrhoea or abdominal pain) are the first line treatments. Intra-articular injection of a corticosteroid or a short course of systemic corticosteroids may be used if necessary. NSAIDs should be avoided in patients with renal insufficiency, recent GI ulceration/bleeding or severe heart failure.

Allopurinol or uricosuric (probenecid, sulphinpyrazone) drugs should not be started until the acute attack has settled for 2–3 weeks because they can prolong the acute attack or trigger further episodes.

Long-term treatment

Prolonged administration of drugs that lower the serum urate level should be considered following complete resolution of the acute attack when:

there have been recurrent attacks
there is evidence of tophi or chronic gouty arthritis
there is associated renal disease
the patient is young with a high serum uric acid and a family history of renal or heart disease
normal levels of serum uric acid cannot be achieved by life-style modifications (gradual weight loss and restriction of intake of alcohol and food with a high purine content).

---

* Avoid aspirin as it causes uric acid retention unless given in very high doses.

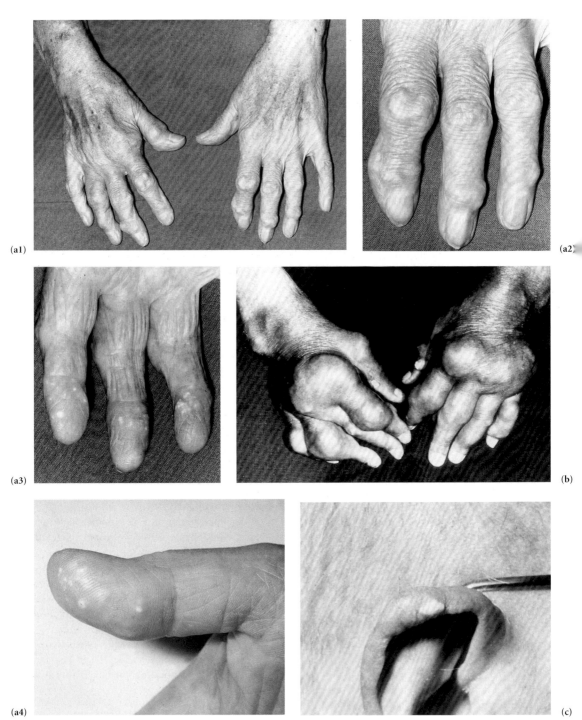

(a1)

(a2)

(a3)

(b)

(a4)

(c)

Figure C5.52 (a1–4) Gouty tophi and arthropathy. (b) An extreme case of tophaceous gout. (c) A tophus on the helix of the ear.

Case 6 | **Ankylosing spondylitis**

Frequency in survey: main focus of a short case in 4% of attempts at PACES station 5, locomotor.

Survey note: in the original, pre PACES, survey candidates were asked to examine either the chest, the back, the neck, to watch the patient walk, or to watch the patient 'look at the ceiling'. One-third of candidates made the point that the diagnosis was not apparent with the patient lying down.

Record

There is (in this male patient) *loss of lumbar lordosis* and *fixed kyphosis* which is compensated for by extension of the cervical spine (to attempt to keep the visual axis horizontal) producing a *stooped*, 'question mark' posture. When I ask the patient to turn his head to look to the side his whole body turns as a block (the spine being rigid with little movement). *Chest expansion* is *reduced*; the patient breathes by increased diaphragmatic excursion which is the cause of the *prominent abdomen*.

The diagnosis is ankylosing spondylitis. (If allowed, look at the *eyes*—iritis; listen to the *heart*—aortic incompetence; and examine the *chest*—apical fibrosis).

Ratio males to females is 8:1.

Complications and extra-articular manifestations

Iritis—30% (acute, deep aching pain, redness, photophobia, miosis, sluggish pupillary reflex, circumcorneal conjunctival injection; may result in synechiae or cataracts)

Aortitis—4% (?collapsing pulse and early diastolic murmur of aortic incompetence; ascending aortic aneurysm)

Apical fibrosis—rare (?apical inspiratory crackles; probably secondary to diminished apical ventilation; there may be calcification and cavitation; may get secondary aspergillus infection)

Cardiac conduction defects—10% (usually AV block; other cardiac abnormalities may occur—pericarditis and cardiomyopathy)

Neurological (atlantoaxial dislocation or traumatic fracture of a rigid spine may injure the spinal cord—tetra/paraplegia; involvement of the sacral nerves at the sacroiliac joints may cause sciatica; rarely cauda equina involvement can cause urinary or rectal sphincter incompetence)

Secondary amyloidosis (kidneys, adrenals, liver—?hepatomegaly).

Other features

There is a strong (87%) association with HLA-B27. There is a familial tendency; 50% of relatives are HLA-B27 and 9% have sacroiliitis, which may be symptomless.* Ankylosing spondylitis usually starts before the age of 45.† It may present as an asymmetrical peripheral arthritis usually of large, weight-bearing joints; the small joints of the hands and feet are only rarely involved.‡ It commonly presents with low back pain:

Ankylosing spondylitis—pain worse on waking, eases with exercise

Compared with

---

* The disease is more severe in sporadic cases (about 80%) than in the familial form (20%). Sibling pairs concordant for the disease tend to have disease of comparable severity.

† In the early stages, loss of lateral flexion of the lumbar spine is usually the first sign of spinal involvement, followed by loss of lumbar lordosis.

‡ Enthesitis may occur (plantar fasciitis, Achilles tenditinitis).

Mechanical back pain—no pain on waking; pain brought on by exercise.

In the *'heels, hips, occiput' test* the patient is asked to demonstrate that he can put all three against a wall at once. *Schober's test* examines lumbar mobility. While the patient stands upright with heels together, a mark is made in the midline at the level of the sacral dimples. Two additional marks are made above and 5 cm below this first mark. On full forward flexion the distance between the upper and lower mark should increase by >5 cm. Movement of <5 cm indicates decreased lumbar spine movement.

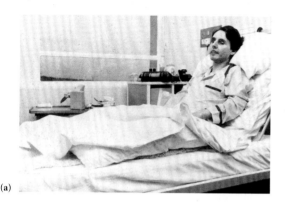

(a)

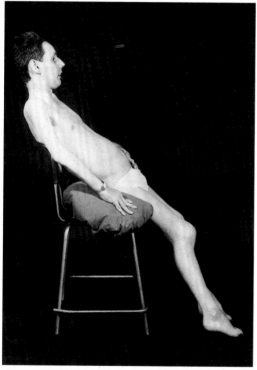

(b)

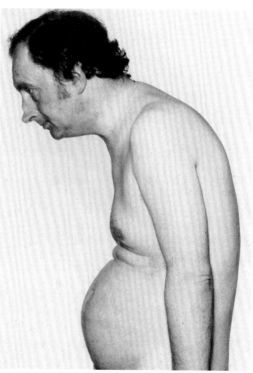

(c)

Figure C5.53 (a) The ankylosing spondylitis is less obvious when reclining in bed. (b) In the same patient as (a), a rigid and immobile spine was revealed by his attempt at sitting up (note the generalized involvement of the joints in this severe case). (c) Patient attempting to look straight ahead (note the kyphosis, loss of lumbar lordosis and protuberant abdomen).

Case 7 | **Paget's disease**

Frequency in survey: did not occur in the initial small survey of PACES station 5, locomotor.

Predicted frequency from older, more extensive MRCP short case surveys: main focus of a short case in 23% of attempts at PACES station 5, locomotor.

Record

There is (in this elderly patient) *enlargement* of the *skull*. There is also *bowing* of the R/L *tibia* (or femur) which is *warmer* (due to increased vascularity) than the other and the patient is (may be) *kyphotic* (vertebral involvement may lead to *loss of height* and kyphosis from disc degeneration and vertebral collapse).

The diagnosis is Paget's disease. (There may be evidence of complications, e.g. a *hearing aid*—see below.)

Paget's disease occurs in 3% (autopsy series) of the population over the age of 40, rising to 10% over the age of 70, though it is not clinically important in the vast majority of these. Though it is often asymptomatic, patients may have symptoms such as bone pain, headaches, tinnitus and vertigo. Serum *alkaline phosphatase* and *urinary hydroxyproline* are elevated except sometimes in very early disease. Serum calcium and phosphate concentrations are usually normal in mobilized patients but may be increased or decreased. Urinary calcium and hydroxyproline rise in immobilized patients. High serum uric acid and ESR may also occur. There is growing ultrastructural and immunohistochemical evidence that Paget's disease may represent a 'slow' virus infection in susceptible individuals—paramyxoviruses (which include respiratory syncytial virus, measles and distemper) have been implicated. Specific therapies which can be considered if indicated* include bisphosphonates, calcitonin and mithramycin.

Complications

Progressive closure of skull foramina may lead to:
1 Deafness (also results from pagetic involvement of the ossicles†)

2 Optic atrophy‡
3 Basilar invagination (platybasia causing brainstem signs).
Other complications include:
1 High output cardiac failure (?bounding pulse—occurs when more than 30–40% of the skeleton is involved)
2 Pathological fractures
3 Urolithiasis
4 Sarcoma (incidence is probably <1%; increase in pain and swelling may occur; 'explosive rise' in alkaline phosphatase occurs only occasionally).

Causes of 'bowed tibia'

True bowing due to soft bone:
Paget's disease (asymmetrical)
Rickets (bilateral, symmetrical—p. 418).
Apparent bowing due to thickening of the anterior surface of the tibia secondary to periostitis:
Congenital syphilis (?saddle nose, bulldog jaw, rhagades, Hutchinson's teeth, Moon's molars, etc.—p. 256)
Yaws.

---

* Bisphosphonates are now the first-line treatment with short courses leading to long-term suppression of disease activity and improvement in bone pain, etc. Indications for specific therapy in Paget's disease are: bone pain; osteolytic lesions in weight-bearing bones; neurological complications (except deafness); delayed or non-union of fractures; immobilization hypercalcaemia; before and after orthopaedic surgery.

† Although hearing loss is frequently attributed to compression of the VIIIth cranial nerve in the canal in the temporal bone, this is unlikely to be the major cause because the facial nerve, which follows the same course, is rarely affected.
‡ The other ophthalmological finding which may occur in Paget's disease is angioid streaks in the retina (see p. 301).

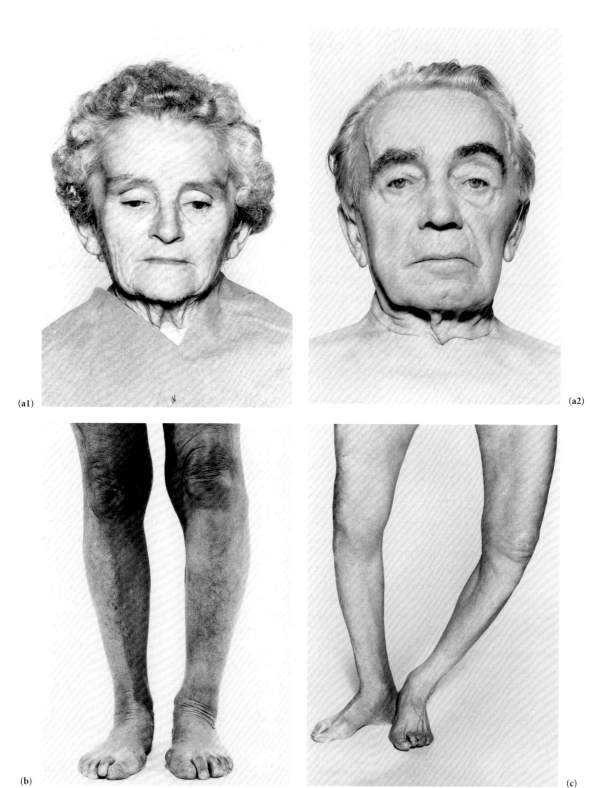

Figure C5.54 (a1,2) Note the hearing aids. (b) Bowing of tibiae. (c) Gross deformity.

Case 8 | **Osteoarthritis**

Frequency in survey: main focus of a short case in 2% of attempts at PACES station 5, locomotor.

Record

There are *Heberden's nodes* present at the bases of the distal phalanges (and less commonly Bouchard's nodes at the proximal interphalangeal joints). There is a 'square hand' deformity due to subluxation of the base of the first metacarpal. Signs of joint inflammation are (generally) absent. There is swelling and deformity of the knee joints with development of varus (or valgus) deformity. There is crepitus in these joints. There is wasting and weakness of the quadriceps and glutei, and there is downward tilting of the pelvis when the patient stands on the affected leg (Trendelenberg's sign).

   This patient has osteoarthritis.

Complications

Pain

Deformity

Ankylosis

Entrapment of nerves (e.g. ulnar nerve palsy or carpal tunnel syndrome)

Cervical spondylosis.

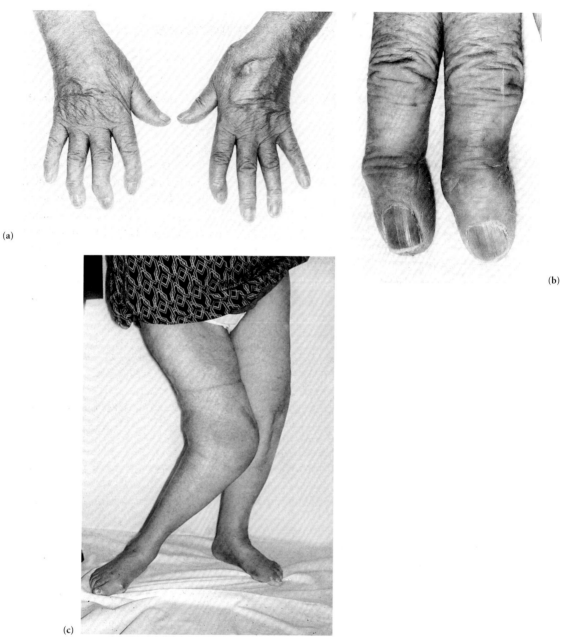

(a)

(b)

(c)

Figure C5.55 (a,b) Note the square hand deformity, Heberden's nodes and lateral bending of the terminal digits. (c) Osteoarthritis of the knee joint with valgus deformity.

Case 9 | Marfan's syndrome

Frequency in survey: main focus of a short case in 2% of attempts at PACES station 5, locomotor.

Record

The patient is *tall* with disproportionately *long extremities* (pubis–sole > pubis–vertex) and elongated fingers and toes (*arachnodactyly*). He has a *high-arched palate* (gothic), long narrow face and his span is greater than his height. His musculature is underdeveloped and hypotonic (and he may have a funnel or pigeon chest, pectus excavatum, kyphoscoliosis, flat feet, genu recurvatum, hyperextensibility of joints and recurrent dislocations). The tremor of the iris (*iridodonesis*) is evidence of *lens dislocation* (50–70% of patients; a slit lamp may be needed for detection in minor cases). He has (may have) a collapsing pulse (auscultate if allowed) suggestive of *aortic incompetence* (cystic necrosis of the aortic media leading to steadily progressive* dilatation of the aorta; aortic dissection can occur).

The diagnosis is Marfan's syndrome.

Autosomal dominant.

Defects in fibrillin (gene responsible is on the long arm of chromosome 15).

Other features which may occur in Marfan's syndrome

Heterochromia of the iris

Blue sclerae

Myopia

Undue liability to retinal detachment

Cystic disease of the lungs (tendency to spontaneous pneumothorax which is often recurrent and may be bilateral; other pulmonary manifestations are bullae, apical fibrosis, aspergilloma and bronchiectasis)

Mitral valve prolapse (common — p. 159; severe mitral incompetence may occur)

Coarctation of the aorta

Bacterial endocarditis even on valves with only minor abnormalities

Inguinal or femoral herniae

Decreased subcutaneous fat

Miescher's elastoma (small nodules or papules in the skin of the neck)

Death due to cardiovascular component (average age is mid-forties).

NB *Homocystinuria* (autosomal recessive) may produce a similar clinical picture to Marfan's except in addition mental retardation, a malar flush and osteoporosis are common and ocular lens dislocation is downwards (in Marfan's it is upwards). Homocystine can be detected in the urine by the cyanide–nitroprusside test.

---

* Prophylactic β-blockade may slow the rate of aortic dilatation and reduce the development of aortic complications in some patients with Marfan's.

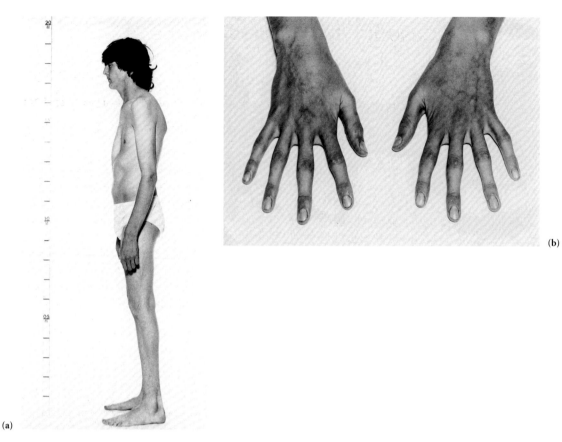

(b)

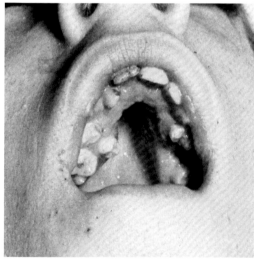

(c)

Figure C5.56 (a–c) Marfan's syndrome.

Case 10 | **Vasculitis**

Frequency in survey: main focus of a short case in 2% of attempts at PACES station 5, locomotor.

Vasculitis is dealt with on p. 332.

Case 11 | **Proximal myopathy**

Frequency in survey: main focus of a short case in 2% of attempts at PACES station 5, locomotor.

Proximal myopathy is dealt with on p. 222.

Case 12 | One leg shorter and smaller than the other

Frequency in survey: main focus of a short case in 2% of attempts at PACES station 5, locomotor.

This case appearing in station 5, locomotor was presumably either old polio (see p. 234) or infantile hemiplegia (see p. 269).

Case 13 | Radial nerve palsy

Frequency in survey: main focus of a short case in 1% of attempts at PACES station 5, locomotor.

Survey note: see experience 1, vol. 2, p. 282.

Radial nerve palsy is dealt with on p. 272.

Case 14 | Arthropathy associated with inflammatory bowel disease

Frequency in survey: main focus of a short case in 1% of attempts at PACES station 5, locomotor.

Record

There is *symmetrical* (may be asymmetrical) *arthropathy* of the *hands* with *swelling* of the *metacarpophalangeal* and *proximal interphalangeal joints*. There is *wasting* of the *small muscles* of the *hand* with *guttering* in between the metacarpals. There are no nodules or arteritic lesions (check for these). She cannot make a complete fist but can pick up a paperclip suggesting a reasonable retention of function. I also noticed an *operation scar* on the *abdomen* (check for extraintestinal signs; see Table C5.3), possibly from a hemicolectomy in the past.

The appearances suggest rheumatoid arthritis but I would also have to consider peripheral arthropathy associated with inflammatory bowel disease.

Enteropathic arthropathies

Two distinct forms of arthritis have been recognized in association with inflammatory bowel disease: peripheral and axial arthropathies.

Peripheral arthropathy

About 15% of patients with Crohn's disease and 10% with ulcerative colitis develop peripheral arthritis. It is commonly non-erosive, reversible and migratory affecting the large joints (i.e. knees, ankles and elbows) but, in chronic cases, it may be indistinguishable from seronegative rheumatoid arthritis. Peripheral arthritis frequently occurs in those who have other extraintestinal manifestations such as erythema nodosum in Crohn's disease. It affects all age groups and both sexes equally. In adults the arthritis usually develops in cases with well-established intestinal inflammation but the converse is true in children. Peripheral arthritis parallels gut inflammation and measures to control the bowel disease may ameliorate the articular activity. Total colectomy is associated with remission of arthritis in half of the patients with ulcerative colitis though sometimes the arthritis may begin after surgery. Septic arthritis in the hip joint has been reported in Crohn's disease.

Axial arthropathy

Spinal involvement may be symptomatic or silent sacroiliitis and it may precede or coincide with the onset of colitis. Axial arthritis is commoner in males and it is clinically and radiologically indistinguishable from ankylosing spondylitis. The course of sacroiliitis and spondylitis is independent of active bowel inflammation. HLA-B27 is found in 50% of patients with spondylitic colitis.

Table C5.3 Extraintestinal signs of inflammatory bowel disease

Area	Sign/manifestation
Joints	Peripheral and axial–sacroiliac arthritides, septic arthritis rarely in Crohn's disease and not reported in ulcerative colitis
Eyes	Uveitis, iritis and scleritis* — all occur in both conditions but are commoner in Crohn's disease
Mouth	Aphthous ulcers and swollen lips in Crohn's disease but never in ulcerative colitis
Hands	Finger clubbing — commoner in Crohn's disease
Skin	Erythema nodosum — up to 9% in Crohn's disease, 20% in ulcerative colitis
	Pyoderma gangrenosum† — 0.5% in Crohn's disease, occurs more often and mostly on the limbs in ulcerative colitis, usually with a bout of acute colitis
	Pallor — resulting from anaemia in either condition
	Erythema multiforme — occurs but is rare in either condition, has some association with erythema nodosum
Abdomen	Fistulae and laparotomy scars in Crohn's disease, operation scar of a colectomy in ulcerative colitis
Vasculitis	Cutaneous polyarteritis nodosa (painful skin nodules) reported in both conditions. Digital ischaemia and gangrene are rare complications
Nutritional status	Weight loss in both conditions

* These changes also occur in rheumatoid arthritis without inflammatory bowel disease.
† Ulcerative colitis should be considered in any patient presenting with diarrhoea and pyoderma gangrenosum. Unfortunately, the latter is often misdiagnosed as a simple ulcer, unrelated to the bowel problem, in such patients.

Case 15 | **Polymyositis**

Frequency in survey: main focus of a short case in 1% of attempts at PACES station 5, locomotor.

Polymyositis is dealt with on p. 254.

Case 16 | Systemic lupus erythematosus

Frequency in survey: did not occur in the initial small survey of PACES station 5, locomotor.

Predicted frequency from older, more extensive MRCP short case surveys: main focus of a short case in 4% of attempts at PACES station 5, locomotor.

Record

There is (in this *young female* patient) a *red, papular butterfly rash* on the face (and else-where—especially light-exposed areas) with *scaling, follicular plugging** and *scarring*.

These features suggest lupus erythematosus (chronic discoid lupus erythematosus if only the skin is affected; SLE if there is evidence of multisystem involvement).

Discoid LE: ratio of males to females is 1 : 2.
SLE: ratio of males to females is 1 : 9.

Look for other features

Buccal mucosa (sharply defined whitish patches with red borders)
Scalp (scarring alopecia)
Hands and joints (arthritis; deformity may occur but is usually mild and non-erosive; Raynaud's in 20%)
Skin (vasculitis—see below)
Lungs† (pleural effusions, or rarely crepitations from interstitial involvement)
Ankles (oedema—SLE is an important cause of nephrotic syndrome)
Heart (for pericardial friction rub, rarely pericardial effusion; cardiac enlargement or failure—myocarditis; or murmurs—Libman–Sachs endocarditis)
Proximal muscles (myalgia is common; polymyositis may occur)

Eyes (Sjögren's syndrome; fundal haemorrhages or white exudates called cytoid bodies; papilloedema)
Reticuloendothelial system (lymph nodes; splenomegaly)
Mucous membranes for pallor—anaemia is normochromic normocytic and/or haemolytic (Coombs' positive or negative); thrombocytopenia often occurs; haematological changes may antedate other features of the disease by years
Hepatomegaly (chronic passive congestion—usually transient‡)
Urine (proteinuria and haematuria).

NB In SLE vasculitic rashes can occur in addition to the classic butterfly rash. They characteristically affect the elbows, knees, hands and feet. The rash may be a punctate erythematous rash, palmar erythema, periungual erythema, or livedo reticularis (see pp. 336–337). Subcutaneous nodules may occur (5%) somewhat resembling those encountered in rheumatoid arthritis.

---

* Very close examination of the butterfly rash reveals that the scales in many areas appear as dots. These dots indicate where the follicle has been plugged by a scale. When the scales are removed (very unlikely to be required in the examination) and the undersurface is inspected, they clearly appear as tiny spicules projecting from the scaly mass. No other scaly condition produces this phenomenon. Healing of the discoid lesions occurs with atrophy, scarring (telangiectasia), hyperpigmentation or hypopigmentation (vitiligo).

† Drug-induced SLE involves the lungs more commonly and kidneys less commonly than classic SLE. The commonest (90%) drugs are hydralazine (slow acetylators), isoniazid, pheny-

toin and procainamide (rapid acetylators). Other drugs include hydrochlorothiazide, oral contraceptives, penicillin, practotol, reserpine, streptomycin, sulphonamides, minocycline and tetracycline.

‡ Liver biopsy may be normal or show fatty infiltration and/or fibrosis. These manifestations in SLE should not be confused with the form of chronic active hepatitis, which often has a positive antinuclear factor, called 'lupoid hepatitis'. The liver biopsy in the latter shows an inflammatory infiltrate extending into the liver lobule, causing erosion of the limiting plate and piecemeal necrosis. Fibrous septa isolate rosettes of cells. Cirrhosis is usually present and eventually hepatic failure may develop.

Autoantibodies and their antigens in systemic lupus erythematosus

Antigen	Autoantibody
Nucleosome	Anti-dsDNA Antihistone antibody
Small nuclear ribonucleoprotein	Anti-RNP Anti-Sm
Small cytoplasmic ribonucleoprotein	Anti-Ro Anti-La
Ribosome	Antiribosomal RNA Antiribosomal P protein

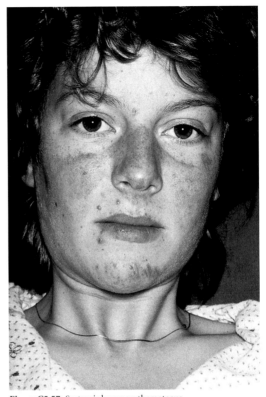

Figure C5.57 Systemic lupus erythematosus.

Case 17 | Old rickets

Frequency in survey: did not occur in the initial small survey of PACES station 5, loco-motor.

Predicted frequency from older, more extensive MRCP short case surveys: main focus of a short case in 0.6% of attempts at PACES station 5, locomotor.

Record

The legs are *bilaterally* and *symmetrically curved laterally* in this *short-statured* patient. The bowing involves both the thighs (femurs) and the lower legs (tibiae). The curved areas are not warmer than the neighbouring areas, joints and feet.

The deformity is probably long standing* and the symmetrical appearance* suggests the diagnosis of old rickets. Although there are many causes of rickets and osteomalacia, the old age (may be 80 years or older) of this patient suggests that he/she may have suffered nutritional deprivation during childhood.†

Main causes of rickets and osteomalacia‡
Decreased availability of vitamin D:
    insufficient sunlight exposure
    low dietary intake
Malabsorption:
    Billroth type II gastrectomy
    coeliac disease
    jejunoileal bypass
    regional enteritis
    pancreatic insufficiency
    biliary cirrhosis
Abnormal metabolism:
    chronic renal failure

liver disease
X-linked hypophosphataemia
renal tubular disorders
anticonvulsants
vitamin D-resistant rickets
Miscellaneous:
    aluminium toxicity
    etidronate
    hypophosphatasia
    nephrotic syndrome (urinary loss)
    total parenteral nutrition.

---

* Unlike Paget's disease (see p. 403) the deformity of old rickets is present from childhood. The bilateral involvement of the tibiae and the symmetrical appearance of the bowing are highly suggestive of old rickets. Bilateral Paget's disease of the legs is very rare and the deformity is very unlikely to be symmetrical.

† Bowing of the long bones results when poor exposure to sunlight and a low dietary intake of vitamin D occur during active skeletal growth, e.g. child refugees of the First and Second World Wars. Rickets with gross bony deformities is also seen in patients with *familial hypophosphataemia*, renal tubular disorders and in Asian immigrants of all ages.

‡ After closure of the epiphyses, vitamin D deficiency manifests as *osteomalacia*. Severe osteomalacia may present with bone pain, proximal muscle weakness, difficulty in climbing stairs and rising from chairs, and waddling gait. Pseudofractures (also known as Looser's zones or Milkman's fractures) on X-ray of pelvis, ribs, clavicles or lateral scapulae are pathognomonic of osteomalacia and rickets. However, osteomalacia is often diagnosed in relatively asymptomatic individuals. A raised alkaline phosphatase with low or low normal calcium should arouse suspicion. The level of vitamin D in the blood may be low, though elevation of serum parathyroid hormone level (secondary rise) is a more sensitive indicator.

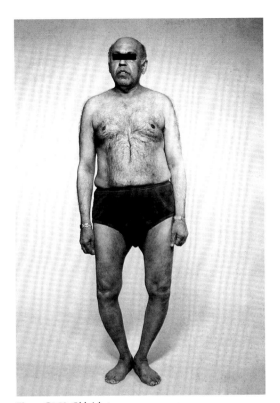

Figure C5.58 Old rickets.

Case 18 | Juvenile chronic arthritis

Frequency in survey: did not occur in the initial small survey of PACES station 5, locomotor.

Predicted frequency from older, more extensive MRCP short case surveys: main focus of a short case in 0.6% of attempts at PACES station 5, locomotor.

Record

This (febrile) *teenager* with painful joints (*polyserositis*) has an evanescent salmon-coloured *rash*, lymphadenopathy and hepatosplenomegaly.

These features are suggestive of Still's disease (juvenile chronic arthritis* (JCA) of systemic onset).

Other features of Still's disease

Twenty per cent of patients with JCA

Rheumatoid factor and antinuclear antibodies not found

Usually a childhood disease but can begin at any age

Anaemia, leucocytosis and thrombocytosis common (can be confused with leukaemia or infection).

Other forms of JCA

Polyarticular onset

Forty per cent of patients with JCA

Female predominance

Usually seronegative† (if seropositive, HLA-DR4 common and follows a course similar to adult rheumatoid arthritis).

Pauciarticular onset

Forty per cent of patients with JCA.

Early age of onset and female preponderance

Antinuclear antibodies positive, rheumatoid factor negative

Risk of chronic iridocyclitis (prophylactic ophthalmological surveillance mandatory)

Arthritis usually resolves without deformity

HLA-DR5 and HLA-DRw8 associated

Strong male predominance and later age of onset

Mostly HLA-DR27

Follows a course consistent with spondyloarthropathy.‡

---

* Also called *juvenile idiopathic arthritis* (JIA). Has been termed in the past juvenile rheumatoid arthritis, though the majority of cases do not resemble adult rheumatoid arthritis.

† No HLA association except small subset with HLA-B27 who develop cervical spine fusion and less often sacroiliitis or ankylosing spondylitis.

‡ The seronegative spondyloarthritides are characterized by sacroiliac joint involvement, peripheral inflammatory arthropathy and the absence of rheumatoid factor. Pathological changes are concentrated around the *enthesis*—at sites of ligamentous inser-

tions into bones (rather than the synovium). Changes may also develop in the eye, aortic valve, lung parenchyma and skin. Types include ankylosing spondylitis (p. 401), Reiter's syndrome (p. 370), psoriatic arthropathy (p. 390) enteropathic sacroiliitis (ulcerative colitis and Crohn's disease—p. 127), reactive arthritides (infections such as with *Yersinia, Salmonella, Helicobacter, Campylobacter*), certain subsets of JCA, and perhaps a group of rarer disorders (Whipple's disorders, Behçet's syndrome and pustular arthroosteitis).

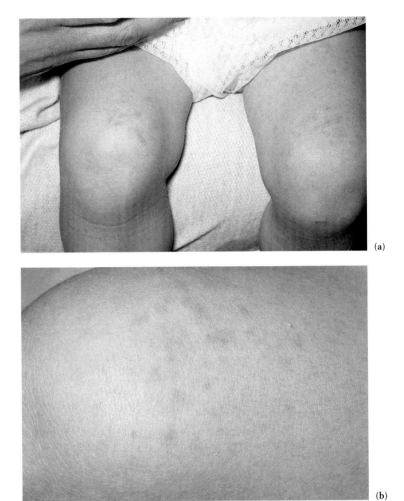

(a)

(b)

Figure C5.59 Juvenile chronic arthritis. (a) Arthropathy affecting the knees. Note a crop of characteristic macular lesions. (b) Close-up view of the rash.

Case 19 | Swollen knee

Frequency in survey: did not occur in the initial small survey of PACES station 5, locomotor.

Predicted frequency from older, more extensive MRCP short case surveys: main focus of a short case in 2% of attempts at PACES station 5, locomotor. Additional feature in a further 3%.

Survey note: half of the cases were due to rheumatoid arthritis.

Record

There is generalized *swelling* of the R/L *knee joint* obscuring the medial and lateral dimples. The *patellar tap sign** is *positive* suggesting the presence of fluid in the synovial cavity. The swelling does not extend to the back in the popliteal fossa (always check).†
The joint is *painful* to move and it is *warm*.

There is an *effusion* in the knee joint. (Now look at the hands for evidence of rheumatoid arthritis—p. 384.)

Causes of a swollen knee

Rheumatoid arthritis (the swelling may be due to synovial thickening—synovium is palpable as boggy tissue around the joint margin)

Osteoarthritis (osteophytes on X-ray)

Rupture of a Baker's cyst (?rheumatoid arthritis—p. 511)

Pseudogout (calcified menisci; birefringent calcium pyrophosphate crystals; associated with a large variety of conditions including hyperparathyroidism, haemochromatosis, acromegaly, diabetes mellitus,

Wilson's disease, hypothyroidism, alkaptonuria and gout; there are also idiopathic and hereditary varieties)

Septic arthritis (purulent fluid, organisms in a smear)

Gout (urate crystals)

Trauma

Charcot's knee (painless, ?tabes dorsalis—p. 265)

Haemarthrosis of haemophilia

Oedematous states (congestive cardiac failure, nephrotic syndrome).

---

* With one hand above the knee joint, exert pressure to drive fluid from the suprapatellar pouch into the knee joint proper. With the index finger of the other hand, depress the patella with a sharp jerky movement. If the patella rebounds this is definite evidence of fluid in the knee joint. The sign may not be positive if there is too much or too little fluid. To test for a small amount of fluid in the knee joint, displace fluid by depressing one of the obliterated hollows on either side of the ligamentum patellae. The hollow will slowly refill.

† Swelling in the popliteal fossa extending down to the upper third of the calf in cases of ruptured Baker's cyst—p. 511.

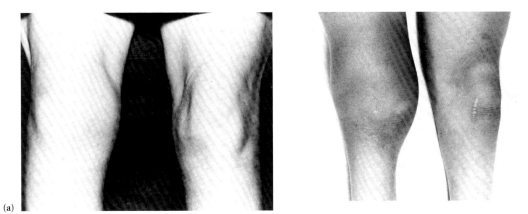

(a)

(b)

Figure C5.60 (a) Osteoarthritis with effusion of the knee joint. (b) Charcot's knee (spina bifida).

Station 5
Endocrine

1 Exophthalmos
2 Acromegaly
3 Graves' disease
4 Goitre
5 Hypothyroidism
6 Cushing's syndrome
7 Addison's disease
8 Hypopituitarism
9 Pretibial myxoedema

10 Gynaecomastia
11 Turner's syndrome
12 Klinefelter's syndrome/hypogonadism
13 Bitemporal hemianopia
14 Charcot's joint
15 Necrobiosis lipoidica diabeticorum
16 Short stature
17 Pseudohypoparathyroidism
18 Pendred's syndrome

Case 1 | Exophthalmos

Frequency in survey: main focus of a short case in 26% of attempts at PACES station 5, endocrine. Additional feature in a further 19%.

Record 1

There is (may be) bilateral *swelling* of the *medial caruncle* and *vascular congestion* of the *lateral canthus* with exophthalmos (protrusion of the eye revealing the *sclera above the lower lid* in the position of forward gaze) which is greater on the R/L side.*

Likely causes include:

1 Hyperthyroid Graves' disease† (?lid retraction or lag, tachycardia, bruit over the goitre; exophthalmos usually symmetrical)

2 Euthyroid Graves' disease (?no lid lag, *normal* pulse rate, no sweating or tremor, etc.)

3 Hypothyroid Graves' disease (?facies, scar of thyroidectomy, hoarse voice, slow pulse, ankle jerks, etc.).

Record 2

There is severe exophthalmos, *chemosis, exposure keratitis, corneal ulceration* and *ophthalmoplegia‡* which is reducing the upward and lateral gaze most and which is responsible for the *diplopia*. Convergence (check for this) is also impaired. Testing the eye movements caused the patient discomfort (or pain).

The diagnosis is Graves' malignant exophthalmos (patient may be hyper-, eu- or hypothyroid).

Graves' malignant exophthalmos (congestive ophthalmopathy) can cause severe pain and the patient is at risk of blindness due to pressure on the optic nerve, if not treated. The condition may require large doses of systemic steroids and sometimes *tarsorrhaphy* (which may be in evidence in the examination patient), or orbital decompression may even be necessary. Radiotherapy has also been successfully used.

Protective measures for the eye with exophthalmos

Eyedrops/lubrication

Stop smoking/avoid smoky atmospheres

'Cataract glasses', i.e. wrap-around glasses

Optimize thyroid status (improves lid lag and retraction but will have little effect on exophthalmos itself).

Other causes of exophthalmos

Bilateral (though asymmetrical) with conjunctival oedema

Cavernous sinus thrombosis (follows infection of the orbit, nose and face; eyeball is painful and there is extreme venous congestion)

Caroticocavernous fistula (pulsating exophthalmos).

---

* Look for pretibial myxoedema (see p. 311) if the legs are exposed and for thyroid acropachy (see pp. 432 and 434) if pretibial myxoedema is present.

† There are some studies that suggest that radioactive iodine therapy for Graves' disease may worsen exophthalmus, though this is a controversial area.

‡ The ophthalmoplegia is due to infiltration, oedema and subsequent fibrosis of the external ocular muscles. It may occur with oedema of the lids and conjunctivae and precede the exophthalmos. For this reason the term 'congestive ophthalmopathy' may be preferable to 'malignant exophthalmos'.

Unilateral

Retro-orbital tumour (the protrusion measured with the Hertel exophthalmometer is usually >5 mm more than the unaffected eye by the time of presentation, whereas Graves' eyes rarely achieve a difference of 5 mm*)

Orbital cellulitis.

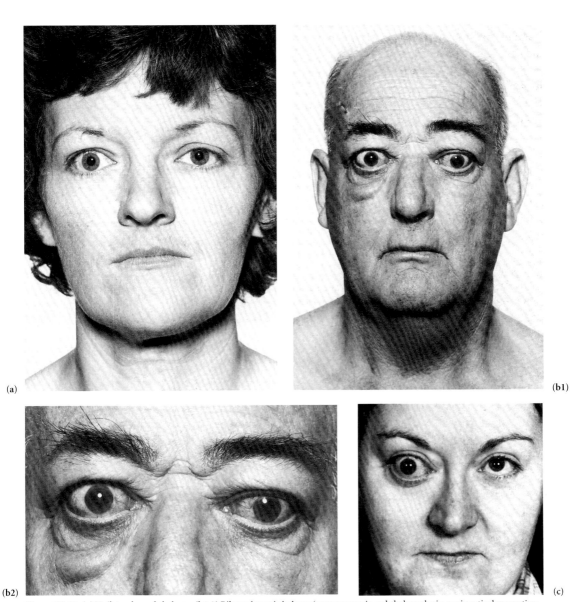

Figure C5.61 (a) Unilateral exophthalmos. (b1,2) Bilateral exophthalmos (note proptosis, ophthalmoplegia, conjunctival congestion, swelling of the medial caruncle and periorbital swelling). (c) Ophthalmoplegia of the right eye.

* Unless the diagnosis is unquestionably Graves' disease, the possibility of a retro-orbital tumour should always be investigated with CT scan, etc., regardless of the Hertel exophthalmometer measurement.

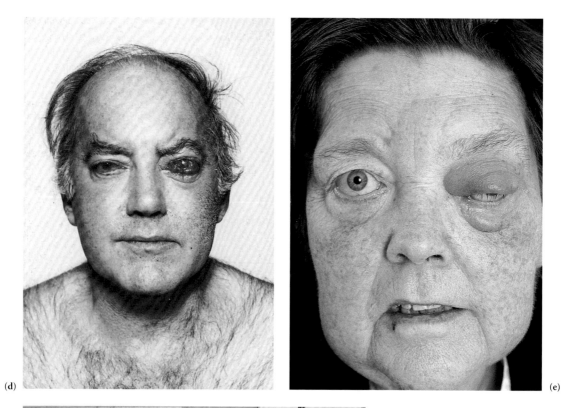

(d)

(e)

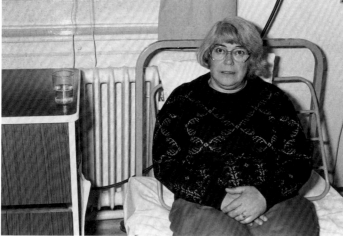

(f)

Figure C5.61 (*continued*) (d) Severe congestive ophthalmopathy, chemosis and corneal ulceration. (e) Severe congestive ophthalmopathy on the left. (f) Tell-tale glass of water (for examination of the goitre) in a patient with exophthalmos.

Case 2 | **Acromegaly**

Frequency in survey: main focus of a short case in 24% of attempts at PACES station 5, endocrine. Additional feature in a further 3%.

Survey note: candidates were sometimes asked questions on subjects such as presentation, investigation and complications.

Record

The patient has prominent *supraorbital ridges* and a *large lower jaw*. The facial wrinkles are exaggerated and the lips are full. There is *malocclusion* of the teeth, the *lower teeth overbiting* in front of the upper (prognathism), and there is an increase in the *interdental spaces*. The *nose, tongue* and *ears* are enlarged and the patient is *kyphotic*. The *hands* are *large*, doughy and spade-shaped,* and the *skin* over the back of them is *thickened* (shake hands and examine the dorsum). There is (may be) loss of the thenar eminence bilaterally with impaired sensation in the median nerve distribution (*carpal tunnel syndrome*). The patient is *sweating* excessively and is mildly *hirsute* (one-third of cases). The *voice* is husky and cavernous.† There is a *bitemporal peripheral visual field defect*.

The diagnosis is acromegaly.

Other physical signs which may be present

Increased foot (shoe) size
Increased head (hat) size
Bowed legs
Rolling gait
Goitre
Gynaecomastia
Galactorrhoea
Large testes
Small testes (if hypogonadal)
Greasy skin
Acne
Multiple skin tags (correlate with the occurrence of colonic polyps)
Acanthosis nigricans

Osteoarthrosis
Prominent superficial veins of extremities
Proximal muscle weakness
Cardiomegaly (hypertension and cardiomyopathy)
Third nerve palsy.

Other features

Diabetes mellitus (glycosuria, glucose intolerance or frank diabetes (10–20%) may occur; it is usually mild and ketoacidosis is rare; it is somewhat resistant to insulin)
Hypertension (20–50%)
Hypercalciuria (common)
Hypercalcaemia‡ (occasionally)
Urolithiasis (5–10%)

---

* Shaking hands with the patient may give the impression of losing one's hands in a mass of dough.
† Thick vocal cords in conjunction with sinus enlargement results in the characteristic deep, resonant voice.
‡ Most likely to be due to associated hyperparathyroidism as part of *multiple endocrine adenopathy (MEA) type I* (Werner's syndrome) which is two or more of:
1 Pituitary tumour (eosinophil or chromophobe)

2 Islet cell tumour (gastrin or insulin)
3 Primary hyperparathyroidism (adenoma or hyperplasia)
4 Adrenocortical adenoma (see also p. 441 and footnote).
MEA type 1 should probably be regarded as a complex of separate genetic abnormalities rather than as a consequence of a single primary disease. It should not be confused with MEA type 2 which is usually an autosomal dominant trait with a high degree of penetrance (see footnote, p. 437).

Hypertriglyceridaemia (20–40%)

Diabetes insipidus (normally due to hypothalamic pressure effect; if there is impaired cortisol secretion symptoms may be masked)

Hypopituitarism (see p. 449).

Symptoms before presentation*

Excessive sweating

Increasing size of shoes, gloves, hats, dentures and rings

Paraesthesiae of hands and feet

Digital pain and stiffness (of slowly expanding fingers and toes)

Arthralgia

Hypogonadism (amenorrhoea, loss of libido)

Headache (may be severe; may occur without clinically detectable enlargement of the pituitary tumour; the mechanism is not clear)

Visual field or acuity disturbance.

Investigations

IGF-I (not diagnostic but good initial screening test)

Glucose tolerance test with GH response (lack of suppression; sometimes a paradoxical rise)

MRI scan of pituitary fossa (CT scan if MRI scan cannot be done)

Visual fields

Comparative study of old photographs of the patient can be useful to date onset

Skull X-ray

Tests of anterior pituitary function (*adrenocorticotroph:* short Synacthen test,† insulin tolerance test; *thyrotroph:* TSH plus total or free T_4; *gonadotroph:* menstrual history plus oestrodiol, LH and FSH (female), potency plus testosterone (male); *lactotroph:* prolactin‡).

Treatment

Trans-sphenoidal hypophysectomy—GH falls to <$5\,\mu g\,l^{-1}$ in >60% (more successful in those with smaller tumours)

Transfrontal hypophysectomy in some cases with large extensive adenomata

External irradiation (especially if surgery fails or patient is unfit for surgery; takes 1–10 years to take effect)

Radioactive gold or yttrium implants (very restricted in terms of availability)

Bromocriptine (70% respond by reducing GH levels but few suppress to <$5\,\mu g\,l^{-1}$; the size of the tumour is not reduced; useful for GH hypersecretion after surgery)

Long-acting somatostatin analogues (require parenteral administration); effective in lowering GH before and (if necessary) after surgery/radiotherapy; tumour may shrink in some cases.

---

* The mean age of onset has been estimated at about 27 years whereas the mean age of presentation is over 40 years, i.e. there is an average pre-presentation lapse of 13–14 years. The prevalence is 40–70 per million; the incidence is 3 per million. Males = females. Ninety-nine per cent are due to pituitary adenomata; <1% due to excess GHRH production from gangliocyomata of the hypothalamus or pituitary or from peripheral tumours (ectopic), especially carcinoid (see p. 125).

† In hypopituitarism, the adrenal cortex does not respond sufficiently in the short Synacthen test. It needs to be primed continually by ACTH from a functioning pituitary in order to be responsive.

‡ The prolactin may be low in hypopituitarism. However, production may also be elevated because (i) some GH-secreting pituitary tumours co-secrete prolactin, and (ii) any pituitary macroadenoma that presses on the pituitary stalk will interfere with dopamine suppression of prolactin production and lead to hyperprolactinaemia.

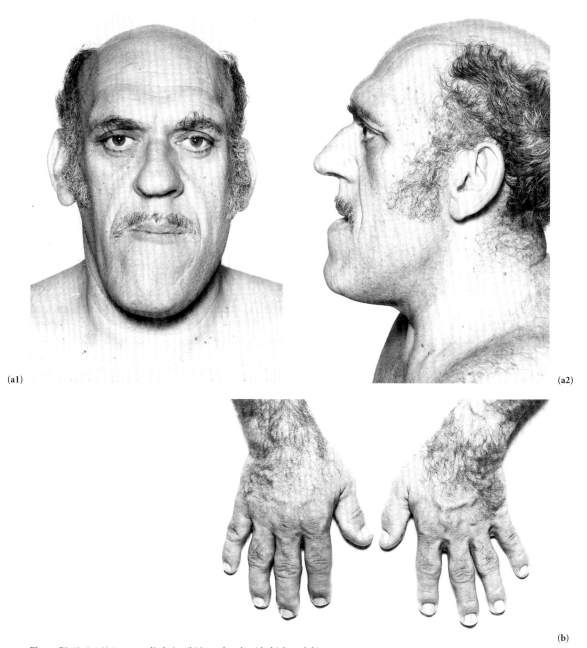

(a1)

(a2)

(b)

Figure C5.62 (a1,2) Acromegalic facies. (b) Large hands with thickened skin.

Case 3 | Graves' disease

Frequency in survey: main focus of a short case in 9% of attempts at PACES station 5, endocrine. Additional feature in a further 9%.

Record 1

The patient (usually female) is *thin*, has *sweaty palms*, a *fine tremor* of the outstretched hands, a *tachycardia*,* and she is *fidgety* and nervous. There is a small diffuse *goitre* with a *bruit*, and she has *exophthalmos* (see p. 494) with *lid lag*.†

This patient is *thyrotoxic* and has Graves' disease.

Record 2

There is *exophthalmos* (?chemosis, ophthalmoplegia, diplopia, lateral tarsorrhaphy), *thyroid acropachy*,‡ and the lesions on the front of the shins are *pretibial myxoedema* (see p. 311). The pulse is regular* and the *pulse rate* is *normal* (give rate), the palms are *not sweaty*, and there is *no hand tremor* or *lid lag*. There is a *thyroidectomy scar*.

The diagnosis is *euthyroid* Graves' disease,§ the patient having been treated by thyroidectomy in the past.

Male to female ratio is 1:5.

Record 3

This patient with *exophthalmos* (?chemosis, ophthalmo-plegia, diplopia, lateral tarsorrhaphy, goitre, thyroidec-tomy scar, pretibial myxoedema, thyroid acropachy) has *hypothyroid facies*, a *hoarse voice, slow pulse** and *slowly relaxing reflexes*.

The patient has Graves' disease and is clinically *hypothyroid*. It is likely that she had hyperthyroidism treated in the past (?thyroidectomy or radioactive iodine) and is probably now on inadequate thyroxine replacement.

(Because of the close links between the autoimmune thyroid diseases—see below—patients with Graves' disease occasionally go on to develop hypothyroidism spontaneously.)

Other signs which may occur

Fever (rarely hyperpyrexia)
Systolic hypertension with wide pulse pressure
Cutaneous vasodilatation
Systolic murmur due to increased blood flow
Proximal muscle weakness (thyrotoxic myopathy)
Hyperactive reflexes

---

* The pulse may be regular or irregular—the patient may have sinus rhythm or atrial fibrillation whatever the thyroid status (hyperthyroid; eu- or hypothyroid due to treatment).

† Graves' disease may be present in the absence of the eye signs and in an elderly male patient. There may be evidence of humoral autoimmunity, more specifically a circulating antibody to the thyrotrophin receptor. The thyroid gland may even have a nodular enlargement but its radioactive iodine uptake is uniformly increased throughout the gland between the nodules in autoimmune disease (Graves' disease). The patient with nodular goitre and thyrotoxicosis due to autonomous hypersecretion of nodule(s) that does not have an autoimmune (thyrotoxicosis) basis, will have some nodules with increased uptake (hot nodules) on the isotope scan. Such patients are more likely to relapse after antithyroid drug therapy than patients with Graves' disease.

‡ Thyroid acropachy may resemble finger clubbing in hypertrophic pulmonary osteoarthropathy (HPOA). However, in thyroid acropachy new bone formation seen on X-ray has the appearance of soap bubbles on the bone surface with coarse spicules. In HPOA new bone is formed in a linear distribution. Sometimes the new bone formation in acropachy is both visible and palpable along the phalanges.

§ Graves' exophthalmos is due to increased retro-orbital fat and enlarged intraorbital muscles infiltrated with lymphocytes and containing increased water and mucopolysaccharide. It may develop in the absence of hyperthyroidism and remit, persist or develop further despite successful treatment of hyperthyroidism. Though there are no hard and fast rules, pretibial myxoedema tends to develop after the hyperthyroidism has been treated—especially with radioactive iodine.

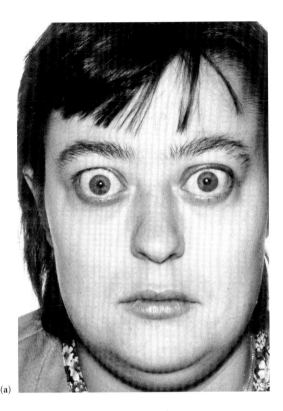

(a)

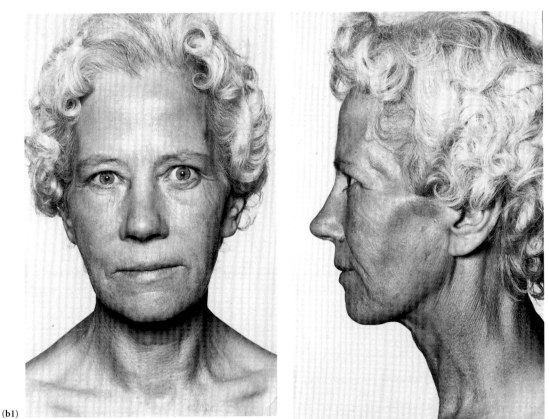

(b1)

(b2)

Figure C5.63 (a) Graves' disease. (b1,2) Hyperthyroidism in a patient who presented with the complaint that she had noticed a staring appearance of her left eye (note thinning of the hair in the temporal region).

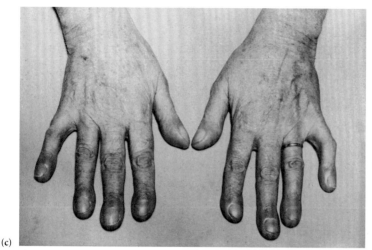

(c)

Figure C5.63 (*continued*) (c) Thyroid acropachy.

Choreoathetoid movements (in children)

Fine thin hair (females may show temporal recession of the hairline)

Onycholysis (Plummer's nails, typically found bilaterally on the fourth finger)

Palmar erythema

Spider naevi

Splenomegaly (minimal)

Hepatomegaly (minimal)

Palpable lymph nodes (especially axillae)

Thyrotoxic osteoporosis (only rarely causes kyphosis or loss of height).

Important symptoms of hyperthyroidism (if asked to ask the patient some questions) are heat intolerance, weight loss, increased appetite, diarrhoea, exertional dyspnoea, undue fatiguability, 'can't keep still', irritability, nervousness and menstrual problems in females.

Other organ-specific autoimmune diseases (see also p. 293) of which autoimmune thyroid disease* is an example include:

1 Pernicious anaemia
2 Atrophic gastritis with iron deficiency anaemia
3 Diabetes mellitus
4 Addison's disease
5 Idiopathic hypoparathyroidism
6 Premature ovarian failure
7 Renal tubular acidosis
8 Fibrosing alveolitis
9 Chronic active hepatitis
10 Primary biliary cirrhosis.

All of these diseases show a *marked female preponderance.* Premature greying of the hair, alopecia areata and vitiligo (see also p. 293) are all associated with this group of diseases. Autoimmune thyroiditis is also associated with:

1 Sjögren's syndrome
2 Myasthenia gravis
3 Systemic sclerosis
4 Mixed connective tissue disease
5 Cranial arteritis
6 Polymyalgia rheumatica.

* Graves' disease is one of the three closely related autoimmune thyroid diseases—the others being Hashimoto's thyroiditis and its atrophic variant, myxoedema. Among patients with one of these three it is typical to find relatives with one of the other two. Some patients appear to have a combination which has been termed 'hashitoxicosis'.

Case 4 | **Goitre**

Frequency in survey: main focus of a short case in 7% of attempts at PACES station 5, endocrine. Additional feature in a further 6%.

Record 1

There is *multinodular* goitre, the R/L lobe being enlarged more than the L/R. There are *no lymph nodes* palpable, there is *no retrosternal* extension, there is *no bruit* and the patient is clinically *euthyroid* (having checked pulse, palms, tremor, lid lag, tendon reflexes).

The diagnosis (in this middle-aged or elderly patient) is likely to be simple multinodular goitre.

Simple multinodular goitre is due to relative iodine deficiency in a susceptible person. The multinodular nature suggests that it is long standing. If there has been no recent rapid increase in size and if the gland is not causing symptoms or worrying the patient then no further investigation or treatment is required. The patient should be observed in 6 months or a year to confirm that there is still no change. Fine-needle aspiration should be undertaken if there is any doubt.

Record 2

There is a *firm, diffusely enlarged* goitre without retrosternal extension (check for bruit and if allowed feel the pulse and assess thyroid status).

Possible causes

Simple goitre (euthyroid, no bruit, relative iodine deficiency, especially females, ?puberty, ?pregnancy)

Treated Graves' disease* (?exophthalmos ± bruit, patient is euthyroid—normal pulse, no tremor or sweatiness—or even hypothyroid—slow pulse, facies, ankle jerks)

Hyperthyroid Graves' disease* (?bruit, tachycardia, exophthalmos, tremor, sweatiness, etc.)

Hashimoto's disease* (goitre usually, but not always, finely micronodular, firm and symmetrical; ?hypothyroid facies, pulse, ankle jerks, etc.)

De Quervain's (viral) thyroiditis (thyroid tender ± constitutional upset; absent radioactive iodine uptake on scan though the serum thyroxine may be elevated with TSH suppressed†)

Goitrogens (e.g. lithium, iodide in large doses, phenylbutazone, para-aminosalicylic acid and others are all rare causes)

Dyshormonogenesis (six different types of congenital enzyme defect, all rare).

Record 3

There is a *solitary nodule* in the thyroid (check for lymphadenopathy).

Possible causes

Only one palpable nodule in a multinodular goitre

Thyroid adenoma (if a scan were done it may show decreased, normal or increased (subclinical toxic nodule) uptake)

Toxic adenoma (hot nodule on scan, tachycardia, sweaty palms, lid lag, etc.)

Thyroid cyst

Thyroid carcinoma (?hard, lymph nodes, recent change, cold on scan).

As well as assessment of thyroid function, fine-needle aspiration to attempt to establish histological diagnosis

---

* Note the possibility of associated autoimmune disease adding extra interest to the case of goitre in the Membership (see experience 18a, vol. 2, p. 328), e.g. diabetes mellitus, rheumatoid arthritis, Addison's disease or pernicious anaemia. About 7% of patients with Graves' disease have vitiligo. About 5% of patients with myasthenia gravis have thyrotoxicosis at some time. (See also pp. 432, 438 and p. 293)

† By contrast, when the goitre and raised serum thyroxine is due to Graves' disease there is high radioactive iodine uptake on scan.

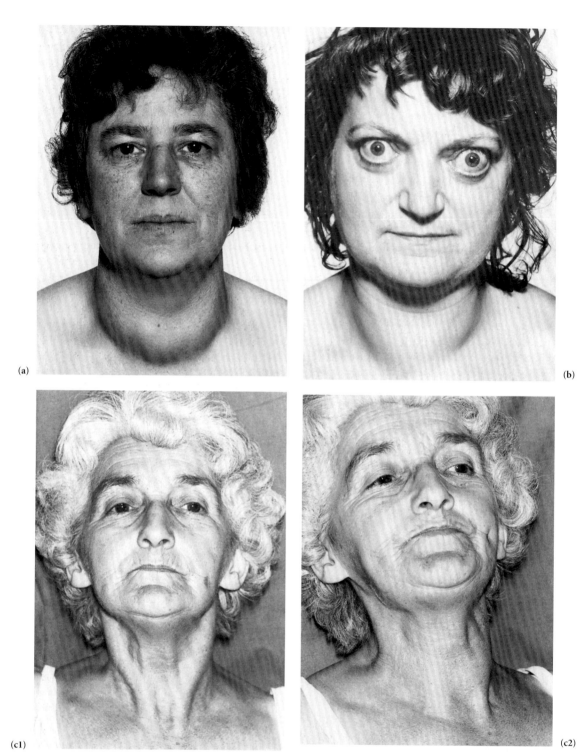

Figure C5.64 (a) Multinodular goitre. (b) Diffusely enlarged thyroid (Graves' disease). (c1,2) A solitary nodule only made obvious by swallowing (right).

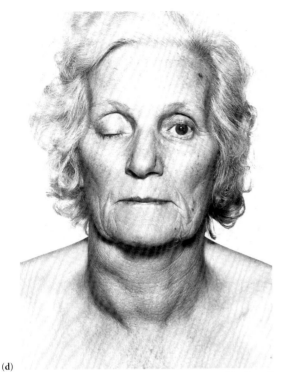

(d)

Figure C5.64 (*continued*) (d) Follicular carcinoma of the thyroid with secondaries in the cavernous sinus (total ophthalmoplegia and absent corneal reflex on the right).

should be undertaken in most cases of solitary thyroid nodule. As an adjunct the nodule may be scanned radioisotopically though this is not usually necessary. If the nodule is hot it is not malignant but if it is cold it may be. In an older patient in whom the nodule has been present without changing for a long time, observation only (perhaps with full dose thyroxine therapy which will reduce some nodules) may sometimes be justified initially. In any case of doubt, exploration of the neck and biopsy of the nodule are indicated, proceeding to subtotal lobectomy if the nodule is benign.

Types of thyroid carcinoma

Papillary carcinoma is the commonest form. It occurs in children and the middle-aged. It spreads to regional lymph nodes but is often resectable and has a good prognosis. It is often TSH-dependent and may respond to thyroxine

Follicular carcinoma is the next commonest and tends to arise later in life. Blood-borne metastases may occur, but following surgery and suppressive thyroxine treatment, the prognosis is fair. It and its secondaries often take up and respond to radioactive iodine

Anaplastic carcinoma tends to arise in the elderly and is highly malignant

Medullary carcinoma* is rare, tends to arise in young adults, secretes calcitonin and sometimes ACTH, but usually carries a good prognosis

Lymphoma generally arises in a gland affected by Hashimoto's thyroiditis. A rapidly enlarging mass in the thyroid of a patient with Hashimoto's should arouse suspicion.

---

* Multiple endocrine neoplasia (MEN) type 2a (Sipple's syndrome, also known as MEA (multiple endocrine adenopathy) syndrome) describes the association of:

1 Medullary cell carcinoma of the thyroid
2 Phaeochromocytoma
3 Parathyroid hyperplasia (50%).

In MEN type 2b, medullary cell carcinoma of the thyroid and sometimes phaeochromocytoma are associated with a variety of neurological abnormalities including mucosal neuromata (lumpy, bumpy lips and eyelids), marfanoid habitus, hyperplastic corneal nerves, skin pigmentation, proximal myopathy and intestinal disorders such as megacolon and ganglioneuromatosis.

Parathyroid hyperplasia is less common. In MEN type 2a medullary carcinoma may occasionally secrete other substances such as ACTH, histaminase, vasoactive intestinal peptide, prostaglandins and serotonin, whereas in MEN type 2b production of hormones other than calcitonin is rare. Both are autosomal dominant. MEN type 2 is associated with *RET gene mutation*. Family members can be screened for this mutation. Those who are RET positive can be offered prophylactic thyroidectomy (or annual calcitonin measurement) and can undertake annual screening of urinary catecholamines and serum calcium. Type 2b is sometimes called type 3.

Case 5 | Hypothyroidism

Frequency in survey: main focus of a short case in 6% of attempts at PACES station 5, endocrine. Additional feature in a further 1%.

Record 1

The patient is *overweight* with myxoedematous facies (*thickened* and *coarse facial features, periorbital puffiness* and pallor). The *skin* is rough, *dry, cold* and inelastic with a distinct yellowish tint (due to carotenaemia), and there is generalized *non-pitting swelling* of the subcutaneous tissues. The patient's voice is *hoarse* and *croaking*, she is somewhat hard of hearing and her movements are *slow*. There is *thinning* of the *hair* which is *dry* and *brittle* and there is (may be) loss of the outer third of the eyebrows (not a reliable sign). The pulse is *slow* (give rate). There is no palpable goitre. The relaxation phase of the *ankle jerks* (and other reflexes) is delayed and *slow*.

This patient has *myxoedema** (?evidence of associated autoimmune disease — see below).

Record 2

As appropriate from the above, plus: in view of the symmetrical, firm, finely micronodular (the typical features of a Hashimoto's goitre though there are many exceptions) *goitre* the likely diagnosis is hypothyroidism due to *Hashimoto's thyroiditis** (?associated autoimmune disease — see below).

Record 3

As appropriate from the above, plus: in view of the *exophthalmos* it is likely that this patient was treated in the past for *Graves' disease* by radioactive iodine (or thyroidectomy if there is a scar) and is now hypothyroid (occasionally Graves' disease progresses spontaneously to hypothyroidism — see p. 494).

Associated autoimmune diseases†
Pernicious anaemia (?spleen, SACD)
Addison's disease (?buccal + scar pigmentation)
Vitiligo
Rheumatoid arthritis (?hands, nodules)
Sjögren's syndrome (?dry eyes and mouth)
Ulcerative colitis
Idiopathic (presumed to be autoimmune) chronic active
   hepatitis (?icterus, etc.)
Systemic lupus erythematosus (?rash)
Haemolytic anaemia

Diabetes mellitus (?fundi)
Graves' disease
Hypoparathyroidism
Premature ovarian failure.

Important symptoms (if asked to ask the patient some questions — NB deafness and hoarse voice):
Cold intolerance
Tiredness and depression
Constipation (may occasionally present to the surgeons
   with faecal impaction)

* In hypothyroidism, accumulation of hyaluronic acid in the dermis as well as other tissues alters the composition of the ground substance. This material binds water, producing the mucinous oedema that is responsible for the thickened features and puffy appearance of full blown hypothyroidism which is termed myx-oedema. Hypothyroidism due to autoimmune thyroiditis may present as primary thyroid atrophy (*record* 1) or Hashimoto's disease (*record* 2).
† See also p. 293

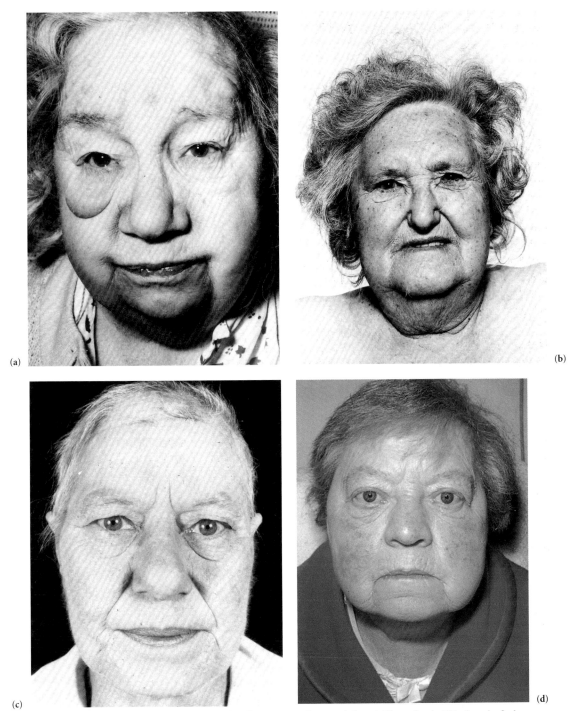

Figure C5.65 (a–d) Note thickened skin, periorbital swelling, sparse eyebrows and alopecia. The patient in (d) had a malar flush.

Angina (treatment may unmask, therefore start with low doses if age >50, or if patient has angina)

Menorrhagia (middle-aged females)

Primary or secondary amenorrhoea (younger patients).

Other features

Anaemia (normochromic, iron deficient—atrophic gastritis, or megaloblastic—frank pernicious anaemia; slight macrocytosis may occur in hypothyroidism without a megaloblastic change in the marrow)

Carpal tunnel syndrome (see p. 217)

Peripheral cyanosis (there may be a malar flush)

Raynaud's phenomenon

Hypertension

Accident proneness (may present to the casualty department)

Hypothermia (especially the elderly living alone)

Hoffman's syndrome (pain, aching and swelling in muscles after exertion together with signs of myotonia)

Psychosis (myxoedematous madness)

Hypothyroid coma.

A variety of other CNS disorders may occur,* such as peripheral neuropathy, cerebellar ataxia, pseudodementia, drop attacks and epilepsy.

---

* Always exclude concomitant vitamin B_{12} deficiency as the association with pernicious anaemia is strong. If you find peripheral neuropathy think also of concomitant diabetes mellitus before putting it down to the hypothyroidism.

Case 6 | Cushing's syndrome

Frequency in survey: main focus of a short case in 5% of attempts at PACES station 5, endocrine. Additional feature in many others in all stations (steroid treatment).

Survey note: almost all cases were secondary to therapeutic steroids—especially for asthma and rheumatoid arthritis, but also for cryptogenic fibrosing alveolitis and chronic active hepatitis, amongst others.

Record

The patient has a *moon face* with *acne* and *truncal obesity* with a *buffalo hump*. The skin is thin (demonstrate by raising a skinfold at the back of the patient's hand) and shows excessive bruising (*purpuric patches*—often at venesection sites), and there are purple *striae* on the abdomen (must be differentiated from the pale pink striae of obese adolescents and the stretch marks of pregnancy and simple obesity). She is *hirsute* with a *deep voice*. There is *proximal muscle weakness* (few patients with Cushing's syndrome can rise normally from the squatting position).

The diagnosis is Cushing's syndrome (?evidence of underlying steroid responsive inflammatory or immunological disorder).

Other features of Cushing's syndrome

Hypertension and peripheral oedema (salt retention)

Irregular menstruation

Impotence

Back pain (osteoporosis and vertebral collapse leading to kyphosis and loss of height)

Diabetes mellitus

Pigmentation (especially ectopic or exogenous ACTH)

Psychiatric disorder (commonly depressive illness).

Causes of Cushing's syndrome*

Therapeutic corticosteroids

Therapeutic ACTH

Cushing's disease—pituitary (basophilic or chromophobe pituitary adenoma) or hypothalamic lesion leading to excessive ACTH

Adrenocortical adenoma (occasionally part of *MEA type 1* with one or more of: primary hyperparathyroidism, islet cell tumour, pituitary tumour—see also p. 429†)

Adrenocortical carcinoma

Ectopic ACTH secreting non-endocrine tumours:

    (a) oat-cell carcinoma of bronchus (weight loss, pigmentation, hypokalaemic alkalosis and oedema)

    (b) bronchial adenoma

    (c) carcinoid tumour (usually bronchial)

    (d) carcinoma of the pancreas

    (e) non-teratomatous ovarian tumour.

Diagnosis of Cushing's syndrome

The best clinical discriminating signs are easy bruising and proximal muscle weakness. There are two stages to diagnosis: (i) establish diagnosis of Cushing's; and (ii) establish the cause.

1 Establishing the diagnosis:

24-hour urinary free cortisol

Overnight or low dose dexamethasone suppression (Table C5.4)

---

* When the syndrome is not iatrogenic, then in about 80% of affected adults the cause is Cushing's disease; whereas adrenal adenoma, carcinoma and ectopic ACTH syndrome contribute equally to the remaining 20%.

† In MEA type 1, the islet cell tumour may secrete gastrin (Zollinger–Ellison syndrome) or insulin (insulinoma). The pituitary tumour may be eosinophilic (acromegaly) or a chromophobe adenoma which is non-secreting (bitemporal hemianopia, headaches, blindness, hypopituitarism and other pressure symptoms—tumour may become very large). Pituitary tumours may also secrete prolactin (impotence, amenorrhoea, galactorrhoea) or ACTH (Cushing's disease).

Table C5.4 Tests for Cushing's syndrome

---

1 *Classic low-dose dexamethasone suppression test*

Dexamethasone, 2 mg day^{-1} administered orally for 2 days in eight divided doses. Normal individuals almost totally suppress cortisol production (24-hour urinary cortisol excretion <10 μg or 100 mmol). Used for the positive diagnosis of Cushing's syndrome

2 *Overnight dexamethasone suppression test*

Dexamethasone, 1 mg administered orally between 2300 and 2400 hours. Plasma cortisol is measured the next morning at 0800 hours. Normal individuals almost totally suppress cortisol production (plasma cortisol <20 ng ml^{-1}, 60 mmol l^{-1}). Used for the positive diagnosis of Cushing's syndrome

3 *Classic high-dose dexamethasone suppression test*

Dexamethasone, 8 mg day^{-1} administered orally for 2 days in eight divided doses. Patients with Cushing's disease show partial suppression of cortisol production (a significant decrease in 24-hour urinary 17-OH steroids or cortisol excretion, usually more than 50%). Patients with other causes of Cushing's syndrome (ectopic ACTH syndrome, adrenal tumours) typically show no significant variation of cortisol production

4 *Corticotrophin-releasing hormone (CRH) test*

Synthetic ovine (or less often human) CRH is administered i.v. 100 μg or 1 μg kg^{-1} body weight, and plasma ACTH and cortisol are measured during the next 60 minutes. Patients with Cushing's disease are typically responsive (ACTH and/or cortisol plasma levels increase by more than 50%) and/or 20% of patients with ectopic ACTH syndrome or adrenal tumour are typically unresponsive

---

Loss of circadian rhythm (measure midnight cortisol — usually done as in-patient)

2 Establishing the cause: see Fig. C5.66.

Treatment of Cushing's disease

Trans-sphenoidal hypophesectomy (usually small microadenoma) is the first line treatment (80% cure). If surgery fails, hypercortisolism can be controlled with antiadrenocortical drugs such as metyrapone. Simultaneous radiotherapy may allow antiadrenocortical therapy to be discontinued later. In rare cases, total bilateral adrenalectomy may eventually become necessary, though it has a low and unpredictable risk of Nelson's syndrome (further development of a pituitary tumour).

Nelson's syndrome

This is due to an ACTH-secreting pituitary tumour in 20% of patients with Cushing's disease who have undergone bilateral adrenalectomy. Untreated, the tumour may enlarge and cause mass effects, in particular visual field defects. May be prevented by external pituitary irradiation at the time of (or prior to) adrenalectomy. The patient is pigmented because of the excess ACTH. The syndrome is rare now that adrenalectomy is no longer a primary treatment for Cushing's disease. Patients with Nelson's syndrome become pigmented due to ACTH causing increased melanin in the skin.

Prophylaxis and treatment of corticosteroid-induced osteoporosis

The therapeutic options for prophylaxis and treatment of corticosteroid-induced osteoporosis are the same: hormone replacement (HRT in women, testosterone in men); bisphosphonates; calcitriol. Consider prophylaxis in all patients taking (or about to commence) prednisolone >7.5 mg day^{-1} (or equivalent) for a period of 3 months or more:

1 Prednisolone dose 7.5–15 mg—offer prophylaxis if there are one or more other risk factors* (in absence of risk factors consider DEXA scan to assess bone mineral density and offer prophylaxis if reduced)

2 Prednisolone dose >15 mg—offer prophylaxis at onset.

---

* Risk factors for osteoporosis:
• long-term steroid treatment
• age greater than 65 years
• premature menopause at less than 45 years
• family history of low trauma fracture
• previous low trauma fracture
• history of amenorrhoea
• slender build
• immobility
• endocrine disorders including Cushing's disease and thyrotoxicosis.

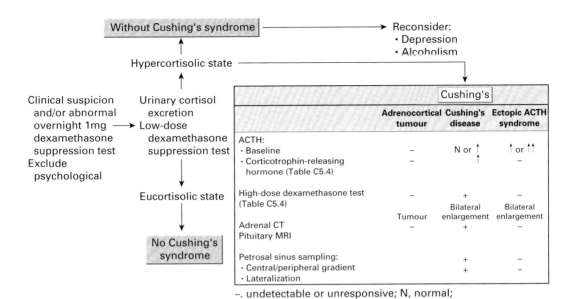

	Cushing's		
	Adrenocortical tumour	Cushing's disease	Ectopic ACTH syndrome
ACTH:			
· Baseline	–	N or ↑	↑ or ↑↑
· Corticotrophin-releasing hormone (Table C5.4)	–	↑	–
High-dose dexamethasone test (Table C5.4)	–	+	–
	Tumour	Bilateral enlargement	Bilateral enlargement
Adrenal CT Pituitary MRI	–	+	–
Petrosal sinus sampling:			
· Central/peripheral gradient		+	–
· Lateralization		+	–

–. undetectable or unresponsive; N, normal;
+, positive or responsive.

Figure C5.66 Diagnosis of Cushings syndrome.

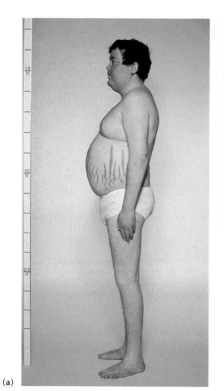

(a)

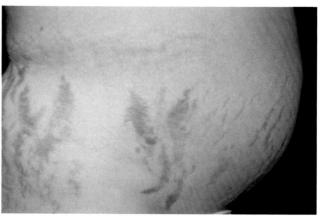

(b)

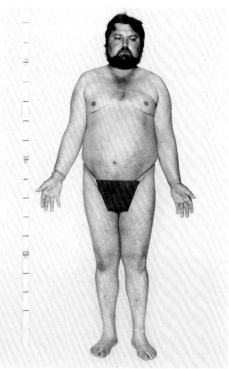

(c)

(d)

Figure C5.67 (a) Cushing's syndrome. (b) Abdominal striae. (c) Cushingoid facies (steroid therapy for cerebral lupus erythematosus). (d) Truncal obesity (Cushing's disease).

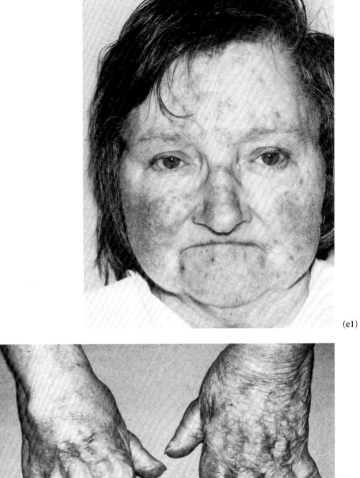

(e1)

(e2)

Figure C5.67 (*continued*) (e1,2) Corticosteroid therapy in a patient with rheumatoid arthritis.

Case 7 | Addison's disease

Frequency in survey: main focus of a short case in 3% of attempts at PACES station 5, endocrine.

Survey note: in the original, pre PACES, survey, often the differential diagnosis of Addison's/Nelson's was given and further differentiation was not required.

Record

There is *generalized pigmentation* (due to the direct action of ACTH causing increased melanin in the skin), which is more marked in the *skin creases* (e.g. palmar), in *scars* (especially more recent ones), in the *buccal mucosa* (look in the mouth), in the *nipples* and at *pressure points*.

This suggests Addison's disease or Nelson's syndrome (?temporal field defect, ?abdominal scar of bilateral adrenalectomy—see p. 442).

Patchy, almost symmetrical, areas of skin depigmentation surrounded by areas of increased pigmentation may occur due to vitiligo (15% of patients with idiopathic Addison's) which is one of the associated organ-specific autoimmune diseases. (For the others, which include autoimmune thyroiditis, diabetes mellitus, pernicious anaemia and hypoparathyroidism, see p. 293. Premature ovarian failure is particularly associated with Addison's disease.)

Common causes of primary hypoadrenalism
Autoimmune adrenalitis
Tuberculosis (?lung signs).

Other causes of primary hypoadrenalism
Bilateral adrenalectomy (malignant disease, e.g. breast cancer; Cushing's syndrome)
Secondary deposits
Amyloidosis (hypoadrenalism preceded by nephrotic syndrome—see footnote, p. 108)
Haemochromatosis
Granulomatous disease (rarely sarcoidosis)
Fungal diseases (e.g. histoplasmosis)
Congenital adrenal hyperplasia*
Meningococcal and pseudomonal septicaemia

AIDS
Adrenal haemorrhage (newborn especially breech delivery; patients on anticoagulants)
Adrenal vein thrombosis after trauma or adrenal venography.

Skin pigmentation is usually racial (including buccal pigmentation) or due to sun-tanning. Other causes of abnormal generalized pigmentation include the following:

Endocrine
ACTH therapy (e.g. asthma)
Cushing's disease (?facies, truncal obesity, striae, etc.—p. 441)
Thyrotoxicosis (?exophthalmos, goitre, etc.—p. 432)
Ectopic ACTH (especially oat cell carcinoma).

Chronic debilitating disorders (also, like Addison's, associated with lassitude and weight loss)
Malignancy (including reticuloses and leukaemias)
Malabsorption syndromes
Chronic infections (especially TB)
Cirrhosis (?icterus, spider naevi, etc.—pp. 106 and 121)
Uraemia (pale, brownish-yellow tinge to skin).

---

* Series of inherited defects in adrenocortical steroidogenesis (e.g. 21-hydroxylase deficiency). Homozygotes present neonatally with salt wasting, hypotension and ambiguous genitalia in females.

Pigments other than melanin such as

Haemochromatosis (slate-grey pigmentation, hepatosplenomegaly, etc. — p. 129)

Argyria

Chronic arsenic poisoning.

Drugs

Phenothiazines (blue–grey pigmentation)

Antimalarials (blue–grey pigmentation)

Amiodarone (grey pigmentation)

Cytotoxics

Minocycline (purple–blue pigmentation; may get blue oral discoloration due to blue–black discoloration of alveolar bone and hard palate — 'black-bone disease').

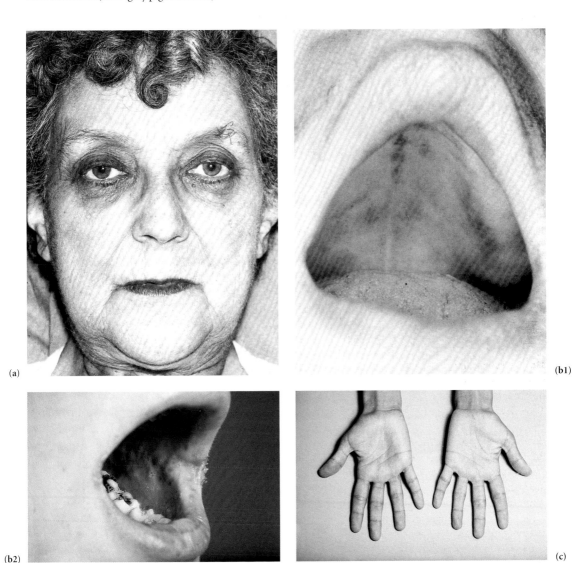

(a)

(b1)

(b2)

(c)

Figure C5.68 Addison's disease. (a) Facial pigmentation, especially periorbitally. (b1,2)Pigmentation of the buccal mucosa. (c)Palmar crease pigmentation.

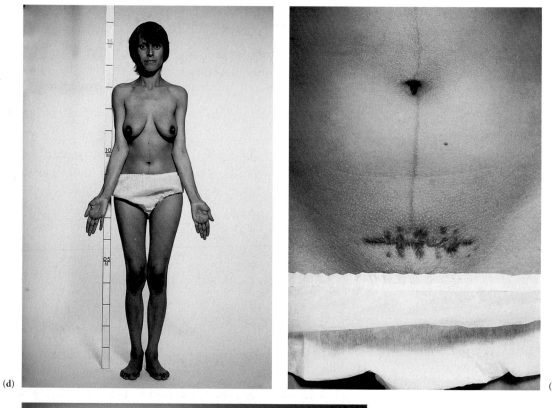

(d)

(e)

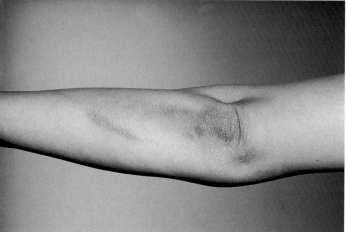

(f)

Figure C5.68 (*continued*) (d) Note pigmentation of the nipples. (e) Pigmentation of the scar and linea alba. (f) Pigmentation of the elbow (a pressure point).

Case 8 | Hypopituitarism

Frequency in survey: main focus of a short case in 2% of attempts at PACES station 5, endocrine. Additional feature in a further 1%.

Record

The patient's *skin* is *soft, wrinkled* and *pale* with a *yellow tint* (the pallor is due to a combination of lack of melanocyte-stimulating hormone and anaemia—marrow hypofunction). The areolae of the breasts are (may be) depigmented. *Pubic, axillary, facial* and *body hair* is *reduced* (and the *genitals* and *breasts* are *atrophied*).

These features suggest hypopituitarism (now check for a bitemporal visual field defect).

With progressing hypopituitarism gonadotrophin secretion is usually impaired first, followed by growth hormone. TSH, ACTH* and antidiuretic hormone, in that order. With the onset of thyroid failure the features of hypothyroidism (see p. 438) are superimposed on those in the above *record*. Lassitude, cold intolerance, dryness of skin and prolongation of the relaxation phase of the tendon reflexes occur, though swelling of the subcutaneous tissues is usually less prominent. The insidious onset of asthenia, nausea, vomiting, postural hypotension, hypoglycaemia, collapse and coma mark progressive ACTH lack. Diabetes insipidus develops with lack of antidiuretic hormone, though impaired glomerular filtration caused by cortisol deficiency may mask the symptoms.

The main causes of adult panhypopituitarism (male to female ratio is 1:2) are:

Sheehan's syndrome (following severe obstetric haemorrhage or shock—much less common nowadays with good obstetric practice)
Pituitary tumour† (especially chromophobe adenoma)
Craniopharyngioma
Pituitary granulomatous lesion (tuberculoma, sarcoidosis, Hand–Schüller–Christian disease, syphilitic gumma)
Iatrogenic (hypophysectomy, radiotherapy to sella or nasopharynx)
Head injury
Idiopathic.

The factors that lead to coma in hypopituitarism include hypoglycaemia, sodium depletion, water intoxication, cerebral anoxia, hypothyroidism, hypothermia and pressure on the midbrain or hypothalamus.

---

*Pituitary hypothyroidism may protect the patient from the effects of failing ACTH secretion. In this situation misdiagnosing the cause of hypothyroidism and waking the patient from hibernation with thyroxine alone may precipitate Addisonian crisis.

†Suprasellar extension may cause compression of the optic chiasm (visual field defect); lateral extension may cause mononeuropathies (IIIrd, IVth, Vth (Va and Vb), VIth).

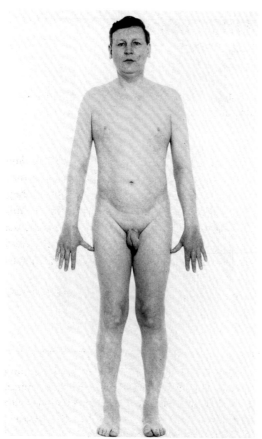

Figure C5.69 Hypopituitarism (8 years after removal of pituitary adenoma).

Case 9 | Pretibial myxoedema

Frequency in survey: main focus of a short case in 2% of attempts at PACES station 5, endocrine. Additional feature in a further 5%.

Record

There are *elevated symmetrical* skin lesions over the anterolateral aspects of the *shins* (may spread onto the feet; may affect other parts of the body, e.g. the face or the dorsa of the hands). The lesions are coarse, *purplish-red* (may be skin colour pink, or rarely, brown) in colour and raised with *well-defined* serpiginous *margins*. The skin is *shiny* and has an *orange peel appearance*. The hairs in the affected areas are coarse and the lesions are *tender* (and itch). The patient has *exophthalmos** (?*thyroid acropachy**) and is likely to have been rendered *euthyroid* (?pulse, etc.) by surgery (?*thyroidectomy scar*) or, more particularly, with *radioactive iodine*.

The diagnosis is pretibial myxoedema (occurs in about 5% of patients with Graves' disease).

The superficial layer of the skin is infiltrated with the mucopolysaccharide, hyaluronic acid. Biopsy scars of the area almost invariably develop keloid.

The latent interval between the treatment for hyperhyroidism and the clinical onset of pretibial myxoedema varies from 4 to 32 months with a mean time of 1 year.

Pretibial myxoedema in its most extreme form clinically resembles lymphoedema. It may be that mucin deposition in the dermis causes compression of the dermal lymphatics which results in dermal oedema and the clinical features of lymphoedema.

---

* Pretibial myxoedema is almost always accompanied by exophthalmos. Thyroid acropachy (see p. 432) is occasionally associated—diffuse thickening of distal extremities, subperiosteal new bone formation simulating clubbing of the digits. Exophthalmos has also been termed *infiltrative ophthalmopathy* and pretibial myxoedema, *infiltrative dermopathy*.

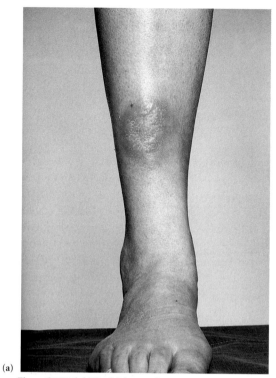

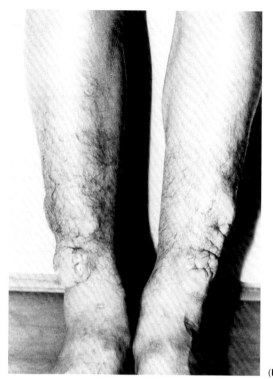

Figure C5.70 (a,b) Pretibial myxoedema.

Case 10 | **Gynaecomastia**

Frequency in survey: main focus of a short case in 2% of attempts at PACES station 5, endocrine. Additional feature in a further 5%, especially station 3, cardiac and station 1, abdominal.

Survey note: all cases were due to either drugs or cirrhosis.

Record

There is gynaecomastia (it may be unilateral). This is confirmed on palpation by the presence of *increased glandular tissue.** (Now look for signs of *cirrhosis, heart failure* (spironolactone), *atrial fibrillation* (digoxin), *clubbing and cachexia* (carcinoma of the lung), *absence of body hair* (hypogonadism, oestrogen therapy) or evidence of an *endocrine disorder*—see below. The *testes* are small and firm in Klinefelter's and asymmetrical with a tumour.)

There may be feminization of the nipples and tenderness of the breasts. Gynaecomastia must be differentiated from tumours of the breast and simple adiposity. Gynaecomastia is due to an imbalance in the free androgen to free oestrogen ratio—an imbalance in production or drug effects on metabolism.

Causes of gynaecomastia
Physiological
Pubertal (very common,† often unilateral—due to transient dominance of circulating oestradiol over testosterone)
Senile (normal rise in oestrogens and fall in androgens with age).

Pathological
Cirrhosis of the liver (?stigmata—p. 106)
Thyrotoxicosis (?exophthalmos, goitre, etc.—p. 432)
Carcinoma of the lung (5% of patients; sometimes with hypertrophic pulmonary osteoarthropathy; HCG secreted by the tumour)

Carinoma of the liver (HCG secreting)
Klinefelter's syndrome (47,XXY, small testes, mental deficiency, incomplete virilization, raised LH and FSH)
Pituitary disease,‡ i.e. acromegaly, hypopituitarism (?visual field defect)
Isolated gonadotrophin deficiency (e.g. Kallman's syndrome—hypogonadotrophic hypogonadism and anosmia, often with harelip or cleft palate)
Testicular tumours (due to HCG secretion, oestrogen secretion or excess aromatase activity in the tumour tissue)
Testicular failure
Addison's disease (?pigmentation—buccal and scar; p. 446)
Adrenal carcinoma
Testicular feminization (androgen insensitivity)
Drug-induced (Table C5.5).§

---

* A disc of tissue arising from beneath the nipple and areolar—concentric, firm and moblie.
† Thirty-nine per cent of 1855 adolescent boys of different ages at one boy scout camp, though other surveys have found it less common.
‡ NB Prolactin excess in the absence of oestrogens produces galactorrhoea rather than gynaecomastia.

§ The letters of the word MADRAS form a useful mnemonic: methyldopa, aldactone, digoxin, reserpine, alkylating agents and stilboestrol—these were the drugs of this mnemonic in the 20th century; today they could be marijuana, ACE inhibitors, digoxin, ranitidine, amiodarone and spironolactone.

Table C5.5 Drugs that may cause gynaecomastia

Hormonal	Oestrogens
	Aromatizable androgens (e.g. testosterone enanthate, testosterone propionate)
	Antiandrogens (cyproterone acetate)
Cardiac	Calcium-channel blockers
	Angiotensin-converting enzyme inhibitors
	Digoxin
	Amiodarone
	Spironolactone
	Methyldopa
CNS	Dopamine receptor antagonists (phenothiazines, metoclopramide)
	Tricyclic antidepressants
	Benzodiazepines
	Opiates
	Marijuana
Gastrointestinal	Omeprazole
	Cimetidine
	Ranitidine
Anti-infective	Isoniazid
	Metronidazole
	Ketoconazole
Cytotoxic	Alkylating agents (cause testicular damage) such as busulphan and nitrosureas
Alcohol	

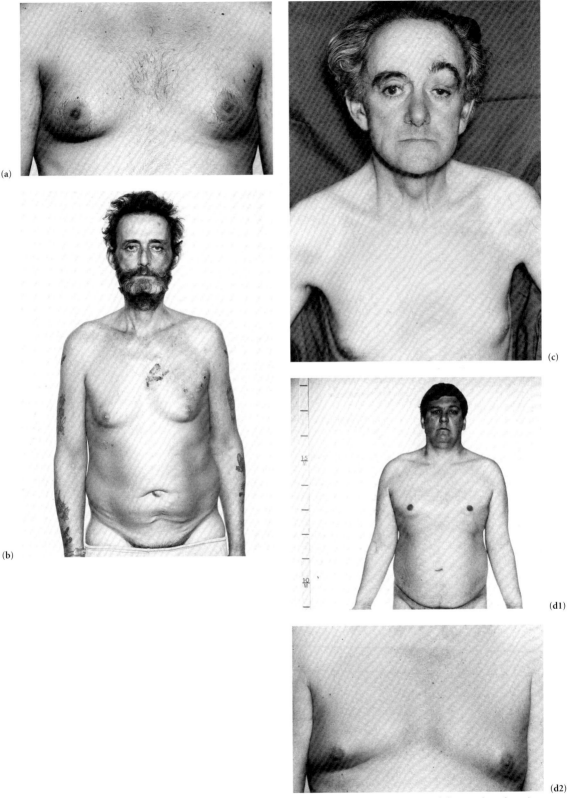

Figure C5.71 (a) Bilateral benign gynaecomastia. (b) Chronic liver disease. (c) Carcinoma of the lung (note left Horner's syndrome). (d1,2) Hypogonadism. (2) is a close-up view of the same patient as (1).

Case 11 | Turner's syndrome

Frequency in survey: main focus of a short case in 2% of attempts at PACES station 5, endocrine.

Record

The patient (who probably presented with primary amenorrhoea) is *short* (usually less than 1.5 m) with a *short webbed neck** (only found in 54%) and shows *cubitus valgus* deformity. She has a *shield-like chest* (and may have widely separated nipples). The *nails* are *hypoplastic* and she has *short fourth metacarpals* (other metacarpals may also be short). The *hairline* is *low*, she has a *high-arched palate* and there are *numerous naevi*. The secondary sexual characteristics are underdeveloped (unless the patient has been treated with oestrogens).

The diagnosis is Turner's syndrome. (If allowed examine the cardiovascular system—abnormal in 20%; especially coarctation of the aorta (p. 165) but also atrial septal defect (p. 175), ventricular septal defect (p. 152) and aortic stenosis (p. 148).

One in 2500–3500 female births.

The patient with Turner's syndrome is likely to have streak gonads and a chromosome constitution which is mostly 45,XO,† though mosaicism (XO,XX) does occur. Red–green colour blindness (an X-linked recessive character) occurs as frequently in Turner's as it does in normal males, and other X-linked conditions may occur.

Other features which sometimes occur

Lymphoedema
Genitourinary abnormality (e.g. horseshoe kidney)
Hypertelorism
Epicanthal fold
Mental retardation is rare

Strabismus
Ptosis
Intestinal telangiectasia
Premature osteoporosis
Premature ageing in appearance
Higher incidence of diabetes mellitus and Hashimoto's thyroiditis.

Noonan's syndrome

May affect both sexes. Females have Turner's phenotype but normal 46,XX, normal ovarian function and normal fertility. Noonan's are more likely to have right-sided cardiac lesions (especially pulmonary stenosis) whereas Turner's are more likely to have left-sided lesions. Mental retardation is frequent.

---

* A feature especially associated with cardiovascular abnormalities in this condition.

† Most 45,XO pregnancies end in spontaneous abortion.

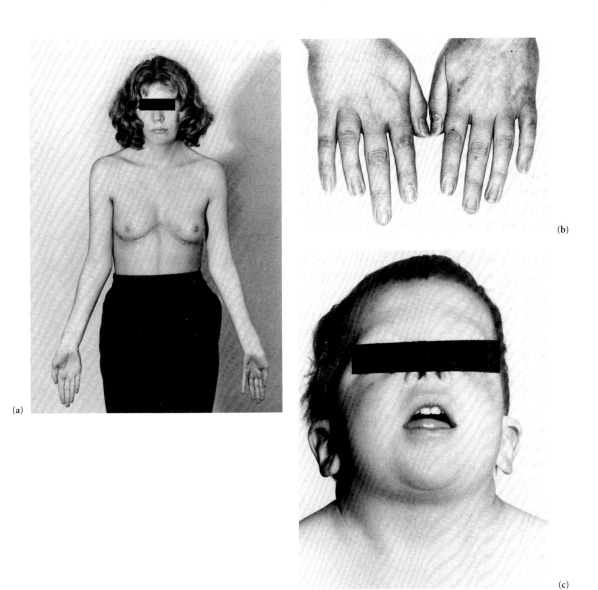

(a)

(b)

(c)

Figure C5.72 (a) XO,XX mosaic. Note the webbed neck, increased carrying angle and scar under the breasts (special incision for atrial septal defect repair). (b) The hands of another patient showing a short fourth metacarpal. (c) Noonan's syndrome.

Case 12 | Klinefelter's syndrome/ hypogonadism

Frequency in survey: main focus of a short case in 2% of attempts at PACES station 5, endocrine.

Survey note: it does not often happen, but occasionally candidates are allowed to examine the testes (see first person experience 10, vol. 2, p. 345 and anecdote 43, vol. 2, p. 365).

Record

He is *tall*, has *gynaecomastia* (may be asymmetrical), sparse body hair and has a *eunuchoid habitus.** He has very small testes (<2 cm length, often termed *pea-sized*; lower limit of normal for adults is 3.5 cm length).

The features suggest Klinefelter's syndrome.

See anecdote 43, vol. 2, p. 365.

Other features of Klinefelter's syndrome

Affects 1 in 400–500 men (1/20 if maternal age >45)

Classically 47,XXY but also XXYY, more than two X (poly X) plus Y and mosaics

Azospermia and raised gonadotrophins

Though the majority have normal intelligence there is a higher than normal incidence of mental retardation (especially if greater than two X chromosomes)

Higher incidence of somatic abnormalities (especially if greater than two X chromosomes) such as hypospadias, cryptorchidism and bony abnormalities of the radius and ulna

If there is an additional Y chromosome, patients tend to be tall with very aggressive antisocial behavioural abnormalities

Less severe manifestations in mosaics (fertility has been recorded in XXY, XY)

Character and personality disorders common (may be in part related to the psychosocial consequences of androgen deficiency)

Slightly increased incidence of certain systemic diseases (diabetes, chronic obstructive airways disease, autoimmune disorders such as SLE and Hashimoto's thyroiditis, malignancy such as breast, lymphoma and germ cell neoplasms, and varicose veins).

Features of eunuchoid appearance

Average height or above (growth until mid-twenties)

Span > height†

Pubis–heel > pubis–crown

Body fat tends to be in feminine contours; broad hips, musculature poor

Sparse body hair/beard

Poorly developed genitalia

Gynaecomastia

Timid behaviour.

Causes of primary hypogonadism (with deficiency of both sperm and androgen production)

Congenital or developmental disorders

Klinefelter's syndrome and variants

Functional prepubertal castrate syndrome (congenital anorchia — no testicular tissue from birth; testes must have been active in fetal life because the phenotype is male; hence sometimes referred to as 'vanishing testis syndrome')

Noonan's syndrome (?short stature, triangular micro-

---

* The degree of eunuchoidism is variable depending on the degree of androgen deficiency which is seldom complete; indeed the occasional Klinefelter's patient may have normal testosterone levels and virilization, the only abnormality being the pea-sized testes and azospermia. The patient treated with exogenous testosterone may also be well virilized.

† In contrast to other conditions which result in prepubertal androgen deficiency, Klinefelter's patients often have a disproportionate increase in lower extremity compared to upper extremity long bone growth.

gnathic facial appearance and posteriorly angulated low-set ears with a thick helix, webbed neck, shield-like chest, pectus excavatum, cubitus valgus, mental retardation, right-sided cardiovascular abnormalities; often cryptorchidism as well as primary testicular dysfunction — see also p. 456)

Myotonic dystrophy — p. 182 (though most cases develop testicular atrophy with maintained androgen production but impaired spermatogenesis in middle age, 20% have manifestations of androgen deficiency as a result of primary testicular failure — testosterone in these patients may help maintain or improve muscle function)

Polyglandular autoimmune disease — p. 293 (though much less common than autoimmune primary ovarian failure, primary testicular failure associated with antitesticular antibodies and androgen deficiency may also occur)

Complex genetic disorders (Alström, ataxia telangiectasia, Sohval–Soffer, Weinstein's and Wermer's syndromes)

NB Normal ageing (in healthy men is associated with a relative fall in testosterone with associated elevation of gonadotrophins).

Acquired disorders

Orchitis (viral, especially mumps; also gonorrhoea, leprosy, TB, brucellosis, glanders, syphilis, filariasis, bilharziasis)

Surgical and traumatic castration

Drugs (which may produce antiandrogen effects include spironolactone, ketoconazole, H_2-blockers such as cimetidine, alcohol, marijuana, digitalis, cytotoxics)

Irradiation.

Systemic disorders

Chronic liver disease — p. 106 (total testosterone low or normal, LH usually elevated, high circulating oestrogens due to impaired hepatic clearance of adrenal androgens leading to increased substrate for peripheral aromatization to oestrogens; treatment with aromatizable androgens may worsen the gynaecomastia)

Chronic renal failure (?uraemic pallor; testosterone replacement may improve the anaemia)

Malignancy (Hodgkin's disease, testicular cancer)

Sickle cell disease

Paraplegia (transient reduction in testosterone initially)

Vasculitis (may involve the testes)

Infiltrative disease (amyloidosis, leukaemia).

Causes of secondary hypogonadism (with deficiency of both sperm and androgen production)

Congenital and developmental disorders

Isolated hypogonadotrophic hypogonadism* (?associated anosmia or hyposmia due to developmental failure of the olfactory lobes in which case *Kallman's syndrome* — may also exhibit other midline defects (e.g. cleft-lip or cleft-palate, colour blindness, renal agenesis, nerve deafness), cryptorchidism and skeletal abnormalities (e.g. syndactyly, short fourth metacarpals, craniofacial asymmetry))

Isolated LH deficiency (*'fertile' eunuch syndrome*; variant of Kallman's syndrome in which FSH secretion is preserved resulting in near normal sized testes and well-advanced, though not normal, spermatogenesis; despite the name patients are not fertile without HCG therapy)

Haemochromatosis — p. 129 (iron deposition in the pituitary selectively inhibits gonadotrophins whilst other anterior pituitary hormone secretion remains unaffected)

Complex genetic syndromes (e.g. Prader–Willi;† Laurence–Moon–Bardet–Biedl — p. 504; familial cerebellar ataxia; familial icthyosis).

Acquired disorders

Hypopituitarism — p. 449

Hyperprolactinaemia (either microprolactinoma,

---

* Differentiation from the much commoner constitutional delayed puberty is difficult. Withdrawal of androgen therapy can eventually be achieved in constitutional delayed puberty but not in hypogonadotrophic hypogonadism. Fertility can be facilitated in hypogonadotrophic hypogonadism by treatment with gonadotrophins or gonadotrophin-releasing hormone instead of androgens.

† *Prader–Labhart–Willi syndrome.* Our survey has raised the possibility that this has occurred rarely as an MRCP short case. The syndrome consists of: poor fetal activity, infantile hypotonia and neonatal failure to thrive. Compulsive hyperphagia with massive obesity in later childhood. May be *cryptorchidism*. Thin turned down upper lips and up-slanting palpebral fissures often seen (*almond-shaped eyes*). Poor dentition is often present. Fair skin and hair darkens with age. Hands and feet characteristically small (*acromicria*). Pickwickian syndrome (p. 94) may occur. Diabetes mellitus is common. Mild to severe *mental retardation* with behaviour and personality problems are usual. Hypothalamic dysfunction and *hypogonadotrophic hypogonadism* are often present. *It should be remembered that low testosterone and gonadotrophins may be found in association with any case of massive obesity.*

macroprolactinoma or other large pituitary tumour causing stalk compression;* prolactin inhibits gonadotrophin secretion; macroadenomata may destroy pituitary gonadotrophs)

Oestrogen excess (therapy for prostatic cancer; oestrogen-producing neoplasms)

Opiate-like drugs (such as morphine, methadone and heroin) inhibit gonadotrophin production.

Systemic disorders

Cushing's—p. 441 (high levels of glucocorticoids suppress gonadotrophin secretion)

Acute stress or illness (high glucocorticoids)

Nutritional deficiency (protein–calorie malnutrition or anorexia nervosa; gonadotrophin production inhibited)

Chronic illness (malnutrition may contribute)

Massive obesity.†

---

* Microprolactinomata are <1 cm in diameter and macroprolactinomata >1 cm. Any pituitary macroadenoma which compresses the pituitary stalk and interferes with the prolactin-inhibiting dopaminergic neurones there may lead to hyperprolactinaemia. Serum prolactin levels >5000 mIU l⁻¹ are not usually associated with stalk compression alone and usually reflect a true prolactinoma. Other causes of hyperprolactinaemia include CNS-active drugs such as phenothiazines and other antipsychotic drugs, opiates, sedatives, antidepressants and stimulants.

† See footnote on Prader–Labhart–Willi syndrome on p. 459.

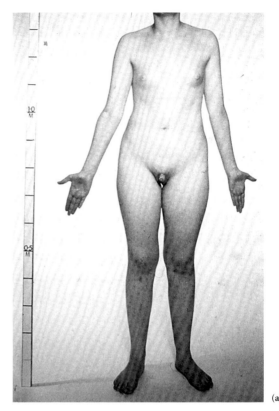

Figure C5.73 Klinefelter's syndrome. (a) Note the disproportionately long lower limbs in relation to the upper torso, the underdeveloped genitalia and the absent axillary and pubic hair. (b) Gynaecomastia.

Case 13 | Bitemporal hemianopia

Frequency in survey: main focus of a short case in 2% of attempts at PACES station 5, endocrine.

Bitemporal hemianopia is dealt with on p. 194.

Case 14 | Charcot's joint

Frequency in survey: main focus of a short case in 2% of attempts at PACES station 5, endocrine.

Charcot's joint is dealt with on p. 396.

Case 15 | **Necrobiosis lipoidica diabeticorum**

Frequency in survey: main focus of a short case in 1% of attempts at PACES station 5, endocrine.

Necrobiosis lipoidica diabeticorum is dealt with on p. 314.

Case 16 | Short stature

Frequency in survey: main focus of a short case in 0.8% of attempts at PACES station 5, endocrine.

Record
The patient is abnormally short (?features of a major systemic disease or of one of the classic syndromes).

Causes of a short adult* include
Genetic
Familial (correlation between a patient's height and the mid-parental height)

Achondroplasia (?short limbs, relatively normal trunk, large head with bulging forehead and scooped nose)

*Turner's syndrome** (?webbed neck, cubitus valgus, short metacarpals, female phenotype, left-sided heart lesions — p. 456)

Noonan's syndrome (?triangular micrognathic facial appearance and posteriorly angulated low-set ears with a thick helix, webbed neck, shield-like chest, pectus excavatum, cubitus valgus, mental retardation, right-sided cardiovascular abnormalities — Fig. C5.72c, p. 457).

Nutritional or general diseases during childhood
Low birth weight and subsequent slow growth (some cases end up as short adults)

Congenital heart disease (?cyanosis, young adult)

Renal disease

---

* The diagnoses in italics represent causes of short stature in adults that our surveys have shown have occurred in the MRCP with the short stature highlighted as a prominent feature. Short stature is a subject more commonly considered in childhood. Shortness which is out of keeping with parental height (familial) can usefully be considered as follows:

1 Child looks normal
(a) **Normal growth velocity:** constitutional delay in growth and adolescence (common; short throughout childhood; pubertal growth spurt delayed; bone age lags behind chronological age; patients usually attain normal height)

(b) **Low growth velocity:**
- *Thin child* (mostly due to a disease of a major system):
  Central nervous system (mental retardation)
  Cardiovascular system (congenital heart disease)
  Respiratory system (cystic fibrosis, asthma, TB)
  Gastrointestinal system (malabsorption, e.g. coeliac disease, Crohn's)
  Renal system (chronic renal failure, renal tubular acidosis)
  Psychosocial problems (emotional deprivation; anorexia nervosa)

- *Fat child* (endocrine causes):
  Hypopituitarism
  Growth hormone deficiency
  Laron's syndrome (same phenotype as growth hormone deficiency but cause is somatomedin deficiency — resting growth hormone levels are high; no response to growth hormone therapy)
  Hypothyroidism
  Cushing's
  Pseudohypoparathyroidism

2 Child looks abnormal
(a) **Dysmorphic features:** recognizable syndrome (e.g. low birth weight, chromosomal abnormality)

(b) **Disproportionate short stature:**

Short limbs (e.g. achondroplasia, hypochondroplasia, dyschondrosteosis, metaphyseal chondroplasia, multiple epiphyseal dysplasia)

Short back and limbs (e.g. metatrophic dwarf, spondyloepiphyseal dysplasia, mucopolysaccharidosis).

Cystic fibrosis* (?clubbing, cyanosis, basal crackles, sputum pot, young person, p. 101)
Chronic infection
Collagenosis
Mental retardation
Coeliac disease
Rickets* (?lateral bowing of legs that is symmetrical, p. 418)
Diabetes
Craniospinal irradiation.

Social
Severe emotional deprivation suppresses growth hormone release.

Endocrine problems during childhood
Isolated growth hormone deficiency
Panhypopituitarism
Hypothyroidism
Cushing's disease
Precocious puberty
Pseudohypoparathyroidism* (?round face, short neck, short metacarpals, decreased intelligence, subcutaneous calcification, see also p. 467).

Case 17 | Pseudohypoparathyroidism

Frequency in survey: main focus of a short case in 0.4% of attempts at PACES station 5, endocrine.

Record

The patient is *short* and *obese* with a *round* face (with frontal bossing of the skull) and a short neck. There is *shortening* of the (most often) fourth and fifth *metacarpals* (ask the patient to make a fist to demonstrate this) and, may be, metatarsals, as well as shortening and broadening of the distal phalanges. There are *subcutaneous calcifications.**

These features suggest the diagnosis of type 1a pseudohypoparathyroidism (Albright's† hereditary osteodystrophy).

Other features which may occur in Albright's hereditary osteodystrophy

Mental retardation (usually slight)
Hypothyroidism (without goitre)
Hypogonadism
Pseudopseudohypoparathyroidism‡ in first-degree relatives
Females affected twice as commonly as males
Parathyroid glands normal or hyperplastic
Usually presents early in life (mental deficiency, epilepsy or tetany)
Treatment is with vitamin D.

In pseudohypoparathyroidism there is target organ resistance to the action of parathyroid hormone. The defect occurs proximal to the formation of the second messenger, cAMP.§

Types of pseudohypoparathyroidism

Type 1a—appearance as described in the above *record*. Deficiency in the Gs protein that couples parathyroid hormone receptors to adenylcyclase, limits the normal cAMP production in response to parathyroid hormone as well as to other hormones such as TSH. As a result patients with type 1a pseudohypoparathyroidism have many abnormalities (e.g. *hypothyroidism, hypogonadism*) as well as hypocalcaemia. The causative mutations in the gene encoding the Gs protein are inherited as *autosomal dominant*

Type 1b—appearance is normal. Gs protein normal—resistance is limited to parathyroid hormone. A defective parathyroid hormone receptor is the postulated cause. Osteitis fibrosa cystica can occur in some subjects suggesting selective renal (but not skeletal) resistance to parathyroid hormone action; this rare combination has been called *pesudohypohyperparathyroidism.*

Other causes of hypoparathyroidism

Autoimmune (there may be an associated endocrine deficiency, most frequently Addison's disease, as well as a

---

* Ectopic deposits of bone may develop in muscles, tendons, connective tissue and skin.
† Albright described pseudohypoparathyroidism as the first example of a hormone-resistance disorder.
‡ Physical features of Albright's osteodystrophy without evidence of hormone resistance.

§ The diagnosis is suggested by the finding of an *elevated* parathyroid hormone in a patient with hypocalcaemia, hyperphosphataemia and normal renal function. Lack of urinary cAMP excretion in response to parathyroid hormone (commercially available 1–34 peptide) infusion confirms the parathyroid hormone resistance.

T-cell defect predisposing to mucocutaneous candidiasis (see p. 293); alopecia and vitiligo may also be seen)

Surgical (incidence varies widely as a function of the skill of the surgeon)

Iron deposition in parathyroids (e.g. repeated transfusions in thalassaemia)

Copper deposition in parathyroids (Wilson's disease)

Failure of development of parathyroids (Di George's syndrome)

Idiopathic (inherited mutations in the parathyroid hormone gene that prevent synthesis and secretion of parathyroid hormone)

Transient (hypomagnesaemia; transient suppression of normal parathyroids by a hyperparathyroid adenoma;* surgical injury to the parathyroids is another postulated cause of transient postoperative hypoparathyroidism).

---

* Though within a week the suppressed parathyroids should be functioning again, the major cause of hypocalcaemia following hyperparathyroidectomy is 'bone hunger'—with removal of the high parathyroid hormone levels, the skeleton rapidly takes in calcium. It may take weeks for the skeleton to recover fully.

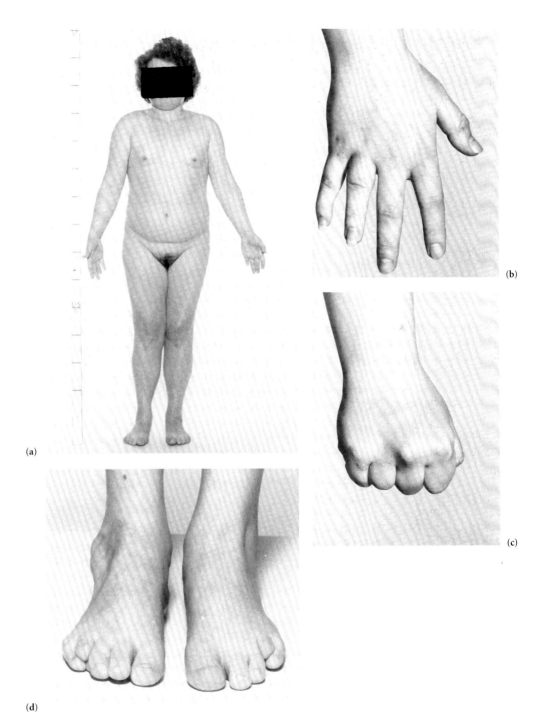

(a)

(b)

(c)

(d)

Figure C5.74 (a) Note the short neck and short fourth finger. (b) Shortening of the fourth finger due to the short metacarpal. (c) Demonstrating the shorter fourth metacarpal. (d) Short fourth toes due to the shorter metatarsals.

Case 18 | Pendred's syndrome

Frequency in survey: did not occur in the initial small survey at PACES station 5, endocrine.

Predicted frequency from older, more extensive MRCP short case surveys: main focus of a short case in 0.6% of attempts at PACES station 5, endocrine.

Record

This *deaf* patient has a smooth, firm, symmetrical *goitre*.

In view of the combination of goitre and deafness one would have to consider the possibility of Pendred's syndrome.*

Congenital goitre (sporadic cretinism)

Goitrous infantile hypothyroidism is due to a defect in any of the steps of thyroid hormone synthesis (Fig. C5.75). Abnormalities that have been identified include defects in: (i) iodide transport; (ii) organification of iodide (defect in the enzyme peroxidase); (iii) synthesis of thyroglobulin; (iv) thyroglobulin proteolysis; or (v) iodotyrosine deiodination. All the defects are rare. The most common is the *inability to organify iodine* due to a defect in the enzyme peroxidase or to the synthesis of an abnormal thyroglobulin molecule. Large amounts of iodide accumulate in the thyroid and this can be demonstrated by the perchlorate discharge test. In some patients this defect is associated with an VIIIth nerve deafness and has the eponym *Pendred's syndrome.*

---

* Hearing impairment may be a manifestation of hypothyroidism *per se*, particularly in the elderly. In the adult with goitre and hy-pothyroidism, the hypothyroidism would be a much commoner cause of hearing impairment than Pendred's syndrome.

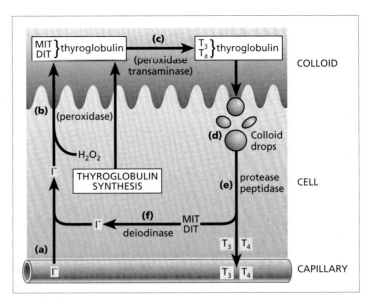

Figure C5.75 Synthesis of thyroid hormones: inorganic iodide (I^-) is concentrated in the thyroid follicles by active transport across the cell membrane (a) and then rapidly transferred across the cell into the colloid lumen. During this process, iodide is oxidized by peroxidase (b) and linked to tyrosine molecules to form monoiodotyrosines (MIT) and diiodotyrosines (DIT) within a large protein, thyroglobulin. These are then coupled by further enzyme action (c) to form thyroxine (T_4) and triiodothyronine (T_3) and, still linked to thyroglobulin, are reabsorbed into the follicular cells in colloid drops by endocytosis (d). T_4 and T_3 are then separated from the thyroglobulin by proteases (e) contained within lysozomes. Any uncoupled MIT and DIT are further deiodinated (f) to release tyrosine and iodide which may be available for recycling. T_4 and T_3 are then secreted into the circulation.

Station 5
Eyes

Case 1 | Diabetic retinopathy

Frequency in survey: main focus of a short case in 41% of attempts at PACES station 5, eyes.

Survey note: this is the commonest short case; it is also one of the easiest to fail. Some candidates who saw haemorrhages failed to note whether there were also micro-aneurysms. The uninitiated failed to recognize photocoagulation scars. The commonest forms reported in the survey were background diabetic retinopathy (40%) and proliferative retinopathy treated with photocoagulation (40%). Most of the rest were fundi with untreated proliferative retinopathy. Advanced diabetic eye disease was only rarely reported.

Record 1

There are *microaneurysms, blot haemorrhages* and *hard exudates* (due to lipid deposition in the retina).*
   The patient has background diabetic retinopathy.

Record 2

The above, plus: in the R/L eye there is a *circinate formation* of *hard exudates* (indicating oedema) *near*† the R/L *macula* suggesting that macular oedema is present or imminent. It would be important to assess the patient's visual acuity.

Record 3

Any of the above, plus: there are *cotton-wool spots, flame-shaped haemorrhages* (both indicating ischaemia) and leashes of *new vessels* (say where). *Photocoagulation scars* are seen (say where).
   The patient has proliferative diabetic retinopathy treated by photocoagulation.

Record 4

Any of the above, plus: *vitreous haemorrhage/vitreous scar/retinal detachment* (widespread and impairing vision) indicate advanced diabetic eye disease.
   NB With diabetic retinopathy there may also be:
1 Cataracts (see. p. 490).
2 AV nipping (indicating either coexistent hypertension or arteriosclerosis).

Indications for photocoagulation are the sight-threatening forms of retinopathy:
1 *Maculopathy* (especially type II = non-insulin-dependent diabetes): warning signs are hard exudates often in rings (indicating oedema) encroaching on the macula, sometimes with multiple haemorrhages (indi-

---

* Say where the lesions are; particularly in relation to the macula — see criteria for referral to an ophthalmologist.
† If you use the tiny spotlight of the ophthalmoscope and ask the patient to *look at* the light while you look in, you will be looking at the macula and this may help you assess whether there are hard exudates or haemorrhages involving the macula.

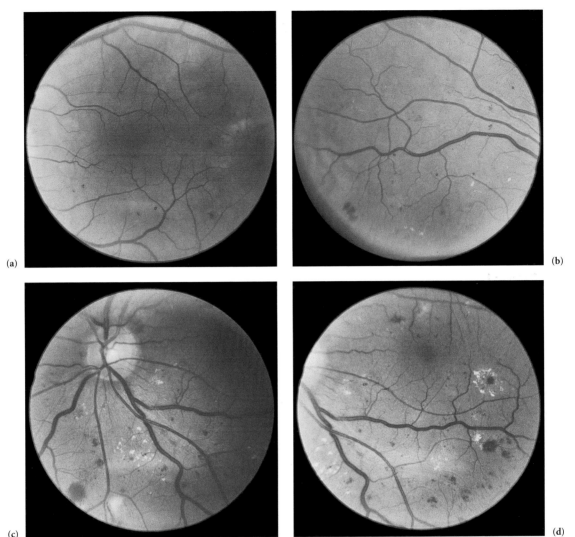

(a)

(b)

(c)

(d)

Figure C5.76 Diabetic retinopathy. (a) Early background changes of microaneurysms and blot haemorrhages. (b) Background retinopathy (note microaneurysms, blot haemorrhages and punctate hard exudates). (c) Extensive background changes and cotton-wool spot 2.5 disc diameters inferior to the disc. (d) More extensive background changes (note small circinate temporal to the macula). (e) The soft exudate in the lower right of the picture indicates ischaemia which is the stimulus to new vessel formation. (f) Note photocoagulation scars. (g) The large circinate temporal to the macula indicates oedema in that area. (h) Haemorrhages and exudates at the macula (maculopathy). (i) Venous irregularity and beading (preproliferative sign). (j) Venous reduplication is seen in the upper part of this picture (a preproliferative sign). (k) The leash of new vessels protruding into the vitreous is in focus, whereas the retina with its photocoagulation scars is further away and therefore slightly out of focus. Note the leash of fibrous tissue accompanying the new vessels (previous haemorrhage). (l) Peripheral new vessels which are haemorrhaging (note photocoagulation scars (same patient as (k)). (m) Advanced diabetic eye disease (note vitreous scar).

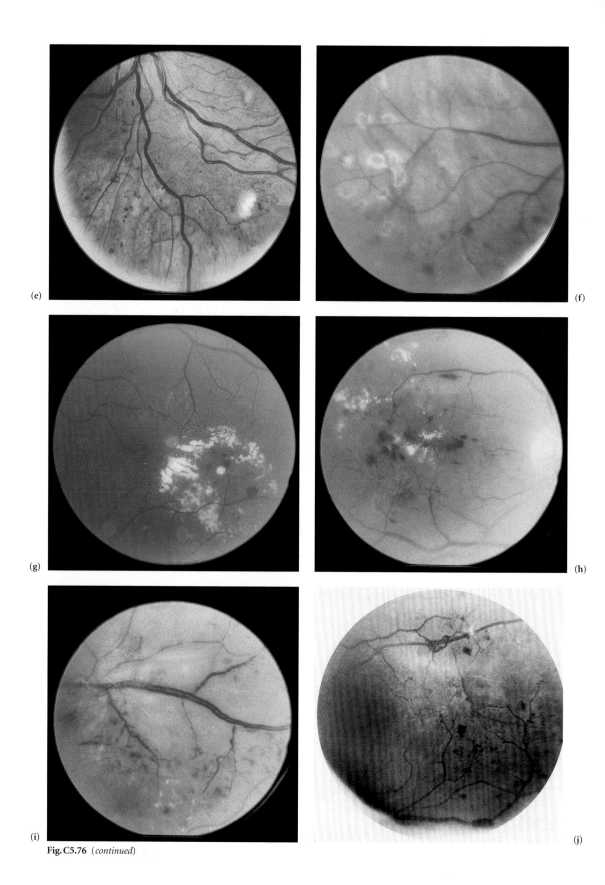

(e)

(f)

(g)

(h)

(i)

(j)

Fig. C5.76 (*continued*)

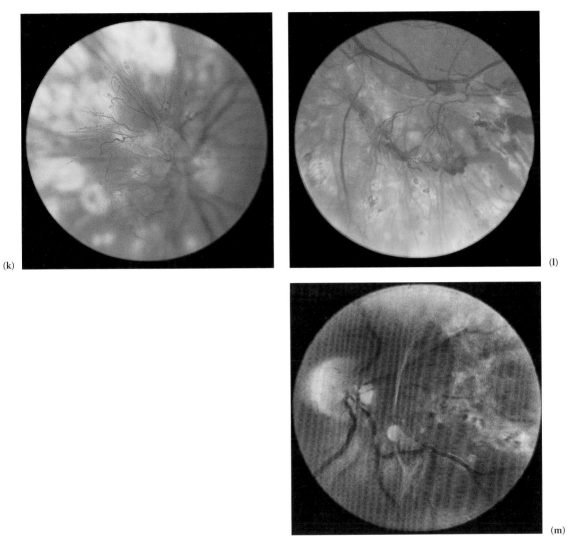

(k) (l)

(m)

Fig. C5.76 *(continued)*

cating ischaemia). Macular oedema itself is recognized by stereo biomicroscopy and not by direct ophthalmoscopy. Even slight visual deterioration is highly significant if there is any suspicion of maculopathy

2 *Preproliferative and proliferative retinopathy* (commonly type I = insulin-dependent diabetes): preproliferative lesions suggesting that neovascularization is imminent are:

Multiple cotton-wool spots

Multiple large blot haemorrhages

Venous beading

Venous loops

Arterial sheathing

Atrophic-looking retina.

Criteria for referral to an ophthalmologist

(according to European diabetic retinopathy screening guidelines):

1 Proliferative retinopathy (new vessels on disc or elsewhere; preretinal haemorrhage; fibrous tissue)

2 Advanced diabetic eye disease (vitreous haemorrhage; fibrous tissue; recent retinal detachment; rubeosis iridis)

3 Preproliferative retinopathy (venous irregularities — beading, reduplication, loops; multiple haemorrhages;

multiple cotton-wool spots; intraretinal microvascular abnormalities (IRMA))

4 Non-proliferative retinopathy with macular involvement (reduced visual acuity not corrected by pinhole, i.e. suggesting macular oedema; haemorrhages and/or hard exudates within 1 disc diameter of the macula, with or without visual loss

5 Non-proliferative retinopathy without macular involvement (large circinate or plaque of hard exudates within the major temporal vascular arcades).

Case 2 | Retinitis pigmentosa

Frequency in survey: main focus of a short case in 16% of attempts at PACES station 5, eyes.

Record

There is *widespread* scattering of *black pigment* in a pattern resembling *bone corpuscles*. The macula is spared. There is *tunnel vision*.

The diagnosis is retinitis pigmentosa.

The patient may well have presented with night blindness. The condition progresses remorselessly with increasing retinal pigmentation, deepening disc pallor of consecutive optic atrophy as the ganglion cells die, and increasing constriction of visual field. It may occur on its own although it is often associated with other abnormalities such as cataracts,* deaf–mutism and mental deficiency. Pigmentary degeneration of the retina may also occur in many conditions such as:

Laurence–Moon–Bardet–Biedl syndrome (autosomal recessive; ?obesity, hypogonadism, dwarfism, mental retardation and polydactyly — p. 504)

Refsum's disease (autosomal recessive; ?pupillary abnormalities, cerebellar ataxia, deafness, peripheral neuropathy, cardiomyopathy and icthyosis)

as well as some of the

Hereditary ataxias

Familial neuropathies

Neuronal lipidoses (ceroid lipofuscinosis).

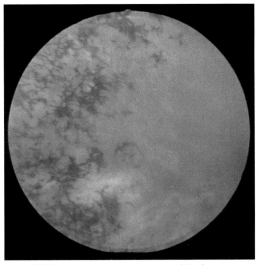

Figure C5.77 Peripheral pigmentation resembling bone corpuscles.

---

* Visual acuity may sometimes be considerably improved by cataract removal.

Case 3 | **Optic atrophy**

Frequency in survey: main focus of a short case in 6% of attempts at PACES station 5, eyes. Additional feature in a further 2%, especially station 3, CNS.

Record

The disc is *pale* and *clearly delineated* and (in the severe case) the *pupil reacts consensually* to light but *not directly*.* Field testing with the head of a hat pin (maybe) reveals a *central scotoma*.

The diagnosis is optic atrophy. The well-defined disc edge suggests that it is not secondary to papilloedema† (yellow/grey disc with blurred margins). Common causes of primary optic atrophy are:

1 Multiple sclerosis (may be temporal pallor only; ?nystagmus, scanning speech, cerebellar ataxia, etc. — p. 209)
2 Compression of the optic nerve by:
    (a) tumour (e.g. pituitary — ?bitemporal hemianopia)
    (b) aneurysm
3 Glaucoma (?pathological cupping).

Other causes

Ischaemic optic neuropathy (abrupt onset of visual loss in an elderly patient; may be painful; thrombosis or embolus of posterior ciliary artery; temporal arteritis is sometimes the cause)
Leber's optic atrophy (males : females = 6 : 1)
Retinal artery occlusion (p. 500)
Toxic amblyopia (lead, methyl alcohol, arsenic, insecticides, quinine)

Nutritional amblyopia (famine, etc., tobacco–alcohol amblyopia, vitamin B_{12} deficiency, diabetes mellitus‡)
Friedreich's ataxia (?cerebellar signs, pes cavus, scoliosis, etc. — p. 220)
Tabes dorsalis (?Argyll Robertson pupils, etc. — p. 255)
Paget's disease (?large skull, bowed tibia, etc. — p. 403)
Consecutive optic atrophy.‡

---

* In early unilateral optic neuritis before the direct reflex is lost, it may simply become more sluggish than the consensual reflex. In this situation it may be possible to demonstrate the *Marcus Gunn* phenomenon. In this the direct reflex may at first appear to be brisk. However, when the light is alternated from one side to the other, the pupil on the affected side may be seen to dilate slowly when exposed to the light. The mechanism is as follows: when the light shines in the healthy eye a rapid constriction occurs in both eyes. As the light then moves to the affected eye, this fails to transmit the message to continue constriction as quickly as normal. As a result the pupils have time to recover and dilate, despite the light shining on the abnormal eye.

† Optic atrophy can be divided into primary, secondary and consecutive. Consecutive optic atrophy follows damage to the parent ganglion cells of the retina as in widespread choroidoretinitis, retinitis pigmentosa and retinal artery occlusion.

‡ Optic atrophy in diabetes mellitus may also occur in the DIDMOAD syndrome — with diabetes insipidus, diabetes mellitus and deafness. It is a rare, recessively inherited disorder.

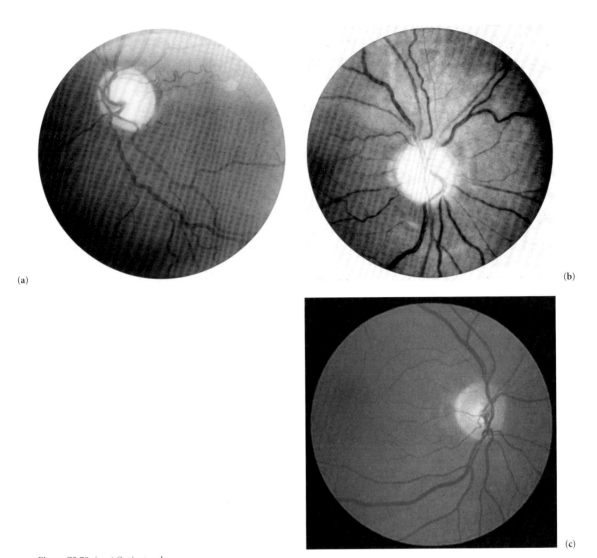

(a)

(b)

(c)

Figure C5.78 (a–c) Optic atrophy.

Case 4 | **Ocular palsy**

Frequency in survey: main focus of a short case in 6% of attempts at PACES station 5, eyes.

Station 5, Eyes, is supposed to be a fundal case. However, it is clear from our initial small PACES survey that ocular palsy has occasionally been used as a case in the Eyes section. Ocular palsy is dealt with on p. 203.

Case 5 | **Visual field defect**

Frequency in survey: main focus of a short case in 4% of attempts at PACES station 5, eyes.

Station 5, Eyes, is supposed to be a fundal case. However, it is clear from our initial small PACES survey that visual field defect has occasionally been used as a case in the Eyes section. Visual field defect is dealt with on p. 194.

Case 6 | Retinal vein occlusion

Frequency in survey: main focus of a short case in 2% of attempts at PACES station 5, eyes.

Record

The veins are *tortuous* and *engorged*. *Haemorrhages* are *scattered riotously* over the whole retina, irregular and superficial, like bundles of straw alongside the veins (*papilloedema* and *soft exudates* may also be seen).

The diagnosis is central retinal vein occlusion (CRVO). There may be *hypertension*, *hyperlipidaemia* or *diabetes mellitus* or there may be an underlying *hyperviscosity syndrome*,* especially *Waldenström's macroglobulinaemia* (?lymphadenopathy, hepatosplenomegaly, bruising and purpura), but also occasionally *myeloma* (?urinary Bence-Jones protein) and *connective tissue disorders*.

The condition is commoner in eyes prone to simple glaucoma (which should, therefore, be excluded in the other eye), in the elderly arteriosclerotic, and the hypertensive and hyperlipidaemic, but may also arise in young adults (especially women—the contraceptive pill is a risk factor). It causes incomplete loss of vision and improvement may be scant. About 3 months after acute CRVO 20% of cases lose the remaining sight in the affected eye because of an acute secondary glaucoma. This is due to new vessels on the iris root developing as a result of retinal hypoxia. Panretinal photocoagulation may decrease the risk of subsequent neovascular glaucoma. A less severe ophthalmoscopic appearance is encountered in younger patients when the terms *partial retinal vein occlusion* and *venous stasis retinopathy* are used; visual acuity in this situation is only slightly reduced and visual prognosis is good.

In occlusion of a branch of the retinal vein (also occurred in our survey) the occlusion usually occurs at an AV crossing with the changes confined to the sector beyond this—haemorrhages and cotton-wool spots spread out in a wedge from the AV crossing. Macula oedema and decreased visual acuity may occur or it may be asymptomatic. Neovascularization is a rare complication. Any loss of sight† mostly recovers and there is no secondary glaucoma, though sometimes the visual outcome is poor. Branch retinal vein occlusion must be distinguished from *viral retinitis* which it resembles ophthalmoscopically (see p. 506). In view of the association with hypertension, hypertensive changes may be visible in the rest of the fundus (thin arterioles, AV nipping, etc.).

---

* The symptoms and signs of a hyperviscosity syndrome are principally neurological due to sluggish cerebral circulation. Cardiac failure may occur in the elderly. Waldenström's macroglobulinaemia is the cause in 90% of hyperviscosity syndromes.

† Think of this diagnosis if you find a quadrantic field defect in one eye only.

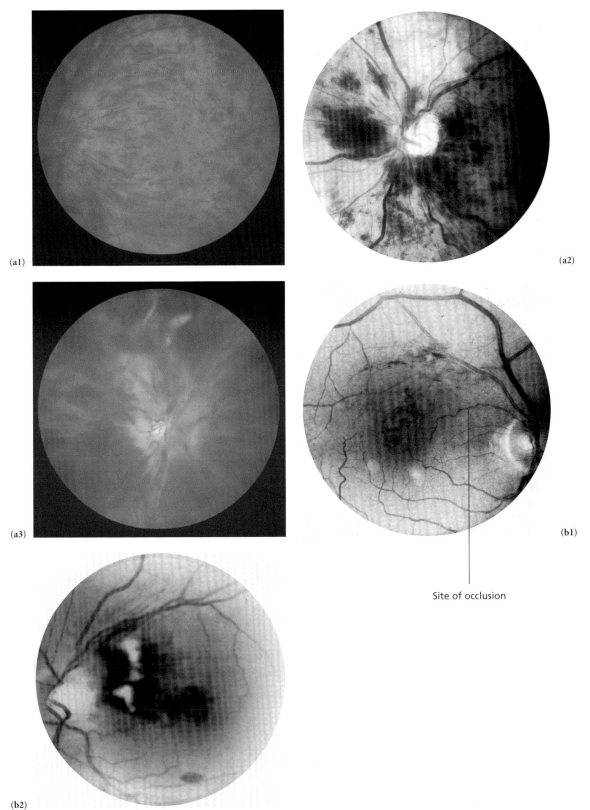

Site of occlusion

Figure C5.79 (a1–3) Three different cases of central retinal vein occlusion. (b1) Branch retinal vein occlusion. (b2) Macular branch retinal vein occlusion.

Case 7 | Old choroiditis

Frequency in survey: main focus of a short case in 2% of attempts at PACES station 5, eyes.

Invigilator's observation: easily confused with laser burn scars in the diabetic fundus.*

Record

There is evidence of old choroiditis in the . . . region of the R/L fundus.

or

In the . . . region of the R/L fundus there is a *patch of white** (or yellow or grey). It suggests exposed sclera due to atrophy of the choroidoretina secondary to old choroiditis. Together with this there are also scattered *pigmented patches* due to proliferation of the retinal pigment epithelium.

In most cases the cause of the choroiditis is unknown but *toxoplasmosis* is commonly implicated.

Other causes

Sarcoidosis (?lupus pernio, chest signs, etc.)

Tuberculosis (often inactive; ?ethnic origin, chest signs)

Syphilis (?tabetic facies and pupils, posterior column signs, extensor plantars, etc.)

Toxocara

Trauma.

---

* Candidates sometimes call laser burns on the diabetic fundus (see. p. 474) old choroiditis, and old choroiditis laser burns, thus diagnosing old choroiditis as diabetic retinopathy. The confusion can be understood when one realizes that laser burn scars are, in a way, a form of old choroiditis. The matter is made worse because the patient with diabetic retinopathy may also happen to have old choroiditis (as diabetics are the main group of people having their fundi carefully examined on a large scale, patients with old choroiditis among them are readily detected). Laser burns can usually be distinguished by their more regular uniform appearance as in Fig. C5.76f, p. 476.

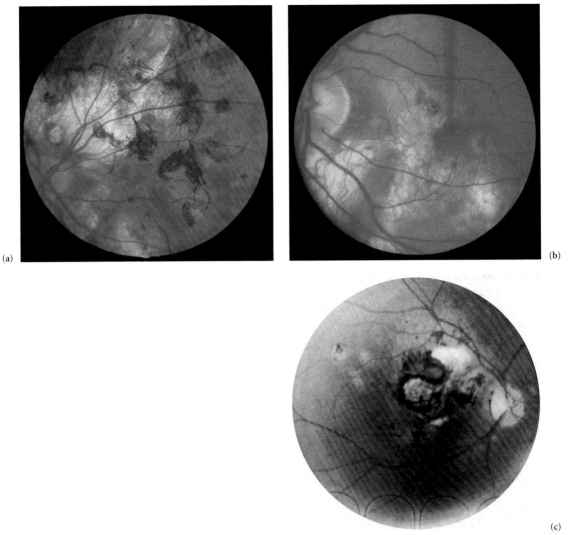

(a)

(b)

(c)

Figure C5.80 (a–c) Three different cases of choroidoretinitis (the artefact on (b) is the shadow cast by the internal fixation device of the fundus camera).

Case 8 | **Papilloedema**

Frequency in survey: did not occur in the initial small survey at PACES station 5, eyes.

Predicted frequency from older, more extensive MRCP short case surveys: main focus of a short case in 4% of attempts at PACES station 5, eyes. Additional feature in a further 2%, especially station 3, CNS.

Record

There is bilateral papilloedema* (search carefully for haemorrhages, exudates and AV nipping).

Possible causes

1 These include:

   (a) *an intracranial space-occupying lesion* (?localizing neurological signs†)

   (b) tumour (infratentorial more often than supratentorial)

   (c) abscess (fever not always present, ?underlying middle ear infection, underlying suppuration elsewhere—e.g. bronchiectasis or empyema)

   (d) haematoma

2 *Accelerated (malignant) hypertension* (check blood pressure—haemorrhages and exudates are not always present; ?narrow tortuous arterioles that vary in calibre, AV nipping—p. 496)

3 *Benign intracranial hypertension‡* (?obese female aged 15–45, no localizing neurological signs).

---

* The disc oedema of papillitis (disc usually pink due to hyperaemia) must be differentiated from developing papilloedema due to raised intracranial pressure. Papilloedema causes enlargement of the blindspot and constriction of the peripheral field, but visual acuity is unaffected. Papillitis (optic neuritis affecting the intraorbital portion of the optic nerve) causes central scotoma, diminished visual acuity, and sometimes tenderness and pain on eye movement during the acute attack. Furthermore, in papillitis there may be a pupillary reflex defect, loss of the central cup and cells may be present in the vitreous over the disc.

† Sixth nerve palsy in the presence of papilloedema may be a false localizing sign due to raised intracranial pressure stretching the nerve during its long intracranial course. A localizing sign may occasionally be rapidly apparent in the case of contralateral optic atrophy—the *Foster–Kennedy syndrome* (a frontal tumour pressing on the optic nerve to cause atrophy and at the same time raising intracranial pressure to cause papilloedema in the other eye). It must be remembered that tumours in and around the frontal lobes can present simply with dementia in the absence of signs and symptoms of raised intracranial pressure (i.e. without papilloedema). A classic lesion to present in this manner is a subfrontal olfac-

tory groove meningioma. These may grow to considerable size, initially causing only memory impairment and marked apathy. On examination and upon closer questioning there is usually a history of diminished or absent sense of smell. Loss of urinary control associated with dementia should be regarded as indicating organic pathology until proven otherwise. A much shorter history of dementia and urinary incontinence together with increasingly severe headache may indicate an underlying malignant glioma of the corpus callosum or of one or other frontal lobe.

‡ This syndrome (also called pseudotumour cerebri, serous meningitis or otitic hydrocephalus) is known to have occurred following middle ear infection which caused lateral sinus thrombosis. It may be that thrombosis of the venous sinuses is the aetiological factor in many other cases. The condition has been associated with the contraceptive pill, long-term tetracycline treatment for acne, corticosteroids (often reduction in dose during long-term therapy), head injury and times of female physiological hormone disturbance such as menarche, pregnancy and puerperium. The CSF pressure is high, frequently above 300 mm, but the composition of the fluid is normal; the protein content is usually low normal, below 20 mg dl^{-1}.

The first sign of raised intracranial pressure is loss of venous pulsation, but recognition of this sign requires much practice and experience (see p. 44). If there is doubt about the normality of the disc, the presence of venous pulsation makes papilloedema and raised intracranial pressure unlikely.

Other causes of papilloedema

Meningitis (especially TB)

Hypercapnoea (cyanosis, flapping tremor of the hands)

Central retinal vein thrombosis (sight affected, usually unilateral, dilated veins, widespread haemorrhages)

(Graves') congestive ophthalmopathy (= malignant exophthalmos though exophthalmos is not always present; prominent eyes, eyelids and conjunctivae swollen and inflamed, marked ophthalmoplegia, often pain)

Cavernous sinus thrombosis (usually becomes bilateral, follows infection of orbit, nose and face; eyeball(s) protrudes, is painful, immobile and there is extreme venous congestion)

Hypoparathyroidism (tetany, epilepsy, cataracts, etc.)

Severe anaemia especially due to massive blood loss and leukaemia (there may be haemorrhages and cotton-wool spots as well)

Guillain–Barré syndrome (papilloedema possibly due to impaired CSF resorption because of the elevated protein content)

Paget's disease (large head, bowed tibiae)

Hurler's syndrome (dwarf, large head, coarse features, hepatosplenomegaly, heart murmurs)

Poisoning with vitamin A, lead, tetracyclines or naladixic acid

Ocular toxoplasmosis.

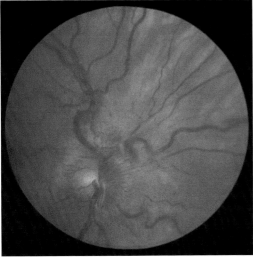
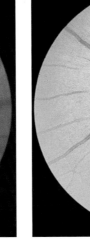

(a)

(b)

Figure C5.81 (a,b) Papilloedema.

Case 9 | Cataracts

Frequency in survey: main focus of a short case in 2% attempts at PACES station 5, eyes. Additional feature in a further 8%.

Record
There are partial cataracts in both eyes (may be localized to the lens nucleus, or seen as flakes, dots or sector-shaped opacities within the lens periphery).

Commonest causes of cataract
1 Old age (usually nuclear, with a brownish discoloration, or of the cortical spoke variety)
2 Diabetic patients develop senile cataracts at younger ages than non-diabetics and this is the commonest type of cataract in diabetes. Rarely* a 'snowflake' (dot cortical opacities) cataract can develop in a young, poorly controlled diabetic, and may progress rapidly to a mature cataract in months or even days (good control may halt and even reverse development).

Other causes of cataract in adults
Trauma
Chronic anterior uveitis
Hypoparathyroidism (Chvostek's and Trousseau's signs, tetany, paraesthesiae and cramps, ectodermal changes, moniliasis, mental retardation and psychiatric disturbances, papilloedema, epilepsy, bradykinetic-rigid syndrome)
Radiation (infrared, ultraviolet, X-rays and possibly microwaves)
Myotonic dystrophy (?frontal balding, ptosis, sternomastoid wasting, myopathic facies, myotonia, etc.—p. 182)
Retinitis pigmentosa (including Refsum's, Laurence–Moon–Bardet–Biedl—pp. 479 and 504)

Steroid therapy (10 mg prednisolone daily for more than 1 year)
Chlorpromazine (500 mg daily for 3 years or more)
Chloroquine.

Causes of cataracts in children
These include: perinatal hypoglycaemia, perinatal hypocalcaemia, maternal rubella, galactosaemia, galactokinase deficiency, genetically inherited, Down's syndrome (trisomy 21), Patau's syndrome (trisomy 13), Edward's syndrome (trisomy 18), Alport's syndrome, Lowe's syndrome.

---

* Rare with modern insulin therapy. A case was seen recently in an insulin-dependent patient who did not take insulin for prolonged periods for personal religious reasons.

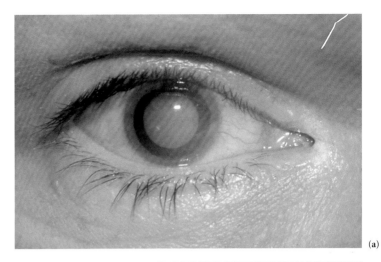

(a)

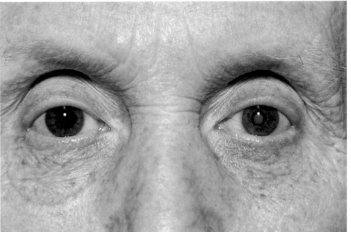

(b)

Figure C5.82 (a) Cataract. (b) A cataract is seen in the left eye.

Case 10 | Myasthenia gravis

Frequency in survey: main focus of a short case in 2% of attempts at PACES station 5, eyes.

Survey note: The following anecdote was reported in our PACES survey. A candidate in the eyes section of station 5 was asked to examine a patient's eye movements. He found unilateral partial ptosis and weakness of abduction of both eyes. When asked the causes he said that cranial nerve lesions could not easily explain the findings and that the likely diagnosis was myasthenia gravis. There then took place a discussion on the other signs of myasthenia.

Station 5, Eyes, is supposed to be a fundal case. However, it is clear from our initial small PACES survey that myasthenia gravis has occasionally been used as a case in the Eyes section. Myasthenia gravis is dealt with on p. 242

Case 11 | Albinism

Frequency in survey: main focus of a short case in 2% of attempts at PACES station 5, eyes.

Record

The (?blind) patient is *very pale* skinned (marked hypomelanosis) and has *very white hair* (or faintly yellow blond). On examination of the eyes there is *nystagmus*, and the *irides* are *translucent*. The *fundus* is *pale*.

The diagnosis is oculocutaneous albinism. (Now look for and comment on the presence (indicate the tyrosinase-positive type) or absence (indicate the tyrosinase-negative type) of *freckles*.*)

Oculocutaneous albinism is a group of autosomal recessive traits recognized by generalized hypomelanosis of the skin, hair and eyes. Albinism can be classified according to the presence or absence of tyrosinase, the enzyme crucial in the synthesis of eumelanin and pheomelanin. Normal plucked hair bulbs darken when incubated *in vitro* with tyrosine. Tyrosinase-positive albinos display some minimal darkening (but not normal) of the hair bulb when incubated with tyrosinase, whereas tyrosinase-negative show no darkening of the hair bulb. These two types of albinism have separate gene loci. Although melanogenesis is deficient in both forms, persons with the tyrosinase-positive form develop some pigmented naevi and have less eye damage than tyrosinase-negative albinos. Patients with phenylketonuria† have diffuse hypopigmentation, with light hair and blue eyes.

---

* Another feature which distinguishes the two types of albinism is the colour of the eyes. The eyes are grey–blue in the tyrosinase-negative. In tyrosinase-positive individuals the eye colour may be brown or blue–yellow.

† *Phenylketonuria* is an autosomal recessive disorder in which the enzyme that converts phenylalanine to tyrosine is deficient. Consequently, melanin synthesis is deficient.

Case 12 | **Exophthalmos**

Frequency in survey: main focus of a short case in 2% of attempts at PACES station 5, eyes.

Station 5, Eyes, is supposed to be a fundal case. However, it is clear from our initial small PACES survey that exophthalmos has occasionally been used as a case in the Eyes section. Exophthalmos is dealt with on p. 426.

Case 13 | Myelinated nerve fibres

Frequency in survey: main focus of a short case in 1% of attempts at PACES station 5, eyes.

Record

There are *bright white*, streaky, irregular patches with frayed margins at the edge of the disc.

These are due to myelinated nerve fibres. They do not affect vision.

Normally the fibres of the optic nerve lose their myelin sheath as they enter the eye. Occasionally the sheath persists for some distance after the fibres leave the optic disc. If this phenomenon is extensive the disc and emerging vessels can be obscured. This appearance may be mistaken for papilloedema and has been termed 'pseudopapilloedema'.

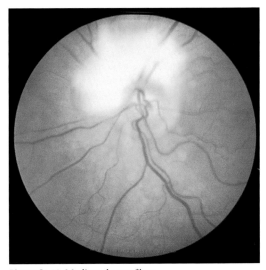

Figure C5.83 Myelinated nerve fibres.

Case 14 | Hypertensive retinopathy

Frequency in survey: main focus of a short case in 1% of attempts at PACES station 5, eyes.

Record

The retinal arterioles are *narrow* (normal ratio of vein to artery is 1.1 : 1), they are (may be) *tortuous* and (may) vary in calibre (localized constriction followed by segments of arteriolar dilatation) with increased light reflex (copper or *silver wiring*) and *AV nipping* (these changes all occurring with ageing and arteriosclerosis as well as with hypertension). There are *flame-shaped* and (less frequently) *blot haemorrhages*, and *cotton-wool exudates* (all indicating grade 3 retinopathy and a diagnosis of malignant (accelerated) hypertension *even without* papilloedema), and there is *papilloedema* (indicating cerebral oedema; papilloedema may occur in malignant hypertension even without haemorrhages and exudates).

This is grade 4 hypertensive retinopathy.

Causes of hypertension

Essential — 94% (cause unknown)

Renal — 4% (renal artery stenosis — ?*bruit*, acute nephritis, pyelonephritis, glomerulonephritis, polycystic disease, systemic sclerosis, SLE, hydronephrosis, renin-secreting tumour and renoprival — after bilateral nephrectomy)

Endocrine — 1%* (Cushing's, Conn's, phaeochromocytoma,† acromegaly, hyperparathyroidism, hypothyroidism and oral contraceptive use)

Miscellaneous — <1% (coarctation of the aorta — ?*radiofemoral delay*, polycythaemia, acute porphyria, pre-eclampsia).

NB Cerebral tumour or raised intracranial pressure from any cause may lead to secondary hypertension (Cushing's reflex).

* The figure 1% does not include hypertension due to oral contraceptive use.
† All patients with phaeochromocytomata should be screened for multiple endocrine neoplasia (MEN) type 2 (p. 437) and von Hippel–Lindau disease (see p. 110) to avert further morbidity and mortality in the patients and their families. All patients in families with MEN-2 or von Hippel–Lindau disease should be screened for phaeochromocytoma even if they are asymptomatic.

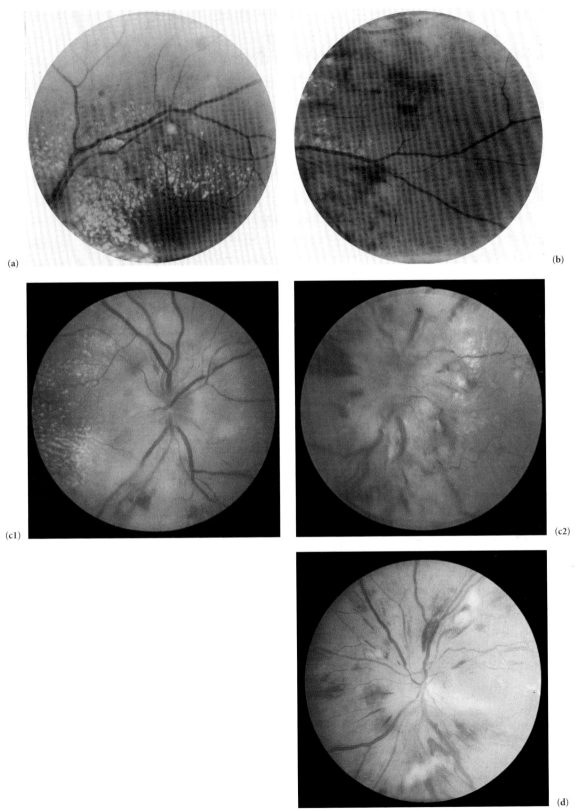

Figure C5.84 (a) Thin, irregular arterioles, AV nipping, haemorrhages and exudates forming a macular star in hypertension. (b) Flame-shaped haemorrhages in hypertension. (c1) Hypertensive retinopathy grade 4, part of a macular star can be seen. (c2) Papilloedema–hypertension. (d) Hypertensive retinopathy grade 4, note papilloedema, flame-shaped haemorrhages and cotton wool spots.

Case 15 | Glaucoma/peripheral field loss

Frequency in survey: main focus of a short case in 1% of attempts at PACES station 5, eyes.

Survey note: in the original, pre PACES, surveys the candidates were usually told that the patient had some difficulty with his vision, and they were asked to examine the visual fields. One candidate reported that he had found unilateral loss of the peripheral field and gave retinitis pigmentosa, extensive choriodoretinitis and diabetes mellitus with laser therapy as the possible causes, and the examiner told him that the patient had chronic glaucoma.

Record 1

There is unilateral R/L nasal visual field defect. This could be due to a space-occupying lesion compressing the lateral part of the optic chiasma* or it could be due to chronic simple glaucoma.* (Ask to examine the fundi.†)

Record 2

The visual fields are grossly constricted and the patient only has central vision (*tunnel vision*).

The most likely causes are retinitis pigmentosa, advanced chronic glaucoma or diffuse choroidoretinitis.

Several mass screening studies have shown a prevalence of 1–2% for glaucoma in the age group of more than 40 years; the greatest incidence of simple glaucoma being between 60 and 70 years. Heredity is an important predisposing factor in 13–25% of cases.

In the early stages a sickle-shaped extension of the blind spot may be demonstrated and some impairment of the nasal field may be apparent on the Bjerrum screen. As the condition progresses there is a contraction of the peripheral field leaving only the central vision intact.

The problem is often one of when to start treatment in a patient suspected of having chronic open angle glaucoma. In general, patients who have a raised intraocular pressure of 24 mmHg or more, especially when it is persistent, those who have a family history of the disease, and those who are in their seventh decade should all be considered. Medical treatment consists of the instillation of miotics (e.g. pilocarpine, neostigmine, carbachol, etc.) in the eyes aiming to reduce the intraocular pressure to a normal level, and thereby to slow the progression of visual failure.

---

* The nasal field loss can be bilateral in chronic glaucoma but would not be bilateral with lateral chiasmal compression. The condition is insidious and asymptomatic in its early stages. It may be discovered accidentally when the vision of one eye is almost lost and of the other seriously impaired. The patient may need to change his/her presbyopic glasses frequently. There is usually accommodative failure. The patient finds it difficult to see in a less illuminated room. Dark and light adaptation are slower than in normal subjects. Periodic eye examinations by an expert are advisable *for those who have a family history of glaucoma.*

†*Cupping of the disc* is an essential feature of chronic glaucoma. The sides of the disc are steep and the retinal vessels have the appearance of *being broken* off at the margin of the disc. The edges of the disc overhang and the course of the vessels, as they climb the sides of the cup, is hidden.

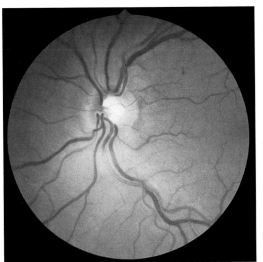

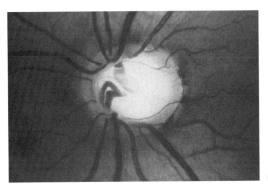

(a)

(b)

Figure C5.85 (a) Early glaucoma with a cup : disc ratio of >0.6. (b) Advanced glaucoma. Note large optic disc with sharply angulated vessels (cupping).

Case 16 | Retinal artery occlusion

Frequency in survey: main focus of a short case in 0.5% of attempts at PACES station 5, eyes.

Survey note: in the original, pre PACES, surveys, it was reported to have occurred as the underlying cause of optic atrophy with attenuated retinal arteries, and as a retinal artery branch occlusion causing a quadrantic field defect. No cherry-red spots were reported!

Record

The eye is blind, the *fundus* is *pale*, the *arterioles* are *thin* and *scanty* and there is a *cherry-red spot* at the macula (because the underlying choroidal circulation is intact).

The diagnosis is central retinal artery occlusion.

Retinal artery occlusion may occur in a central (CRAO) or branch (BRAO) form.

CRAO: in the acute phase the whole fundus (except for the cherry-red spot) is milky white due to retinal oedema. By the time the retinal oedema has faded optic atrophy is generally apparent. The cherry-red spot is usually only seen for about 5–10 days.

BRAO: in retinal artery branch occlusion the fundoscopic appearances of thin arterioles and pale retina are limited to one area and there is a corresponding field defect (e.g. an inferior temporal field defect due to infarction of the superior nasal fundus).

The condition occurs most commonly in the elderly arteriosclerotic patient. It may be due to thrombosis, embolus (?carotid bruits, atrial fibrillation, heart murmurs) or spasm. Transient retinal artery occlusions associated with contralateral hemiparesis may occur from recurrent carotid emboli.

Occlusion of the central retinal artery may also follow giant cell arteritis involving the arterioles around the optic disc (?headaches and temporal artery tenderness).

(a)

(b)

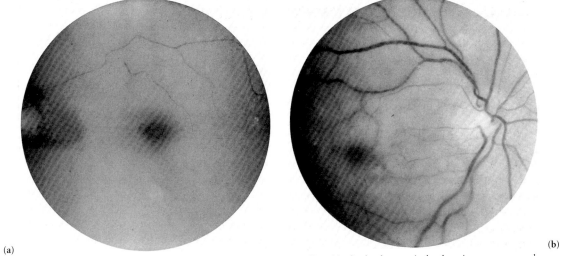

Figure C5.86 (a,b) Acute CRAO. Note the macular cherry-red spots. The milky-white fundus due to retinal oedema is very pronounced in (a).

Case 17 | Asteroid hyalosis

Frequency in survey: did not occur in the initial small survey at PACES station 5, eyes.

Predicted frequency from older, more extensive MRCP short case surveys: main focus of a short case in 0.6% of attempts at PACES station 5, eyes.

Record

With the ophthalmoscope focused in front of the retina, the vitreous is seen to be filled with a *myriad* of *tiny, white,* discrete, shiny *opacities,* like a galaxy of stars.

The diagnosis is asteroid hyalosis.

Asteroid hyalosis is usually diagnosed in patients aged between 60 and 65 years. It may be more common in males. It is *unilateral* in the majority of patients. Biomicroscopically there are *white* bodies of *oval* shape and varying size that are adherent to the framework of the vitreous gel. The opacities consist mainly of *calcium soaps.* Visual function is not disturbed and patients are unaware of the bodies which may be scattered throughout the entire vitreous cavity or may be accumulated in one part of it. Although it has been suggested by some authors that this condition is related to diabetes (approximately 30% of patients with asteroid hyalosis have diabetes), it is now generally agreed that the two are probably not connected. It probably reflects the fact that diabetic patients have their eyes looked into more than others. It has also been suggested that the incidence of hypercholesterolaemia is higher and that of posterior vitreous detachment lower than expected for the age group concerned.

Synchysis scintillans appears to be rarer than asteroid hyalosis. Most descriptions relate it to injury or inflammation involving the vitreous cavity. In contrast to asteroid hyalosis it is usually *bilateral* and the opacities, which are *cholesterol crystals,* appear more *golden.* The opacities do not appear to be attached to the collagen fibrils and float freely in the vitreous fluid with ocular motion; they settle together at the bottom of the vitreous when the eye ceases to move. They have a *flat, angular, crystalline* appearance in contrast to the white spheres of asteroid hyalosis.

Case 18 | **Drusen**

Frequency in survey: did not occur in the initial small survey at PACES station 5, eyes.

Predicted frequency from older, more extensive MRCP short case surveys: main focus of a short case in 0.4% of attempts at PACES station 5, eyes.

Record

Multiple, discrete, round, yellow–white dots of variable size scattered around the macula and posterior pole of the eye.

These are retinal drusen.

Retinal drusen represent abnormal accumulations in the retinal pigment epithelium basement (Bruch's) membrane in subjects usually over the age of 40 years. Drusen in the macular region are often precursors to visual loss from *senile macular degeneration*. The latter may lead to impairment of central vision early in its course — noncongruent central scotoma.

Once drusen have been discovered, the patient needs to be told to screen one eye at a time regularly for possible signs of neovascular macular degeneration. Such screening involves checking lines on a piece of graph paper or between tiles in a bathroom. Blank spots or distortion may be a sign of neovascularisation. Photodynamic therapy using the drug verteporfin reduces the risk of vision loss.

Retinal drusen need to be distinguished from optic disc drusen (also called hyaline bodies) which are bright excrescences at the optic disc which may be calcified. These are sometimes obvious but may be difficult to see in young persons, in whom the disc elevation they produce can be mistaken for papilloedema (*pseudopapilloedema*). Occasionally, these may be associated with tuberous sclerosis.

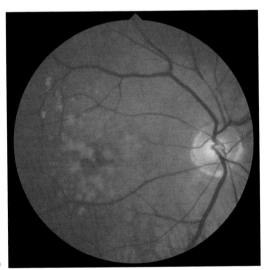

(a)

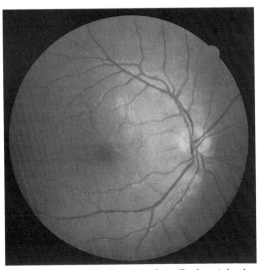

(b)

Figure C5.87 (a) Retinal drusen in the macular area. (b) Optic disc drusen in a young person leading to pseudopapilloedema (when he presented to casualty with headache, the optic disc changes were noted and an urgent CT scan was ordered; this was normal and ultrasonography of the optic disc showed up the drusen as the only abnormality).

Case 19 | Laurence–Moon–Bardet–Biedl syndrome

Frequency in survey: did not occur in the initial small survey at PACES station 5, eyes.

Predicted frequency from older, more extensive MRCP short case surveys: main focus of a short case in 0.7% of attempts at PACES station 5, eyes. Additional feature in some others.

Record

On examination of the fundi of this *blind** patient, there is a pigmentary retinopathy suggestive of *retinitis pigmentosa.** There is truncal *obesity, short stature* (not always) and *polydactyly.†*

These features suggest the diagnosis of the Laurence–Moon–Bardet–Biedl syndrome. (There is likely to be *mental retardation†* of variable severity, and *hypogonadism†*.)

Autosomal recessive

Renal structural and functional abnormalities are very common. Interstitial nephritis may lead to renal failure.

The 'splitters' and the 'lumpers'

Some investigators (the 'splitters') consider the Bardet–Biedl syndrome and the Laurence–Moon syndrome to be distinct; the Laurence–Moon syndrome being characterized by the absence of polydactyly and obesity and the presence of spastic paraparesis. Other investigators (the 'lumpers') believe these distinctions relate to variable expression of a single disorder.

Related disorders

Alström's syndrome: autosomal recessive; retinal dystrophy and obesity; blindness in early childhood; moderate deafness before the age of 10; diabetes mellitus and slowly progressive chronic nephropathy in early adulthood; *mental retardation and digital abnormalities do not occur*

Carpenter's syndrome (acrocephalopolysyndactyly): autosomal recessive; acrocephaly; syndactyly; characteristic facial appearance associated with obesity, mental retardation, hypogonadism and polydactyly of the feet. In view of the characteristic skeletal findings there should not be diagnostic difficulty.

---

* The retinal dystrophy of the Laurence–Moon–Bardet–Biedl syndrome is usually pigmentary. Though retinitis pigmentosa is commonly cited in this syndrome, the preferred term is *rod-cone dystrophy*, because it more accurately describes the pathological process and in the early stages no pigmentary changes may be seen despite significant visual disturbance. In one study mean age of night blindness was 9 years and of blindness registration was 15 years.

†Hypogonadism, mental retardation and polydactyly are less frequently found in females.

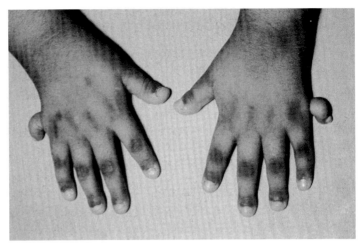

Figure C5.88 Polydactyly.

Case 20 | Cytomegalovirus choroidoretinitis (AIDS)

Frequency in survey: did not occur in the initial small survey at PACES station 5, eyes.

Predicted frequency from older, more extensive MRCP short case surveys: main focus of a short case in 0.1% of attempts at PACES station 5, eyes.

Record

The fundi show discrete areas of *white or yellow retinal opacification* with associated *haemorrhage* and *vascular sheathing* (the appearance resembles branch retinal vein occlusion—p. 484, but is distinguished because one eye often has multiple foci, and there is a tendency for both eyes to be affected).

The appearance ('*scrambled egg and tomato sauce*' and '*cottage cheese and jam*' are both terms that have been used to describe the typical appearance) is suggestive of cytomegalovirus choroidoretinitis in an *immunosuppressed patient*. The diagnosis could be substantiated by culture of throat and urine.

Natural history of HIV infection

Primary infection

Leads to transient fall in CD4+ cells and may lead to opportunistic infection (usually oesophageal candidiasis) and an increase in cytotoxic CD8+ T lymphocytes

Self-limiting (2–4 weeks), febrile myalgic illness often associated with oral and oesophageal ulceration, a maculopapular rash on the trunk and elsewhere, generalized lymphadenopathy (CD8+ lymphocytes), 'aseptic meningitis-like' picture; conventional HIV antibody tests positive 2–6 weeks after onset of illness

Seroconversion at a median of 2 months after exposure, 6 months in over 95%

At least 50% progress to severe immunodeficiency over a variable period—on average 10 years

After infection, despite immune response which results in an approximately 1000-fold decrease in the amount of HIV, a slow but relentless destruction of CD4+ T lymphocytes occurs rendering the patient susceptible to opportunistic infections.

Early HIV disease (asymptomatic phase)

Attacks usually mild: generalized lymphadenopathy (B lymphocytes), irregular and unpredictable fevers, hypersensitivity reactions, reactivation or worsening of eczema, psoriasis or folliculitis. Polyclonal hypergammopathy (IgG, IgA) is usual. CD8+ titre elevated; CD4+ normal. Less common features: thrombocytopaenia; vasculitis.

Intermediate stage (AIDS-related complex)

Number of CD4+ lymphocytes starts to fall,* delayed-type hypersensitivity to common antigens (*Trichophyton*, mumps, *Candida*, tetanus, tuberculin) lost

Increased susceptibility to pathogens not usually considered opportunistic (e.g. *Pneumococcus*, *Shigella*, *Salmonella*, *Haemophilus*) with more serious illness

Increased vaginal thrush, pelvic inflammatory disease and cervical intraepithelial neoplasia (due to human papillomavirus infection)

Shingles more common

Kaposi's sarcoma at this stage or later.

Late phase HIV infection

Fall in CD4+ lymphocytes,* sometimes to zero, leads to profound immunodeficiency. CD8+ lymphocytes start to fall. Oral thrush common. Significant opportunistic infections depending on level of CD4+ count:

* CD4+ count gives the most consistent predictive measure of the risk of progression. CD4+ < 250 cells μl^{-1} or CD4+ to CD8+ ratio <0.3 indicates 2:3 chance of progression to AIDS in the next 2 years. Oral thrush and serum HIV p[24] antigen are also predictors of progression.

CD4+ level <300 cells μl⁻¹ — reactivation of tuberculosis and syphilis

CD4+ level <200 cells μl⁻¹ — *Pneumocystis carinii* pneumonia, cerebral toxoplasmosis, fungal infections (including cryptococcal meningitis)

CD4+ level<100 cells μl⁻¹ — *Mycobacterium avium*

CD4+ level <50 cells μl⁻¹ — cytomegalovirus retinitis, GI disease.

In late phase HIV infection, direct HIV CNS involvement may occur (dementia, myelopathy); Kaposi's may be extensive and aggressive; high grade B-cell lymphomata are more likely to occur.

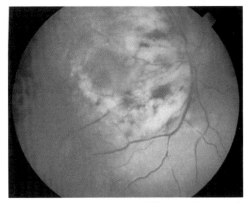

Figure C5.89 Cytomegalovirus retinitis: 'scrambled egg and tomato sauce' appearance.

Case 21 | Normal fundus

Frequency in survey: did not occur in the initial small survey of PACES station 5,*
eyes.

On pp. 103, 135 and 177 the reasons why normal short cases may appear in PACES in stations 1 and 3* have been discussed. In the case of the examination of the fundus there is an additional reason and the College have particularly highlighted the possibility of using a normal fundus with their statement in the guide notes to examination centres: '. . . the inclusion of a normal optic fundus in station 5 is permissible'. The reason for this is that the College have also recommended that in the case scenario, if the patient has diabetes, this may be stated. This is on the grounds that, in 'real life', when examining the fundi, it would be known whether or not the patient had diabetes. The College have accepted also that in 'real life', when the fundus of a person with diabetes is being examined, it is often normal.† Hence they wish that some normal cases are included.

From the pre PACES surveys it was clear that the commonest reason for finding no abnormality is missing the physical signs that are present (probably anecdote on p. 177 and possibly anecdote 2 on p. 135; see also experience 49, vol. 2, p. 331). Other reasons for cases of 'normal' will be either because the physical signs are no longer present by the time the patient comes to the examination (see anecdote on p. 277), or that the examiners and candidate disagree with the selectors of the cases about the presence of physical signs (this may have happened in the anecdote below; see also experience 87b, vol. 2, p. 335 and anecdote 55, vol. 2, p. 367). The following anecdote is from the original, pre PACES, surveys.

Anecdote

A candidate was asked to examine the fundi. He found no abnormality and diagnosed a normal fundus. He reports that the patient had multiple sclerosis and that he knows one of the examiners who has since confirmed that her fundi were considered to be normal. He passed the examination but he felt he would have failed if he had said 'bitemporal pallor'.

---

* It is unlikely that that 'normal' would be a case in station 5, skin, locomotor or endocrine (except perhaps via 'Examine this patients thyroid status' in the latter). If there were a shortage of patients in one subsection of station 5 it seems more likely that patients from another subsection might be deployed. This may account for the cases where more than one from a subsection occurred in our survey—see experiences 3 and 19, vol. 2, pp. 287 and 310.

† It is worth remembering that in 'real life' patients with diabetes can have all the other possible fundal abnormalities—diabetes is common and people with diabetes are as prone to any of the other conditions which affect the eye as anybody else. Furthermore, since people with diabetes are the only ones having their fundi regularly checked, they are more likely to be found to have conditions such as myelinated nerve fibres or old choroiditis. Hence the instruction 'This patient has diabetes, please examine the fundus' could readily be associated with the finding of any retinal abnormality—as well as no abnormality!

Station 5
Other

Case 1 | Bilateral parotid enlargement/ Mikulicz's syndrome

Frequency in survey: 2% of attempts at MRCP short cases, in the original, pre PACES, surveys.

Survey note: all patients with sicca symptoms (dry eyes and dry mouth) in our survey had parotid enlargement.

Record

There is *bilateral parotid enlargement*.* The conjunctivae are injected (the patient complains of *gritty eyes*—the dry eyes of keratoconjunctivitis sicca) and the tongue (touch it) is dry (or the patient complains of a *dry mouth*).†

This is Mikulicz's syndrome (diffuse swelling of lachrymal and salivary glands) which is most likely to be produced by:

1 Sarcoidosis (?lupus pernio, chest signs) but may also be caused by
2 Lymphoma (?lymph nodes, hepatosplenomegaly—both signs, of course, may also occur in sarcoid)
3 Leukaemia (?pallor, hepatosplenomegaly).

Reduction in tear secretion can be demonstrated with *Schirmer's test* in which a 5 mm wide strip of filter paper is folded 3 mm from one end and hooked into the lower conjunctival sac. Normal tear secretion moistens more than 15 mm of strip within 5 minutes.

Secondary Sjögren's syndrome (*Mikulicz's disease*) is the triad of dry mouth (xerostomia), keratoconjunctivitis sicca and a connective tissue disease—most commonly rheumatoid arthritis (50%) but also including autoimmune liver disease and fibrosing alveolitis. Bronchial, pancreatic and vaginal secretions may also be diminished. The lachrymal and salivary glands are not swollen as in *Mikulicz's syndrome* (the issue is complicated, though, by the fact that there is a high incidence of lymphoma in Sjögren's syndrome!).

Primary Sjögren's syndrome (30%) does not have the associated connective tissue disease. It is some-

times referred to as the *sicca syndrome*. Antinuclear antibody (ANA) is positive in 80% of patients. Antibodies to Ro (SS-A) and La (SS-B) should be looked for and identify patients at risk of extraglandular manifestations.

Extraglandular manifestations of primary Sjögren's syndrome

Arthralgia/arthritis	60%
Raynaud's phenomenon	37%
Lymphadenopathy	14%
Vasculitis	11%
Kidney involvement	9%
Liver involvement	7%
Splenomegaly	3%
Peripheral neuropathy	2%
Myositis	1%

---

*Painless parotid enlargement can also occur in bulimia nervosa.

† Look for lack of a pool of saliva under the tongue. A helpful finding in the history is a positive *cracker test*: the patient reports difficulty chewing and swallowing a packet of crackers without fluids.

Case 2 | Deep venous thrombosis/ Baker's cyst/cellulitis

Frequency in survey: 2% of attempts at MRCP short cases in the original, pre PACES, surveys.

Record 1

There is *unilateral* swelling of the R/L leg up to the knee joint which looks normal in appearance* (extension into the thigh suggests femoral or iliac vein thrombosis) associated with an erythematous or a cyanotic hue to the skin, and (feel gently) tenderness to palpation in the calf. The affected calf feels indurated† and is *warmer than the other leg.*

The patient has a deep venous thrombosis.‡

Record 2

The R/L leg is *swollen, painful on movement* and *tender* on palpation. Both the knee joint and the upper, posterior compartment of the calf are swollen, and the normal contours of the joint are obscured by effusion (demonstrate the patellar tap—p. 422).§ A 'fullness' is (may be) palpable in the popliteal space.

The diagnosis is a ruptured Baker's (popliteal) cyst (now check hands for rheumatoid arthritis—p. 384).¶

Record 3

There is an *erythematous, warm swelling* of the R/L leg. There are (may be) vesicles/bullae and crusts on the surface of the erythematous area (look for the portal of bacterial entry).** There is (may be) a puncture mark on the foot (say where exactly) perhaps caused by a thorn (or there may be fungal intertrigo of the feet with secondary bacterial infection).

These features suggest cellulitis. There is (may be) *lymphangitis* (look for the reddish streaky lines running up the leg), and the inguinal lymph nodes are swollen and tender.

---

* If there was associated swelling of the knee it would bring ruptured popliteal cyst and disease of the joint (infection, gout and pseudogout) into the differential diagnosis.

† The calf in DVT feels bulky and indurated and moves *en mass* causing discomfort when gently swayed from side to side. This method is preferable to testing for the *Homan's sign* in which a sudden dorsiflexion of the corresponding foot can cause considerable pain. In the normal calf the muscle contours are clearly visible and a part of the muscle can be moved from side to side without pain or affecting the rest of the calf.

‡ The definitive diagnosis can usually be made by Doppler ultra-sonography which is non-invasive, quick and less expensive than venography, though the latter remains the gold standard.

§ The popliteal cyst may rupture and dissect into the calf muscles causing pain and acute swelling involving the upper part of the calf. The cyst may cause compression of the popliteal vein leading to oedema of the entire leg or a secondary DVT.

¶ Ultrasound scanning has the advantage of being non-invasive but arthrography is the most definitive way to identify a popliteal cyst. The latter procedure also provides the opportunity for aspiration to rule out infection, gout and pseudogout.

** Group A streptococci and *Staphylococcus aureus* are the most commonly responsible organisms.

Record 4

The skin on the R/L leg is *swollen* and *erythematous with a sharply demarcated, irregular border* which is tender to touch, and has an 'orange-peel' epidermal surface.

These features suggest erysipelas.*

The thrombophilia syndromes which predispose to DVT include:

Antiphospholipid syndrome (?livedo reticularis; see p. 336)

Resistance to activated protein C (up to 7% of the population)

Deficiency of antithrombin III (up to 1 per 2000 of population)

Deficiency of protein C and protein S (vitamin K-dependent factors that act together to neutralize factors V and VIII).

---

* Erysipelas is an acute infection of the skin and subcutaneous tissues caused by group A streptococci. It is most commonly seen on the face but may affect other parts of the body. The disease usually affects the two extremes of age.

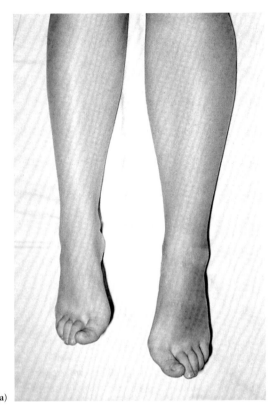

(a)

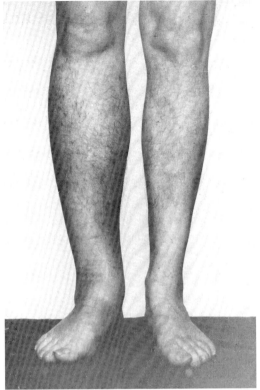

(b1)

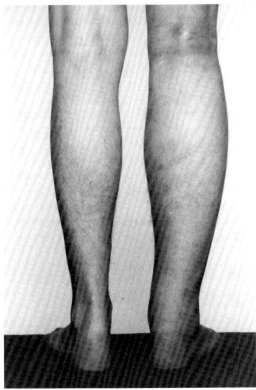

(b2)

Figure C5.90 (a) Left DVT. (b1) Ruptured Baker's cyst; (b2) posterior view.

Case 3 | Peripheral vascular disease

Frequency in survey: main focus of a short case in 0.8% of attempts at MRCP short cases in the original, pre PACES, surveys. Additional feature in others.

Record

The lower leg(s) are pale (pregangrenous areas may be pink), the toes bluish-red (there may be digital gangrene) and the *skin* is *atrophic* (may be stretched and *shiny*) and *hairless*. There are *no pulses** palpable below the femorals (if allowed, listen for a bruit) and the lower legs and feet are *cold* to touch. There is often asymmetry of signs.

These signs suggest peripheral vascular disease (?arcus senilis, ?xanthelasma, ?tendon xanthomata, ?nicotine-stained fingers, ?diabetes†).

Arteriosclerosis obliterans

This, the usual cause of peripheral vascular disease, is due to atheromatous plaques involving the intima of the arteries. As a rule there is superimposed thrombus formation. Degenerative changes occur in the media which frequently calcifies.† The superficial femoral artery is most commonly affected leading to calf claudication. The next most common sites are the popliteal and aortic bifurcation, the latter leading to Leriche's syndrome.

Leriche's syndrome—claudication of low back, buttocks, thigh and calf; limb and buttock atrophy and pallor; impotence, weak or absent femoral pulses, systolic bruits over the lower abdomen and femorals; signs may be asymmetrical; may present as 'sciatica'.

Buerger's postural test

When the legs are lifted to 45° above the horizontal plane, cadaveric pallor devlops if the arterial supply is poor. If, while the clinician supports the legs, the patient flexes and extends the ankles to the point of mild fatigue, this enhances the sign. The patient now sits with his feet lowered to the ground for 2–3 minutes and an impaired arterial supply is indicated by a ruddy, cyanotic hue which spreads over the affected foot (*Buerger's sign*). This sequence indicates occlusion of a major lower limb artery.

The ankle : arm Doppler pressure index uses a

Doppler ultrasonic flow probe to determine the ratio of the peak systolic pressure at the ankle to that in the arm. Symptoms are unlikely to be due to arterial disease if the index is above 0.8. Measurements made immediately after exercise give a good index of disease but are more difficult to perform reliably. In diabetic patients with calcified arteries† the test is unreliable as the pressure in the sphygmomanometer cuff may not reflect that in the artery.

Takayasu's disease‡

This is an arteritis which affects chiefly, but not exclusively, young women from Japan and the Far East. It involves mainly the aortic arch and the large brachiocephalic arteries. Mononuclear cell infiltrates and fibrous proliferation produce progressive narrowing of the lumen and reduced flow in the upper extremities and to the brain. It develops slowly so that although the pulses gradually vanish (hence the alternative name—*pulseless disease*), collateral circulation opens up allowing it to remain un-

---

* The patient with intermittent claudication may have few signs other than reduced or absent pulses in the affected limb. As the atheromatous disease advances, signs of ischaemia appear: low skin temperature, pallor or cyanosis, trophic changes including dry, scaly and shiny skin; the hair may disappear and the toenails can become brittle, ridged and deformed; ischaemic damage may cause persistent reddish or reddish-blue discoloration; ischaemic ulcers and gangrene may develop.

† Peripheral vascular disease in diabetic patients is more progressive, with greater involvement of the more distal vessels which are of smaller calibre; medial calcification is twice as common. See also p. 396.

‡ There were one or two anecdotes in our surveys to suggest that this may have appeared on rare occasions in the MRCP short cases.

noticed for some time. Eventually the patient presents with symptoms such as fainting on turning the head suddenly or rising from supine to sitting, atrophy of the face, headaches, cataracts, optic atrophy, weakness and paraesthesiae of the upper extremities, hemiplegia and convulsions.

Buerger's disease (thromboangiitis obliterans)

An obstructive arterial disease with segmental inflammation and proliferative lesions in medium and small arteries* and veins of limbs. Mostly affects young males aged 20–40 years, especially in Israel, the Orient and India. Patients are almost always moderate to heavy smokers; there may be an autoimmune mechanism triggered by tobacco products. Clinically the disease is characterized by ischaemia of the extremities* and *migratory thrombophlebitis*. Raynaud's phenomenon (see p. 322) is common. If the patient continues to smoke the disease will progress with increasing ischaemia leading to gangrene and amputation of the extremities which is required in a high percentage of patients.

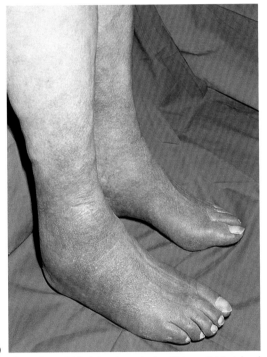
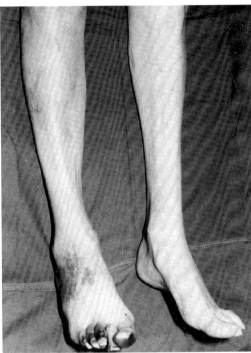

(a)   (b)

Figure C5.91 (a) Peripheral vascular insufficiency. (b) Peripheral vascular disease with gangrenous toes.

* The features which distinguish this *thromboangiitis obliterans* from the common atheromatous arterial disease (*arteriosclerosis obliterans*), are the younger age of the patient, the relative sparing of larger arteries, the presence of migratory superficial thrombophlebitis, the increased involvement of the upper extremities, and more rapid progression. The diagnosis can be confirmed by biopsy of an early lesion showing a characteristic inflammatory and proliferative lesion on histology.

Case 4 | Osteogenesis imperfecta

Frequency in survey: 0.5% of attempts at MRCP short cases in the original, pre PACES, surveys.

Record

The *sclerae* are *slaty-blue*. (Look for evidence of *deformity* from poor fracture healing; ask the patient if he has been particularly prone to *fractures* in the past.)

The diagnosis is osteogenesis imperfecta (the patient may be deaf due to *otosclerosis*).

Osteogenesis imperfecta is due to defects in collagen. In the adult the diagnosis is likely to be the milder tarda type* (usually dominant). In this type the sclerae are more likely to be blue and the fragile bones of childhood become stronger after adolescence though they remain abnormal. The blueness is due to the thin sclerae allowing choroid pigment to show through. Though blue sclerae are not always present, some patients manifest only blue sclerae or otosclerosis without clinical bone disease. Deafness from otosclerosis does not usually develop before the third decade and may occur even later still. Laxity of ligaments, hypotonia of muscles and muscle wasting (partly disuse atrophy) are other features which may occur. Serum alkaline and acid phosphatases are often elevated and the urine often contains hydroxypro-line, pyrophosphate and glycosaminoglycans. Though no specific treatment is known, favourable responses to calcitonin have been reported. Aminobisphosphonates offer promise, while bone marrow transplants remain experimental. Osteogenesis imperfecta may be confused with idiopathic juvenile osteoporosis but in the latter condition osteoporosis is typically confined to the vertebral column, there is no family history of fractures and the sclerae are normal in colour.

Other conditions in which blue sclerae may occur

Marfan's syndrome (see p. 156)
Ehlers–Danlos syndrome (see p. 334)
Pseudoxanthoma elasticum (see p. 299).

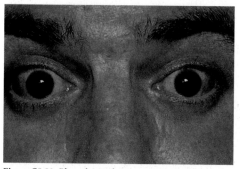

Figure C5.92 Blue sclerae of osteogenesis imperfecta.

---

* Other types are:
1 The severe prenatal type which causes intrauterine death or life for only a few days after birth.
2 The severe type in which the baby survives but is extremely sus-ceptible to fractures. The bones are soft as well as brittle and may therefore bow. Deformities are common and walking may induce fractures. Blue sclerae are less common.

Case 5 | Down's syndrome

Frequency in survey: main focus of a short case in 0.5% of attempts at MRCP short cases in the original, pre PACES, surveys. Additional feature in a further 0.6%.

Record

This short-statured patient has *low-set ears*, a *flattened nasal bridge*, *slanting eyes*, *epicanthus*, white '*Brushfield spots*' in the iris and a small *mouth which hangs open* revealing a large heavily fissured tongue. There is an over-rolled helix of each ear. There is a single *transverse palmar crease* (not pathognomonic) and a short inward curving little finger. The axial triradius is situated towards the centre of the palm (normally should be near the wrist). There is generalized hypotonia and hyperextensibility of the joints.

The patient has Down's syndrome.

Trisomy 21 (occasionally translocation between 21 and 14).

Other features which may occur

Congenital heart lesions (septal defects, Fallot's tetralogy)

Lenticular opacities

Mental retardation which varies from very mild (author of an autobiography) to very severe

Dementia of Alzheimer type

Hypothyroidism.

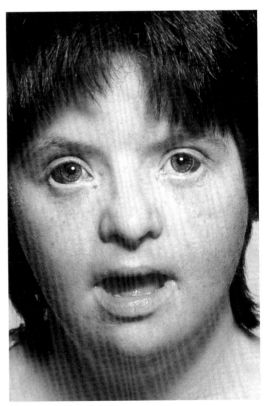

Figure C5.93 Down's syndrome.

Case 6 | Pernicious anaemia

Frequency in survey: 0.4% of attempts at MRCP short cases in the original, pre PACES, surveys.

Record

The patient has *pallor* (may be a pale lemon yellow tinge), a *smooth tongue** and *angular stomatitis.** *Vitiligo*† is (may be) present.

The likely diagnosis is pernicious anaemia (splenomegaly and pyrexia‡ may both occur).

Other general clinical features of megaloblastic anaemias*

Gastrointestinal symptoms
Weight loss
Hyperpigmentation
Infertility
Orthostatic hypotension.

Haematological abnormalities associated with megaloblastic anaemias*

Anaemia
Reticulocytopenia
Macrocytosis
Neutropenia
Thrombocytopenia
Neutrophil hypersegmentation
Poikilocytosis
Anisocytosis
Raised lactate dehydrogenase
Raised bilirubin
Raised serum iron
Decreased haptoglobin
Hypercellular bone marrow with megaloblastic morphology, giant bands and metamyelocytes.

Neuropsychiatric abnormalities associated with vitamin B₁₂ deficiency

(See also p. 223)
Paraesthesiae
Peripheral neuropathy (absent ankle jerks; impaired touch and pain perception; impaired vibration sense and joint position sense (may be Romberg's positive) may also be due to dorsal column involvement)
Ataxia (posterior column involvement; ?joint position sense; ?Romberg's)
Decreased reflexes (peripheral neuropathy—pp. 180 and 223)
Increased reflexes (pyramidal tract involvement—pp. 199 and 223)
Spasticity (pyramidal tract involvement)
Weakness
Dementia (memory loss, disorientation, obtundation)
Incontinence (urinary or faecal)
Impotence
Optic atrophy
Abnormal smell or taste
Lhermitte's phenomenon (p. 223)
Psychiatric abnormalities (depression, paranoia, listlessness, acute confusional state, hallucinations, delu-

---

* Most patients with folate or vitamin B₁₂ deficiency do not have many of the features listed. Even anaemia and raised mean corpuscular volume may be absent in a patient with otherwise severe folate or vitamin B₁₂ deficiency; in one prospective study of patients with vitamin B₁₂ deficiency, 44% did not have anaemia, 36% had a mean corpuscular volume equal to or less than 100, 86% had a normal white cell count, 79% a normal platelet count, 33% had a normal peripheral blood film, 43% had a normal lactate dehydrogenase and 83% a normal bilirubin.

† The cutaneous marker of organ-specific autoimmune diseases (p. 293) creates the suspicion of addisonian pernicious anaemia rather than any other cause of megaloblastic anaemia leading to pallor and a smooth tongue.
‡ Why were you not previously aware that untreated pernicious anaemia may be associated with fever? Perhaps it should be called *hypo-cyanocobalimic fever*? — see Appendix 5, p. 545).

sions, insomnia, apprehensiveness, psychosis, slow mentation, paraphrenia, mania, panic attacks, suicide).

Causes of megaloblastic anaemia

Vitamin B$_{12}$ deficiency

Decreased ingestion (poor diet, lack of animal products, strict vegetarianism)

Impaired absorption:

(a) failure of release of B$_{12}$ from food protein (old age; partial gastrectomy)

(b) intrinsic factor deficiency (pernicious anaemia; total gastrectomy; destruction of gastric mucosa by caustics; congenital abnormality or absence of intrinsic factor)

(c) chronic pancreatic disease

(d) competitive parasites (bacteria in bowel diverticula, blind loops, fish tapeworm)

(e) intrinsic intestinal disease (ileal resection, Crohn's disease, radiation ileitis; tropical sprue, coeliac disease; infiltrative intestinal disease such as lymphoma or scleroderma; drug-induced malabsorption; congenital selective malabsorption — Imerslund–Grasbeck syndrome)

Impaired utilization (congenital enzyme deficiencies; lack of transcobalamin II; nitrous oxide administration).

Folate deficiency

Decreased ingestion (poor diet, lack of vegetables; alcoholism; infancy)

Impaired absorption (intestinal short circuits; tropical sprue, coeliac diseaes; drugs such as anticonvulsants and sulphasalazine; congenital malabsorption)

Impaired utilization (folic acid antagonists such as methotrexate, triamterene, trimethroprim, pyrimethamine, ethanol; congenital enzyme deficiencies)

Increased requirement (pregnancy, infancy, hyperthyroidism, chronic haemolytic disease, neoplastic disease, exfoliative skin disease)

Increased loss (haemodialysis).

Drugs—metabolic inhibitors

Purine synthesis (methotrexate, 6-mercaptopurine, 6-thioguanine, azathioprine)

Pyrimidine synthesis (methotrexate, 5-fluorouracil)

Deoxyribonucleotide synthesis (hydroxyurea, cytosine arabinoside).

Miscellaneous

Inborn errors (e.g. Lesch–Nyhan syndrome, hereditary orotic aciduria)

Unexplained disorders (pyridoxine-responsive megaloblastic anaemia, thiamine-responsive megaloblastic anaemia, some cases of myelodysplastic syndrome, some cases of acute myelogenous leukaemia).

Case 7 | Klippel–Feil syndrome

Frequency in survey: 0.3% of attempts at MRCP short cases in the original, pre PACES, surveys.

Record

The patient has a *short neck*, with *limited rotation* of the head, a low hairline and a webbed neck.*

The limited rotation of the head suggests Klippel–Feil syndrome.

In Klippel–Feil syndrome the number of cervical vertebrae is reduced and two or more may be fused. This bony deformity leads to shortening of the neck, but this does not in itself cause neurological symptoms. There may, however, be neurological complications from coexisting anomalies of the CNS. Basilar impression and syringomyelia (see p. 249) are problems which may be associated.

Other problems which may be associated

Hearing loss

Heart defects

Sprengel's deformity (upward displacement of the scapula)

Genitourinary anomalies (e.g. aplasia of the müllerian structures).

---

*Webbing of the neck is usually associated with Turner's syndrome (short stature, increased carrying angle, shield-like chest, short metacarpals, amenorrhoea, coarctation of the aorta) but is not pathognomonic. The limited rotation of the head is the pointer to the Klippel–Feil syndrome.

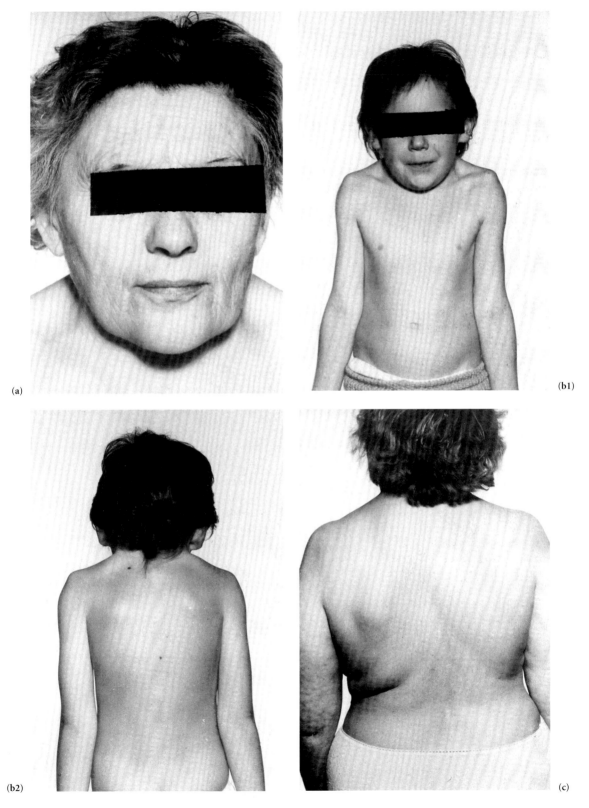

Figure C5.94 (a) Shortening of the neck demonstrated by a reduced ear lobe to shoulder distance. (b) Note (1) webbed neck and (2) low hairline. (c) Scoliosis and low hairline resulting from deficiency of cervical vertebrae.

Case 8 | **Leg oedema**

Frequency in survey: main focus of a short case in 0.3% of attempts at MRCP short cases in the original, pre- PACES, surveys. Additional feature in many others.

Record 1

There is *swelling* of the lower limbs which *pits on pressure*. The patient is (may be) breathless at rest, the *venous pressure* is *raised* and oscillating the ear lobe, and there is *sacral oedema*.

These features suggest the ankle oedema is due to congestive cardiac failure (now consider offering to extend the examination to look for features of the cardiac and/or pulmonary disease and hepatomegaly).

Record 2

This *elderly* female (or male) has bilateral lower limb oedema (check for pitting) up to the mid-calf (look for the presence of a walking aid, engorged jugular veins and, if allowed, sacral oedema).

Her *zimmerframe* suggests a degree of poor mobility and, in the absence of any other signs of cardiovascular disease, it is likely to be dependent oedema though the patient may be on some *salt-retaining drugs* such as steroids or NSAIDs.

Causes of leg oedema
Local causes
Dependent oedema

Venous disorders (chronic venous insufficiency)—
pigmentation, induration and inflammation (lipodermatosclerosis)

Occlusion of a large vein:
phlebothrombosis—*unilateral* (see p. 511)
extrinsic compression

Popliteal (Baker's) cyst—*unilateral* (see p. 511)

Cellulitis—*unilateral* (see p. 511)

Lymphoedema—non-pitting, thickened and indurated skin ('pigskin'). May be idiopathic or secondary to proximal lymphatic obstruction (metastatic carcino-ma, surgical removal of the regional lymph nodes, irradiation or chronic infection)

Gastrocnemius rupture—swelling and ecchymosis around the ankle joint and foot

Lipomatosis—in some cases of obesity the fat may be preferentially deposited in the lower limbs.

Systemic causes
Congestive cardiac failure

Hypoproteinaemia—nephrotic syndrome, liver cirrhosis, Kwashiorkor, protein-losing enteropathy

Hypo- and hyperthyroidism

Drugs—corticosteroids, NSAIDs, vasodilators.

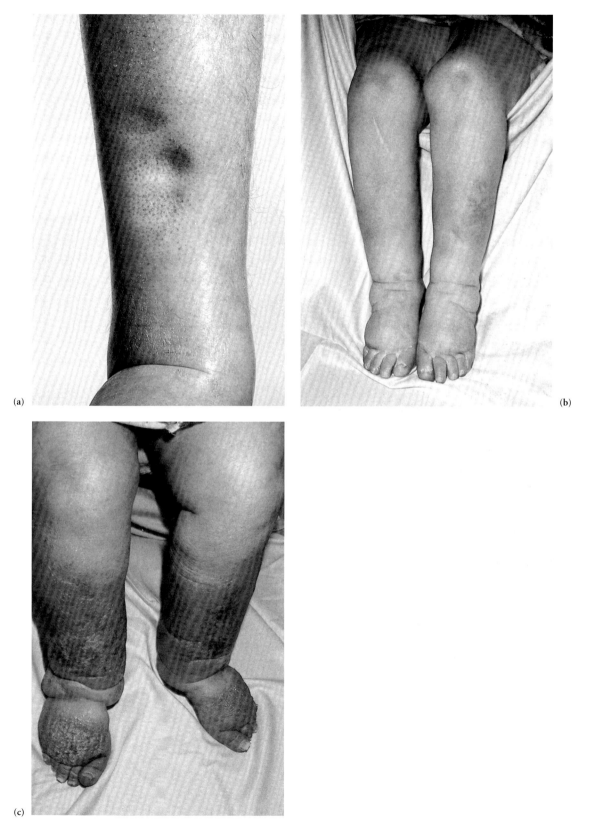

Figure C5.95 (a) Oedema which has pitted with finger pressure. (b) Bilateral leg oedema in an elderly patient. (c) Lymphoedema of the legs.

Appendices

1 | Checklists

1 Pulse

Observe

1 Face (malar flush, thyroid facies).
2 Neck (Corrigan's pulse, raised JVP, thyroidectomy scar, goitre) and chest (thoracotomy scar).

Palpate and assess

3 Pulse.
4 Rate.
5 Rhythm (?slow atrial fibrillation).
6 Character (normal, collapsing, slow rising, jerky).
7 Carotid.
8 Opposite radial.
9 Radiofemoral delay.
10 All the other pulses.
11 Additional diagnostic features.

2 Heart

1 *Visual survey*:
  (a) breathlessness
  (b) *cyanosis*
  (c) pallor
  (d) *malar flush*
  (e) carotids
  (f) jugulars
  (g) *valvotomy scar*, midline scar
  (h) ankle oedema
  (i) clubbing; splinter haemorrhages.
2 Pulse (rate and rhythm).
3 Lift up the arm (?collapsing).
4 Radiofemoral delay.
5 Brachials and carotids (?slow rising).
6 Venous pressure.
7 Apex beat.
8 Tapping impulse.
9 Right ventricular lift.
10 Other pulsations, thrills, palpable sounds.
11 Auscultation (time heart sounds, etc.; turn patient onto left side; lean patient forwards).
12 Sacral oedema (?ankle oedema).
13 Lung bases.
14 Liver.
15 Blood pressure.

3 Chest

1 *Visual survey*—general appearance (cachexia, superior vena cava obstruction, systemic sclerosis, lupus pernio, kyphoscoliosis, *ankylosing spondylitis*).
2 Dyspnoea.
3 Lip pursing.
4 Cyanosis.
5 Accessory muscles.
6 Indrawing (intercostal muscles, supraclavicular fossae, lower ribs).
7 Chest wall (upward movement, asymmetry, scars, radiotherapy stigmata).
8 Clubbing (tobacco staining, coal dust tattoos, rheumatoid deformity, systemic sclerosis).
9 Pulse (flapping tremor).
10 Venous pressure.
11 Trachea (deviation, tug, notch–cricoid distance).
12 Lymphadenopathy.
13 Apex beat.
14 Asymmetry.
15 Expansion.
16 Percussion (do not forget clavicles, axillae).
17 Tactile vocal fremitus.
18 Breath sounds.
19 Vocal resonance.
20 Repeat 14–19 on back of chest (feel for lymph nodes in the neck).

4 Abdomen

1 *Visual survey* (pallor, jaundice, spider naevi, etc.).
2 Pigmentation.
3 Hands (Dupuytren's contracture, clubbing, leuconychia, palmar erythema, flapping tremor).
4 Eyes (anaemia, icterus, xanthelasma).
5 Mouth (cyanosis, etc.).
6 Cervical lymph nodes.
7 Gynaecomastia.
8 Spider naevi.
9 Scratch marks.
10 Body hair.
11 Look at the abdomen (pulsation, distension, swelling, distended abdominal veins).
12 Palpation (light palpation, internal organs, inguinal lymph nodes).
13 Percussion.

14 Shifting dullness.
15 Auscultation.
16 Genitalia.
17 Rectal.

5 Visual fields
Observe
1 *Visual survey* (acromegaly, hemiparesis, cerebellar signs).

Test
2 Peripheral visual fields by confrontation.
3 Central scotoma with a red-headed hat pin.
4 Additional features.

6 Cranial nerves
1 Look.
2 Smell and taste (I, VII, IX).
3 Visual acuity (II).
4 Visual fields (II).
5 Eye movements (III, IV, VI).
6 Nystagmus (VIII, cerebellum and its connections).
7 Ptosis (III, sympathetic).
8 Pupils (light, accommodation — III).
9 Discs (II).
10 Facial movements (VII, V).
11 Palatal movement (IX, X).
12 Gag reflex (IX, X).
13 Tongue (XII).
14 Accessory nerve (XI).
15 Hearing (Weber, Rinné — VIII).
16 Facial sensation (including corneal reflex — V).

7 Arms
Observe
1 Face (hemiplegia, nystagmus, wasting, Parkinson's, Horner's).
2 Neck (pseudoxanthoma elasticum, lymph nodes).
3 Elbows (psoriasis, rheumatoid nodules, scars, deformity).
4 Tremor.
5 Hands (joints, nails, skin).
6 Muscle bulk.
7 Fasciculation.

Test
8 Tone.
9 Arms out in front (winging, myelopathy hand sign, sensory wandering).
10 Power:
    (a) arms out to the side (C5)

(b) bend your elbows (C5,6)
(c) push out straight (C7)
(d) squeeze fingers (C8,T1)
(e) hold the fingers out straight (radial nerve, C7)
(f) spread fingers apart (ulnar nerve)
(g) piece of paper between fingers (ulnar nerve)
(h) thumb at ceiling (median nerve)
(i) opposition (median nerve).
11 Coordination (rapid alternate motion, finger–nose).
12 Reflexes.
13 Sensation (light touch, pinprick, vibration, joint position).

8 Legs
Observe
1 *Visual survey* (*Paget's disease*, hemiparesis, exophthalmos, nystagmus, thyroid acropachy, rheumatoid hands, nicotine-stained fingers, wasted hands, muscle fasciculation).
2 Obvious lesion (see group 1 diagnoses).
3 Bowing of the tibia.
4 Pes cavus.
5 One leg smaller than the other.
6 Muscle bulk.
7 Fasciculation.

Test
8 Tone.
9 Power:
    (a) lift your leg up (L1,2)
    (b) bend your knee (L5,S1,2)
    (c) straighten your leg (L3,4)
    (d) bend your foot down (S1)
    (e) cock up your foot (L4,5).
10 Coordination (heel–shin).
11 Tendon reflexes (clonus).
12 Plantar response.
13 Sensation (light touch, pinprick, vibration, joint position).
14 Gait (ordinary walk, heel-to-toe, on toes, on heels).
15 Rombergism.

9 Legs and arms
As appropriate from *checklists* 7 and 8.

10 Gait
1 *Visual survey* (cerebellar signs, Parkinson's, Charcot–Marie–Tooth, ankylosing spondylitis).
2 Check patient can walk.

3 Observe ordinary walk (ataxia, spastic, steppage, parkinsonian).
4 Arm swing (Parkinson's).
5 Turning (ataxia, Parkinson's).
6 Heel-to-toe (ataxia).
7 On toes (S1).
8 On heels (L5).
9 Romberg's test (sensory ataxia).
10 Gait with eyes closed.
11 Additional features.

11 Ask some questions

1 *Visual survey* (from top to toe, ?obvious diagnosis).
2 Specific questions (Raynaud's, systemic sclerosis/CRST, hypo- or hyperthyroidism, Crohn's, nephrotic syndrome).
3 General questions (name, address).
4 Questions with long answers (last meal).
5 Articulation ('British Constitution', 'West Register Street', 'biblical criticism').
6 Repetition.
7 Additional signs.
8 Comprehension ('put out your tongue', 'shut your eyes', 'touch your nose').
9 Nominal dysphasia (keys).
10 Orofacial dyspraxia.
11 Higher mental function.

12 Fundi
Observe
1 *Visual survey* (medic-alert bracelet, etc.).

Ophthalmoscopy
2 Lens.
3 Vitreous.
4 Disc (optic atrophy, papillitis, papilloedema, myelinated nerve fibres, new vessels).
5 Arterioles and venules (silver wiring, AV nipping).
6 Each quadrant and macula (haemorrhages, microaneurysms, exudates, new vessels, photocoagulation scars, choroidoretinitis, retinitis pigmentosa, drusen).
7 Do not stop until you have finished and are ready.

13 Eyes
Observe
1 Face (e.g. myasthenic, tabetic, hemiparesis).
2 Eyes (exophthalmos, strabismus, ptosis, xanthelasma, arcus senilis).
3 Pupils (Argyll Robertson, Horner's, Holmes–Adie, IIIrd nerve).

Test
4 Visual acuity.
5 Visual fields.
6 Eye movements (ocular palsy, diplopia, nystagmus, lid lag).
7 Light reflex (direct, consensual).
8 Accommodation reflex.
9 Fundi.

14 Face
1 *Visual survey* of patient.
2 Scan the head and face.
3 Break down and scrutinize the parts of the face:
   (a) eyelids (ptosis, rash)
      eyelashes (scanty)
      cornea (arcus, interstitial keratitis)
      sclerae (icteric, congested)
      pupils (small, large, irregular, dislocated lens, cataracts)
      iris (iritis)
   (b) face (erythema, infiltrates)
      mouth (tight, shiny, adherent skin; pigmented patches, telangiectasia, cyanosis).
4 Additional features.

15 Hands
Observe
1 Face (*systemic sclerosis*, Cushing's, acromegaly, arcus senilis, icterus and spider naevi, exophthalmos).
2 Inspect the hands (rheumatoid, sclerodactyly, wasting, psoriasis, claw hand, clubbing).
3 Joints (swelling, deformity, Heberden's nodes).
4 Nails (pitting, onycholysis, clubbing, nail-fold infarcts).
5 Skin (colour, consistency, lesions).
6 Muscles (wasting, fasciculation).

Palpate and test
7 Hands (Dupuytren's contracture, nodules, calcinosis, xanthomata, Heberden's nodes, tophi).
8 Sensation (pinprick, light touch, vibration, joint position).
9 Tone.
10 Power.
11 Pulses.
12 Elbows.

16 Skin
1 *Visual survey* (regional associations: scalp, face, mouth, neck, trunk, axillae, elbows, hands, nails, genitalia, legs, feet).

2 Distribution (psoriasis on extensor areas, lichen planus in flexural areas, etc.).

3 Lesions—look for characteristic features (scaling, Wickham's striae, etc.).

4 Associated lesions (arthropathy, etc.).

17 Rash

1 *Visual survey* (scalp to sole).

2 Distribution.

3 Surrounding skin (?scratch marks).

4 Examine the lesion (colour, size, shape, surface, character, secondary features).

5 Additional features.

18 Neck

1 *Visual survey* of patient (eyes, face, legs).

2 Look at the neck (swallow).

3 Palpate the thyroid (swallow; size, consistency, etc.; pyramidal lobes, percuss over upper sternum).

4 Lymph nodes (supraclavicular, submandibular, postauricular, suboccipital, axillae, groins, spleen).

5 Auscultate the thyroid (distinguish from venous hum and conducted murmurs).

6 Assess thyroid status.

19 Thyroid status

1 *Visual survey* (exophthalmos, goitre, thyroid acropachy, pretibial myxoedema, myxoedematous facies).

2 Composure (fidgety, normal, immobile).

3 Pulse.

4 Ankle jerks.

5 Palms.

6 Tremor.

7 Eyes (lid retraction, lid lag).

8 Thyroid (look, palpate, auscultate).

9 Questions.

20 Knee

1 Observe (*rheumatoid, psoriasis*, gout).

2 Ask (pain).

3 Inspect (valgus, varus, flexion deformity, quadriceps, knee).

4 Palpate (temperature, tender).

5 Effusion (bulge sign, patellar tap).

6 Movement (flex knee).

7 Crepitus over the joint as flexion occurs.

8 Feel behind the knee for a Baker's cyst.

9 Instability (cruciate, McMurray's sign).

10 Other joints (psoriasis, inflammatory bowel disease, reactive arthritis, tophi).

21 Hip

1 Inspect (flexed, shortening, externally rotated, scars, rheumatoid).

2 Ask (pain).

3 Movement (flex, rotate, abduction, adduction, Thomas's test).

4 Straight leg raise (nerve root entrapment, neurological assessment).

5 Tenderness (trochanteric bursitis).

6 Length inequality.

7 Walk (antalgic gait, waddling gait).

22 'Spot' diagnosis

1 *Visual survey*.

2 Retrace the same ground more thoroughly:

(a) head (*Paget's, myotonic dystrophy*)

(b) face (*acromegaly, Parkinson's, hemiplegia*, myotonic dystrophy, tardive dyskinesia, hypopituitarism, Cushing's, hypothyroidism, systemic sclerosis)

(c) eyes (*jaundice, exophthalmos*, ptosis, Horner's, xanthelasma)

(d) neck (*goitre*, Turner's, spondylitis, torticollis)

(e) trunk (pigmentation, ascites, purpuric spots, spider naevi, wasting, pemphigus)

(f) arms (choreoathetosis, psoriasis, Addison's, spider naevi, *syringomyelia*)

(g) hands (acromegaly, *tremor*, clubbing, sclerodactyly, arachnodactyly, claw hand, etc.)

(h) legs (bowing, purpura, pretibial myxoedema, necrobiosis)

(i) feet (pes cavus).

3 Abnormal colouring (*pigmentation, icterus*, pallor).

4 Break down and scrutinize (especially face).

5 Additional features.

2 | Examination frequency of MRCP PACES short cases

Station 1, respiratory

Short case	Main focus in PACES survey (%)	Predicted main focus in PACES from original surveys (%)	Predicted additional feature (%)
1 Interstitial lung disease (fibrosing alveolitis)	21	15	2
2 Pneumonectomy/lobectomy	16	18	1
3 Bronchiectasis	12	6	3
4 Dullness at the lung bases	10	21	3
5 Chronic bronchitis and emphysema	8	8	2
6 Rheumatoid lung	8	1	—
7 Carcinoma of the bronchus	0	8	6
8 Old tuberculosis	6	12	0
9 Stridor	4	0	—
10 Kartagener's syndrome	2	0	—
11 Marfan's syndrome	2	0	—
12 Lung transplant	2	0	—
13 Chest infection/consolidation/pneumonia	1	2	?
14 Superior vena cava obstruction	0	3	—
15 Cor pulmonale	0	2	—
16 Obesity/pickwickian syndrome	0	1	?
17 Tuberculosis/apical consolidation	0	1	—
18 Pneumothorax	0	0.5	—
19 Cystic fibrosis	0	0.5	—
20 Normal chest	0		

Station 1, abdominal

Short case	Main focus in PACES survey (%)	Predicted main focus in PACES from original surveys (%)	Predicted additional feature (%)
1 Chronic liver disease	21	14	5
2 Hepatosplenomegaly	17	25	6
3 Polycystic kidneys	14	13	2
4 Splenomegaly (without hepatomegaly)	13	15	2
5 Transplanted kidney	9	0.8	0
6 Hepatomegaly (without splenomegaly)	5	11	4
7 Ascites	4	3	6
8 Polycythaemia rubra vera	4	0.5	0
9 Generalized lymphadenopathy	0	4	6
10 Single palpable kidney	0	3	3
11 Primary biliary cirrhosis	0	3	—

Continued p. 532

Abdominal contd.

Short case	Main focus in PACES survey (%)	Predicted main focus in PACES from original surveys (%)	Predicted additional feature (%)
12 Abdominal mass	2	4	1
13 Carcinoid syndrome	2	0	—
14 Crohn's disease	1	2	—
15 Idiopathic haemochromatosis	0	1	—
16 Nephrotic syndrome	0	0.7	—
17 Hereditary spherocytosis	0	0.3	—
18 Felty's syndrome	0	0	0.8
19 Normal abdomen	0	0	—

Station 3, cardiovascular

Short case	Main focus in PACES survey (%)	Predicted main focus in PACES from original surveys (%)	Predicted additional feature (%)
1 Prosthetic valves	17	2	?
2 Mitral incompetence (lone)	13	7	—
3 Mixed aortic valve disease	9	10	—
4 Mixed mitral valve disease	9	15	—
5 Other combinations of mitral and aortic valve disease	8	10	—
6 Mitral stenosis (lone)	7	19	—
7 Aortic stenosis (lone)	7	8	—
8 Aortic incompetence (lone)	5	9	1
9 Ventricular septal defect	3	3	1
10 Irregular pulse	2	3	13
11 Hypertrophic cardiomyopathy	2	0	—
12 Marfan's syndrome	2	0	—
13 Eisenmenger's syndrome	0	2	1
14 Mitral valve prolapse	0	2	—
15 Patent ductus arteriosus	0	2	—
16 Tricuspid incompetence	0	2	?
17 Fallot's tetralogy with a Blalock shunt	0.9	0.9	—
18 Raised jugular venous pressure	0	0.9	?
19 Coarctation of the aorta	0	0.9	1
20 Slow pulse	0	0.9	—
21 Dextrocardia	0	0.5	—
22 Pulmonary stenosis	0	0.5	—
23 Cannon waves	0	0.5	—
24 Pulmonary incompetence	0	0.3	—
25 Infective endocarditis	0	0.3	—
26 Atrial septal defect	0	0.1	—
27 Normal heart	0	0	—

Station 3, central nervous system

Short case	Main focus in PACES survey (%)	Predicted main focus in PACES from original surveys (%)	Predicted additional feature (%)
1 Peripheral neuropathy	9	5	8
2 Myotonic dystrophy (dystrophia myotonica)	8	4	—
3 Hemiplegia	6	8	2
4 Cerebellar syndrome	6	5	6
5 Charcot–Marie–Tooth disease (hereditary motor and sensory neuropathy)	5	0.9	—
6 Motor neurone disease	5	6	1
7 Ulnar nerve palsy	5	6	—
8 Visual field defect	5	5	2
9 Spinal cord compression	5	0	—
10 Spastic paraparesis	4	9	?
11 Abnormal gait	4	3	4
12 Ocular palsy	3	7	1
13 Parkinson's disease	3	4	—
14 Multiple sclerosis	3	0	?
15 Lower motor neurone VIIth nerve palsy	2	3	—
16 Drug-induced extrapyramidal syndrome	2	2	—
17 Choreoathetosis	2	0.9	3
18 Carpal tunnel syndrome	2	0.4	3
19 Diabetic foot	1	3	1
20 Friedreich's ataxia	1	2	—
21 Proximal myopathy	1	0.8	—
22 Subacute combined degeneration of the cord	1	0.7	1
23 Muscular dystrophy	0.4	2	—
24 Wasting of the small muscles of the hand	0	4	?
25 Nystagmus	0	3	2
26 Horner's syndrome	0	3	—
27 Old polio	0	3	1
28 Cervical myelopathy	0	2	2
29 Bulbar palsy	0	0.9	—
30 Dysarthria	0	0.9	1
31 Dysphasia	0	0.9	1
32 Myasthenia gravis	0	0.9	1
33 Guillain–Barré syndrome (acute inflammatory demyelinating polyradiculopathy)	0	0.9	—
34 Pseudobulbar palsy	0	0.8	—
35 Syringomyelia	0	0.8	—
36 Holmes–Adie–Moore syndrome	0	0.7	—
37 Jugular foramen syndrome	0	0.6	—
38 Polymyositis	0	0.5	—
39 Argyll Robertson pupils	0	0.4	?
40 Congenital syphilis	0	0.4	—
41 Cerebellopontine angle lesion	0	0.4	—
42 Absent ankle jerks and extensor plantars	0	0.4	1
43 Lateral popliteal (common peroneal) nerve palsy	0	0.4	—

Continued p. 534

Short case	Main focus in PACES survey (%)	Predicted main focus in PACES from original surveys (%)	Predicted additional feature (%)
44 Ptosis	0	0.4	4
45 Tabes	0	0.3	0.8
46 Subclavian-steal syndrome	0	0.3	—
47 Infantile hemiplegia	0	0.3	—
48 Thalamic syndrome	0	0.3	—
49 Radial nerve palsy	0	0	—
50 Lateral medullary syndrome (Wallenberg's syndrome)	0	0	—
51 Psychogenic/factitious	0	2 anecdotes	—
52 Normal central nervous system	0	0	—

Station 5, skin

Short case	Main focus in PACES survey (%)	Predicted main focus in PACES from original surveys (%)	Predicted additional feature (%)
1 Systemic sclerosis/CRST syndrome	15	11	1
2 Neurofibromatosis (von Recklinghausen's disease)	13	5	4
3 Osler–Weber–Rendu syndrome	11	9	—
4 Psoriasis	11	9	1
5 Rash of uncertain cause	6	0	—
6 Dermatomyositis	3	2	—
7 Xanthomata	2	4	2
8 Vitiligo	2	2	—
9 Tuberous sclerosis/adenoma sebaceum	2	2	—
10 Pseudoxanthoma elasticum	2	1	—
11 Lichen planus	2	0.9	—
12 Yellow nail syndrome	2	0.5	—
13 Gouty tophi	2	0	—
14 Alopecia	2	0	—
15 Eczema	2	0	—
16 Pretibial myxoedema	2	0	—
17 Clubbing	2	4	14
18 Necrobiosis lipoidica diabeticorum	2	5	—
19 Lupus pernio	2	4	—
20 Tinea	2	0	—
21 Koilonychia	2	0	—
22 Raynaud's phenomenon	0.5	0.9	2
23 Erythema nodosum	0	5	—
24 Sturge–Weber syndrome	0	5	—
25 Purpura	0	4	?
26 Peutz–Jeghers syndrome	0	4	—
27 Vasculitis	0	4	?
28 Ehlers–Danlos syndrome	0	2	—
29 Livedo reticularis	0	2	—

Continued

Skin contd.

Short case	Main focus in PACES survey (%)	Predicted main focus in PACES from original surveys (%)	Predicted additional feature (%)
30 Pemphigus/pemphigoid	0	2	—
31 Radiation burn on the chest	0	1	?
32 Herpes zoster	0	1	—
33 Henoch–Schönlein purpura	0	1	—
34 Mycosis fungoides	0	0.9	—
35 Morphoea	0	0.9	—
36 Kaposi's sarcoma (AIDS)	0	0.9	—
37 Porphyria	0	0.9	—
38 Lupus vulgaris	0	0.9	—
39 Dermatitis herpetiformis	0	0.5	—
40 Urticaria pigmentosa (mastocytosis)	0	0.5	—
41 Tylosis	0	0.5	—
42 Secondary syphilis	0	0.5	—
43 Ectodermal dysplasia	0	0.5	—
44 Partial lipodystrophy	0	0.5	—
45 Fabry's disease	0	0.5	—
46 Reiter's syndrome/keratoderma blenorrhagica	0	0.5	—
47 Malignant melanoma	0	0.5	—
48 Acanthosis nigricans	0	0.5	—
49 Keratoacanthoma	0	0.5	—
50 Pyoderma gangrenosum	0	0.2	—
51 Psychogenic/factitious	0	1 anecdote	—

Station 5, locomotor

Short case	Main focus in PACES survey (%)	Predicted main focus in PACES from original surveys (%)	Predicted additional feature (%)
1 Rheumatoid arthritis	31	33	13
2 Psoriatic arthropathy	12	12	1
3 Systemic sclerosis/CRST syndrome	12	14	1
4 Diabetic foot/Charcot's joint	7	0	—
5 Tophaceous gout	6	2	—
6 Ankylosing spondylitis	4	6	—
7 Paget's disease	0	23	—
8 Osteoarthritis	2	2	—
9 Marfan's syndrome	2	2	—
10 Vasculitis	2	0	—
11 Proximal myopathy	2	0	—
12 One leg shorter and smaller than the other	2	0	—
13 Radial nerve palsy	1	0	—
14 Arthropathy associated with inflammatory bowel disease	1	0	—
15 Polymyositis	1	0	—

Continued p. 536

Locomotor contd.

Short case	Main focus in PACES survey (%)	Predicted main focus in PACES from original surveys (%)	Predicted additional feature (%)
16 Systemic lupus erythematosus	0	4	—
17 Old rickets	0	0.6	—
18 Juvenile chronic arthritis	0	0.6	—
19 Swollen knee	0	2	3

Station 5, endocrine

Short case	Main focus in PACES survey (%)	Predicted main focus in PACES from original surveys (%)	Predicted additional feature (%)
1 Exophthalmos	26	23	19
2 Acromegaly	24	17	3
3 Grave's disease	9	17	9
4 Goitre	7	15	6
5 Hypothyroidism	6	11	1
6 Cushing's syndrome	5	4	8
7 Addison's disease	3	4	—
8 Hypopituitarism	2	2	1
9 Pretibial myxoedema	2	2	5
10 Gynaecomastia	2	1	5
11 Turner's syndrome	2	1	—
12 Klinefelter's syndrome/hypogonadism	2	0.6	—
13 Bitemporal hemianopia	2	0	—
14 Charcot's joint	2	0	—
15 Necrobiosis lipoidica diabeticorum	1	0	—
16 Short stature	0.8	1	—
17 Pseudohypoparathyroidism	0.4	1	—
18 Pendred's syndrome	0	0.6	—

Station 5, eyes

Short case	Main focus in PACES survey (%)	Predicted main focus in PACES from original surveys (%)	Predicted additional feature (%)
1 Diabetic retinopathy	41	47	—
2 Retinitis pigmentosa	16	8	—
3 Optic atrophy	6	19	2
4 Ocular palsy	6	0	—
5 Visual field defect	4	0	—

Continued

Eyes contd.

Short case	Main focus in PACES survey (%)	Predicted main focus in PACES from original surveys (%)	Predicted additional feature (%)
6 Retinal vein occlusion	2	3	—
7 Old choroiditis	2	4	—
8 Papilloedema	0	4	—
9 Cataracts	2	1	8
10 Myasthenia gravis	2	1	—
11 Albinism	2	0	—
12 Exophthalmos	2	0	—
13 Myelinated nerve fibres	1	1	—
14 Hypertensive retinopathy	1	8	—
15 Glaucoma/peripheral field loss	1	0	—
16 Retinal artery occlusion	0.5	1	—
17 Asteroid hyalosis	0	0.6	—
18 Drusen	0	0.4	—
19 Laurence–Moon–Bardet–Biedl syndrome	0	0.7	—
20 Cytomegalovirus choroidoretinitis (AIDS)	0	0.1	—
21 Normal fundus	0	0	—

Station 5, other

Short case	Main focus in PACES survey (%)	Predicted main focus in PACES from original surveys (%)	Predicted additional feature (%)
1 Bilateral parotid enlargement/Mikulicz's syndrome	0	2	—
2 Deep venous thrombosis/Baker's cyst/cellulitis	0	2	—
3 Peripheral vascular disease	0	0.8	?
4 Osteogenesis imperfecta	0	0.5	—
5 Down's syndrome	0	0.5	0.6
6 Pernicious anaemia	0	0.4	—
7 Klippel–Feil syndrome	0	0.3	—
8 Leg oedema	0	0.3	?

3 | Pocket Snellen's chart

This pocket Snellen's chart held 2 m from the patient's eyes (i.e. just beyond the end of the bed) can be used to gain some bedside information about the visual acuity. It gives only an approximation because 6 m is the least distance at which the effects of accommodation can be ignored (hence visual acuity is normally tested at 6 m with a Snellen's chart three times as big as this). Remember that the commonest cause of diminished visual acuity is a refractive error so that to gain information about other pathology in the eye (e.g. diabetic maculopathy), the corrected visual acuity needs to be assessed (with glasses on or through a pinhole).

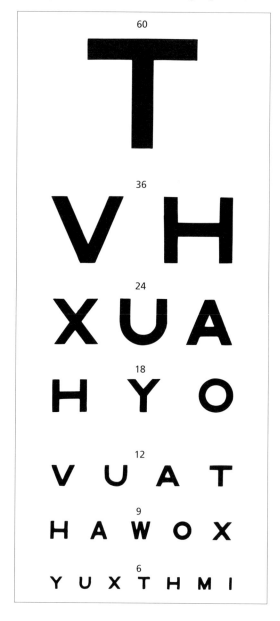

4 | Mark sheets used by the examiners in PACES Stations 1, 3 and 5

ROYAL COLLEGES OF PHYSICIANS OF THE UNITED KINGDOM
MRCP(UK) PACES EXAMINATION - CLINICAL MARKSHEET
STATION ONE: Respiratory System Examination

CANDIDATE NAME (PLEASE PRINT)

Examination Number	Centre Number	Sheet No.
c0ɔ c0ɔ c0ɔ c0ɔ	c0ɔ c0ɔ c0ɔ c0ɔ	
c1ɔ c1ɔ c1ɔ c1ɔ	c1ɔ c1ɔ c1ɔ c1ɔ	I
c2ɔ c2ɔ c2ɔ c2ɔ	c2ɔ c2ɔ c2ɔ c2ɔ	
c3ɔ c3ɔ c3ɔ c3ɔ	c3ɔ c3ɔ c3ɔ c3ɔ	
c4ɔ c4ɔ c4ɔ c4ɔ	c4ɔ c4ɔ c4ɔ c4ɔ	c2ɔ
c5ɔ c5ɔ c5ɔ c5ɔ	c5ɔ c5ɔ c5ɔ c5ɔ	c3ɔ
c6ɔ c6ɔ c6ɔ c6ɔ	c6ɔ c6ɔ c6ɔ c6ɔ	c4ɔ
c7ɔ c7ɔ c7ɔ c7ɔ	c7ɔ c7ɔ c7ɔ c7ɔ	c5ɔ
c8ɔ c8ɔ c8ɔ c8ɔ	c8ɔ c8ɔ c8ɔ c8ɔ	c6ɔ
c9ɔ c9ɔ c9ɔ c9ɔ	c9ɔ c9ɔ c9ɔ c9ɔ	c7ɔ

Examiners are required to make a judgement of the candidate's performance in each of the sections (1, 2 and 3) by filling in the appropriate box like this: ▬ . Please use 2B pencil only.

Brief description of case:

Examiner Number:

EXAMINER
(PLEASE PRINT NAME AND SIGN BELOW)

c0ɔ	c0ɔ	c0ɔ	c0ɔ
c1ɔ	c1ɔ	c1ɔ	c1ɔ
c2ɔ	c2ɔ	c2ɔ	c2ɔ
c3ɔ	c3ɔ	c3ɔ	c3ɔ
c4ɔ	c4ɔ	c4ɔ	c4ɔ
c5ɔ	c5ɔ	c5ɔ	c5ɔ
c6ɔ	c6ɔ	c6ɔ	c6ɔ
c7ɔ	c7ɔ	c7ɔ	c7ɔ
c8ɔ	c8ɔ	c8ɔ	c8ɔ
c9ɔ	c9ɔ	c9ɔ	c9ɔ

_____

_____

1. Physical examination
- general inspection
- confirms position of trachea, assesses chest wall movement
- correctly percusses over both sides of the chest
- assesses tactile vocal fremitus when applicable
- auscultates over both sides of chest
- auscultates vocal fremitus/whispering pectoriloquy and added sounds when applicable

clear pass ▢	pass ▢	fail ▢	clear fail ▢

2. Identification and interpretation of physical signs
- identifies abnormal physical signs correctly
- interprets signs correctly
- makes correct diagnosis

clear pass ▢	pass ▢	fail ▢	clear fail ▢

3. Discussion related to the case
- familiar with appropriate investigation and sequence
- familiar with appropriate further therapy and management

clear pass ▢	pass ▢	fail ▢	clear fail ▢

Now record your overall judgement of the candidate's performance taking into account the above: please grade as clear pass/pass/fail/clear fail, (a fail or clear fail grade must be accompanied by clearly written explanatory comments).

Counselling Recommended ▢

COMMENTS (PLEASE PRINT)

overall judgement

clear pass ▢	pass ▢	fail ▢	clear fail ▢

please continue in the unshaded area overleaf if necessary

DRS Data & Research Services plc/U41410201/BMRV

ROYAL COLLEGES OF PHYSICIANS OF THE UNITED KINGDOM
MRCP(UK) PACES EXAMINATION - CLINICAL MARKSHEET
STATION ONE: Abdominal System Examination

CANDIDATE NAME (PLEASE PRINT)

Examination Number				Centre Number				Sheet No.
[0]	[0]	[0]	[0]	[0]	[0]	[0]	[0]	2
[1]	[1]	[1]	[1]	[1]	[1]	[1]	[1]	
[2]	[2]	[2]	[2]	[2]	[2]	[2]	[2]	[1]
[3]	[3]	[3]	[3]	[3]	[3]	[3]	[3]	
[4]	[4]	[4]	[4]	[4]	[4]	[4]	[4]	[3]
[5]	[5]	[5]	[5]	[5]	[5]	[5]	[5]	[4]
[6]	[6]	[6]	[6]	[6]	[6]	[6]	[6]	[5]
[7]	[7]	[7]	[7]	[7]	[7]	[7]	[7]	[6]
[8]	[8]	[8]	[8]	[8]	[8]	[8]	[8]	[7]
[9]	[9]	[9]	[9]	[9]	[9]	[9]	[9]	

Examiners are required to make a judgement of the candidate's performance in each of the sections (1, 2 and 3) by filling in the appropriate box like this: ▬ . Please use 2B pencil only.

Brief description of case:

Examiner Number:

EXAMINER
(PLEASE PRINT NAME AND SIGN BELOW)

[0]	[0]	[0]	[0]
[1]	[1]	[1]	[1]
[2]	[2]	[2]	[2]
[3]	[3]	[3]	[3]
[4]	[4]	[4]	[4]
[5]	[5]	[5]	[5]
[6]	[6]	[6]	[6]
[7]	[7]	[7]	[7]
[8]	[8]	[8]	[8]
[9]	[9]	[9]	[9]

_____

_____

	clear pass	pass	fail	clear fail
1. Physical examination • inspection, nutrition status • correctly palpates for organomegaly/masses • percusses and assesses for ascites if appropriate • auscultates for bowel sounds/bruit • comments on further features	▭	▭	▭	▭
2. Identification and interpretation of physical signs • identifies abnormal physical signs correctly • interprets signs correctly • makes correct diagnosis	▭	▭	▭	▭
3. Discussion related to the case • familiar with appropriate investigation and sequence • familiar with appropriate further therapy and management	▭	▭	▭	▭

Now record your overall judgement of the candidate's performance taking into account the above: please grade as clear pass/pass/fail/clear fail, (a fail or clear fail grade must be accompanied by clearly written explanatory comments).

Counselling Recommended ▭

COMMENTS (PLEASE PRINT)

overall judgement

clear pass	pass	fail	clear fail
▭	▭	▭	▭

please continue in the unshaded area overleaf if necessary

DRS Data & Research Services plc/U41380201/SVRD

ROYAL COLLEGES OF PHYSICIANS OF THE UNITED KINGDOM
MRCP(UK) PACES EXAMINATION - CLINICAL MARKSHEET
STATION THREE: Cardiovascular System Examination

CANDIDATE NAME (PLEASE PRINT)

Examination Number

[0] [0] [0] [0]
[1] [1] [1] [1]
[2] [2] [2] [2]
[3] [3] [3] [3]
[4] [4] [4] [4]
[5] [5] [5] [5]
[6] [6] [6] [6]
[7] [7] [7] [7]
[8] [8] [8] [8]
[9] [9] [9] [9]

Centre Number

[0] [0] [0] [0]
[1] [1] [1] [1]
[2] [2] [2] [2]
[3] [3] [3] [3]
[4] [4] [4] [4]
[5] [5] [5] [5]
[6] [6] [6] [6]
[7] [7] [7] [7]
[8] [8] [8] [8]
[9] [9] [9] [9]

Sheet No.

4

[1]
[2]
[3]
[5]
[6]
[7]

Examiners are required to make a judgement of the candidate's performance in each of the sections (1, 2 and 3) by filling in the appropriate box like this: ▬ . Please use 2B pencil only.

Brief description of case:

Examiner Number:

EXAMINER
(PLEASE PRINT NAME AND SIGN BELOW)

_____

_____

[0] [0] [0] [0]
[1] [1] [1] [1]
[2] [2] [2] [2]
[3] [3] [3] [3]
[4] [4] [4] [4]
[5] [5] [5] [5]
[6] [6] [6] [6]
[7] [7] [7] [7]
[8] [8] [8] [8]
[9] [9] [9] [9]

	clear pass	pass	fail	clear fail
1. Physical examination • general inspection • checks pulses, notes blood pressure, inspects JVP, palpates carotids • inspects, palpates precordium, localises apex beat, auscultates valve areas with correct positioning • examines for peripheral pulses and ankle oedema when applicable	▢	▢	▢	▢
2. Identification and interpretation of physical signs • identifies abnormal physical signs correctly • interprets signs correctly • makes correct diagnosis	▢	▢	▢	▢
3. Discussion related to the case • familiar with appropriate investigation and sequence • familiar with appropriate further therapy and management	▢	▢	▢	▢

Now record your overall judgement of the candidate's performance taking into account the above: please grade as clear pass/pass/fail/clear fail, (a fail or clear fail grade must be accompanied by clearly written explanatory comments).

Counselling Recommended ▢

COMMENTS (PLEASE PRINT)

overall judgement

clear pass	pass	fail	clear fail
▢	▢	▢	▢

please continue in the unshaded area overleaf if necessary

DRS Data & Research Services plc/U41430201/XVRD

CANDIDATE NAME (PLEASE PRINT)

Examination Number	Centre Number	Sheet No.
c0ɔ c0ɔ c0ɔ c0ɔ	c0ɔ c0ɔ c0ɔ c0ɔ	5
c1ɔ c1ɔ c1ɔ c1ɔ	c1ɔ c1ɔ c1ɔ c1ɔ	
c2ɔ c2ɔ c2ɔ c2ɔ	c2ɔ c2ɔ c2ɔ c2ɔ	c1ɔ
c3ɔ c3ɔ c3ɔ c3ɔ	c3ɔ c3ɔ c3ɔ c3ɔ	c2ɔ
c4ɔ c4ɔ c4ɔ c4ɔ	c4ɔ c4ɔ c4ɔ c4ɔ	c3ɔ
c5ɔ c5ɔ c5ɔ c5ɔ	c5ɔ c5ɔ c5ɔ c5ɔ	c4ɔ
c6ɔ c6ɔ c6ɔ c6ɔ	c6ɔ c6ɔ c6ɔ c6ɔ	▬
c7ɔ c7ɔ c7ɔ c7ɔ	c7ɔ c7ɔ c7ɔ c7ɔ	c6ɔ
c8ɔ c8ɔ c8ɔ c8ɔ	c8ɔ c8ɔ c8ɔ c8ɔ	c7ɔ
c9ɔ c9ɔ c9ɔ c9ɔ	c9ɔ c9ɔ c9ɔ c9ɔ	

Examiners are required to make a judgement of the candidate's performance in each of the sections (1, 2 and 3) by filling in the appropriate box like this: ▬ . Please use 2B pencil only.

Brief description of case:

Examiner Number:

EXAMINER
(PLEASE PRINT NAME AND SIGN BELOW)

c0ɔ	c0ɔ	c0ɔ	c0ɔ
c1ɔ	c1ɔ	c1ɔ	c1ɔ
c2ɔ	c2ɔ	c2ɔ	c2ɔ
c3ɔ	c3ɔ	c3ɔ	c3ɔ
c4ɔ	c4ɔ	c4ɔ	c4ɔ
c5ɔ	c5ɔ	c5ɔ	c5ɔ
c6ɔ	c6ɔ	c6ɔ	c6ɔ
c7ɔ	c7ɔ	c7ɔ	c7ɔ
c8ɔ	c8ɔ	c8ɔ	c8ɔ
c9ɔ	c9ɔ	c9ɔ	c9ɔ

_____

_____

	clear pass	pass	fail	clear fail
1. Physical examination • where appropriate, assesses higher cortical function, tests cranial nerves in sequence including optic fundi and visual fields • appropriately assesses motor function in limbs (tone, power, reflexes inc. plantar response), sensory function (light touch, pinprick, vibration sense, proprioception, temperature) and co-ordination/cerebellar function • assesses gait if appropriate	▭	▭	▭	▭
2. Identification and interpretation of physical signs • identifies abnormal physical signs correctly • interprets signs correctly • makes correct diagnosis	▭	▭	▭	▭
3. Discussion related to the case • familiar with appropriate investigation and sequence • familiar with appropriate further therapy and management	▭	▭	▭	▭

Now record your overall judgement of the candidate's performance taking into account the above: please grade as clear pass/pass/fail/clear fail, (a fail or clear fail grade must be accompanied by clearly written explanatory comments).

Counselling Recommended ▭

COMMENTS (PLEASE PRINT)	**overall judgement**			
	clear pass	pass	fail	clear fail
please continue in the unshaded area overleaf if necessary	▭	▭	▭	▭

ROYAL COLLEGES OF PHYSICIANS OF THE UNITED KINGDOM
MRCP(UK) PACES EXAMINATION - CLINICAL MARKSHEET
STATION 5: Examination of Skin/Locomotor/Endocrine/Eyes

CANDIDATE NAME (PLEASE PRINT)

Examination Number	Centre Number	Sheet No.
c0ɔ c0ɔ c0ɔ c0ɔ	c0ɔ c0ɔ c0ɔ c0ɔ	**7**
c1ɔ c1ɔ c1ɔ c1ɔ	c1ɔ c1ɔ c1ɔ c1ɔ	
c2ɔ c2ɔ c2ɔ c2ɔ	c2ɔ c2ɔ c2ɔ c2ɔ	c1ɔ
c3ɔ c3ɔ c3ɔ c3ɔ	c3ɔ c3ɔ c3ɔ c3ɔ	c2ɔ
c4ɔ c4ɔ c4ɔ c4ɔ	c4ɔ c4ɔ c4ɔ c4ɔ	c3ɔ
c5ɔ c5ɔ c5ɔ c5ɔ	c5ɔ c5ɔ c5ɔ c5ɔ	c4ɔ
c6ɔ c6ɔ c6ɔ c6ɔ	c6ɔ c6ɔ c6ɔ c6ɔ	c5ɔ
c7ɔ c7ɔ c7ɔ c7ɔ	c7ɔ c7ɔ c7ɔ c7ɔ	c6ɔ
c8ɔ c8ɔ c8ɔ c8ɔ	c8ɔ c8ɔ c8ɔ c8ɔ	
c9ɔ c9ɔ c9ɔ c9ɔ	c9ɔ c9ɔ c9ɔ c9ɔ	

Examiners are asked to examine on a case from each of the four systems. They are required to make a judgement of the candidate's performance by filling in the appropriate box like this: ▬ . Please use 2B pencil only.

EXAMINER (PLEASE PRINT NAME AND SIGN)   **Examiner Number:**

c0ɔ	c0ɔ	c0ɔ	c0ɔ
c1ɔ	c1ɔ	c1ɔ	c1ɔ
c2ɔ	c2ɔ	c2ɔ	c2ɔ
c3ɔ	c3ɔ	c3ɔ	c3ɔ
c4ɔ	c4ɔ	c4ɔ	c4ɔ
c5ɔ	c5ɔ	c5ɔ	c5ɔ
c6ɔ	c6ɔ	c6ɔ	c6ɔ
c7ɔ	c7ɔ	c7ɔ	c7ɔ
c8ɔ	c8ɔ	c8ɔ	c8ɔ
c9ɔ	c9ɔ	c9ɔ	c9ɔ

	Brief description of case(s)	clear pass	pass	fail	clear fail
Skin • physical examination • identification of physical signs • discussion related to case		▭	▭	▭	▭
Locomotor • physical examination • identification of physical signs • discussion related to case		▭	▭	▭	▭
Endocrine • physical examination • identification of physical signs • discussion related to case		▭	▭	▭	▭
Eyes • physical examination • identification of physical signs • discussion related to case		▭	▭	▭	▭

Now record your overall judgement of the candidate's performance taking into account the above: please grade as clear pass/pass/fail/clear fail, (a fail or clear fail grade must be accompanied by clearly written explanatory comments).

Counselling Recommended	▭

COMMENTS (PLEASE PRINT)	**overall judgement**			
	clear pass	pass	fail	clear fail
please continue in the unshaded area overleaf if necessary	▭	▭	▭	▭

DRS Data & Research Services plc/U41400201/BVFT

5 | Texidor's twinge and related matters

The following excerpt from Richard Asher's book* is surely compulsory reading for all prospective members of the Royal College of Physicians. No physician's training is complete until the messages contained therein have been assimilated:

'It is pleasant to believe that the facts of medical science are there whether or not we name them; that the truth about clinical medicine exists quite independently of the names we bestow upon it. If that were so, our only responsibility would be to agree upon symbols or words for facts that already existed. That theoretical ideal is hardly ever fulfilled. A little patient thinking will soon convince the enquirer that it is not just a simple matter of finding words to fit the facts, but just as often of finding facts to fit the words. When christening a baby we wait for the child to be born and then we find a name for it. When christening a disease we sometimes wait for the name to be born and then we try to find a disease to suit it. With children we announce their names in the birth columns of The Times and with diseases we announce their names in the original articles of the medical journals. The only difference is that children's names have to be registered. There is no such procedure with medical terms. There is no Medical Registrar-General of Terminological Births and Deaths. Only medical dictionaries and the international list of classified diseases. These do not include every living medical term, and they list many that have died or that ought to be painlessly put away. There is something about a name, particularly an eponymous term, which brings into being things which never seemed to be there before. In creation the word may come first: the opening sentence of the Gospel of Saint John is— "In the beginning was the Word."

Take, for instance, Pel Ebstein fever. Every student and every doctor knows that cases of Hodgkin's disease may show a fever that is high for one week and low for the next week, and so on. Does this phenomenon really exist at all? If you collect the charts of 50 cases of Hodgkin's disease and compare them with the charts of 50 cases of disseminated malignant fever, do you really believe you could pick out even one or two cases because of the characteristic fever? I think it is very unlikely indeed. Yet if, by the vagaries of chance, one case of Hodgkin's did run such a temperature,

the news would soon travel round: "There's a good case of Hodgkin's disease in Galen Ward. You ought to have a look. It shows the typical Pel Ebstein fever very well."

The chart might be copied for teaching purposes, or even put in a book. The mere description and the naming of a mythical fever leads inevitably to its occurrence in textbooks. One popular textbook for nurses depicts particularly classical temperature charts, attributed to various fevers. I asked the author how many hospital notes she had combed before she found such beautiful examples: "Oh, there was no trouble about that," she replied, "I made them up out of my head."

I wonder whether any examples of Pel Ebstein and other fevers in textbooks have similar origins. It does not matter whether or not Pel Ebstein fever exists, my contention remains the same: the bestowal of a name upon a concept, whether real or imaginary, brings it into clinical existence.

Out of curiosity I looked up the original papers, and Dr Burrows kindly translated them for me. Both describe patients with chronic relapsing fever and splenomegaly but there is nothing in either paper to suggest any of them had Hodgkin's disease. Both describe cases of undulant fever and Ebstein suggested the name chronic relapsing fever, but it was very probably one of abortus fever.

An important example of the creation of a thing beginning with the word is gallstone colic. There is no such thing. Colic is a pain continuously waxing and waning, like the colonic cramps of food poisoning. Gallstone pain after its onset steadily climbs to an agonizing peak without any fluctuation, and then passes off. But the label colic has been so firmly stuck on to this pain that the pain is expected to be colic, assumed to be colic, believed to be colic and finally bullied into being colic, so that a man with gallstone pain will be described as having colicky pain, however steady it may be.

Contrariwise, if something has no individual descriptive term it has far less chance of clinical acceptance or clinical recognition. A rose without a name may smell as sweet, but it has far less chance of being smelt. Supposing we take an unnamed fever and an unnamed pain to contrast with the examples I have given. In untreated pernicious anaemia there is often quite a high fever. Sixty per cent of cases with red cell counts under 1.5 million show a fever over 101°F. This invariably settles to normal levels within a week of one adequate injection of B_{12}. I make no assertion that this fever

* From the book Talking Sense, edited by Sir Francis Avery Jones (Pitman Medical, 1972).

is of great importance. What I do assert is that had it been called the Addison–Castle fever or hypo-cyanocobalminic fever there is not a medical student in the land who would not have heard of it, many doctors would be afraid to diagnose pernicious anaemia without its presence, and the proportion of patients showing the fever would rise sharply once the name got into nurses' textbooks (because if they did not show the fever they would have their thermometers put back in their mouths until they behaved themselves).

Now for a pain without a name. Have any of you ever had a very brief, sharp needle-like pain near the apex of the heart: acutely localized to one point seemingly inside the chest wall, but feeling as if something was adherent to it? Breathing sharpens it, so there is often a disinclination to take a deep breath while it lasts. It comes out of the blue, it passes off in a few minutes, and although acute it is not at all distressing.

Enquiries among my friends showed that quite a lot of them occasionally had this pain, but, till they knew other people had it too, they did not mention it; especially because it has no official name, and also because it did not bother them.

I circulated various doctors I knew, and also circularized 50 recently elected Fellows of the College of Physicians — to see if it was reasonably common. It was . . . So if any of you happen to have it, you are not branding yourselves as either grievously neurotic or grossly hypochondriacal if you admit to having it.

[In the second of the Lettsomian lectures, on which this essay is based, with the permission of the President of the Medical Society of London, Dr Asher asked his audience of medical men whether any of them had encountered anything closely resembling this pain in either themselves or their friends, and if they had, to raise their hands. Over a third of the audience held up their hands.]

There seems no doubt that this condition exists, yet, because it has no name, it has no official clinical existence. We cannot discuss it or investigate it or write about it. Whether or not the condition should be named I am unable to say.* Though the naming of disease is not in any way restricted or supervised it ought not to be undertaken lightly. A fertile medical author can easily beget a large number of clinical progeny by describing and naming them, but some of his youngsters may turn out to be illegitimate, and with others there may be much doubt about their paternity if others claim to have begotten them years ago.'

---

* In a foreword to *Sense and Sensibility* the author explained that the pain had been described and named four years previously by A.J. Miller and T.A. Texidor (1955) in the *Journal of the American Medical Association*, and that it might in future be known as *Texidor's twinge*.

6 | Abbreviations

A&E	accident and emergency
ABE	acute bacterial endocarditis
ABPA	allergic bronchopulmonary aspergillosis
ACE	angiotensin-converting enzyme
ACTH	adrenocorticotrophic hormone
ADPKD	autosomal dominant polycystic kidney disease
AFB	acid-fast bacilli
AIDP	acute inflammatory demyelinating polyradiculopathy
AIDS	acquired immune deficiency syndrome
ANA	antinuclear antibody
ANCA	antineutrophil cytoplasmic antibodies
APAS	antiphospholipid antibody syndrome
ARDS	adult respiratory distress syndrome
ARPKD	autosomal recessive polycystic kidney disease
ASD	atrial septal defect
AV	arteriovenous
BMI	body mass index
BRAO	branch retinal artery occlusion
BOS	bronchiolitis obliterans syndrome
cAMP	cyclic adenosine monophosphate
cANCA	cytoplasmic ANCA
CFA	cryptogenic fibrosing alveolitis
CHD	coronary heart disease
CML	chronic myeloid leukaemia
CNS	central nervous system
CO_2	carbon dioxide
COPD	chronic obstructive pulmonary disease
COX	cyclo-oxygenase
CPEO	chronic progressive external ophthalmoplegia
CRAO	central retinal artery occlusion
CREST	calcinosis, Raynaud's, oesophageal involvement, sclerodactyly and telangiectasia
CRH	corticotrophin-releasing hormone
CRST	calcinosis, Raynaud's, sclerodactyly and telangiectasia
CRVO	central retinal vein occlusion
CSF	cerebrospinal fluid
CT	computed tomography
DEXA	Dual Energy X-ray Absorptiometry
DIDMOAD	diabetes insipidus, diabetes mellitus, optic atrophy and deafness
DMARDs	disease-modifying antirheumatic drugs
2,3-DPG	2,3-diphosphoglycerate
DVT	deep venous thrombosis
ECG	electrocardiogram
EMG	electromyograph
ENT	ears, nose and throat
ESR	erythrocyte sedimentation rate
FET	forced expiratory time
FEV_1	forced expiratory volume in 1 second
FFA	free fatty acids
FSH	follicle-stimulating hormone
FVC	forced vital capacity
G6PD	glucose-6-phosphate dehydrogenase
GFR	glomerular filtration rate
GH	growth hormone
GHRH	growth hormone-releasing hormone
GI	gastrointestinal
GPI	general paresis of the insane
HBsAg	hepatitis B surface antigen
HBV	hepatitis B virus
HCG	human chorionic gonadotrophin
HCM	hypertrophic cardiomyopathy
HCV	hepatitis C virus
HDL	high density lipoprotein
5-HIAA	5-hydroxyindole-acetic acid
HIV	human immunodeficiency virus
HLA	human leucocyte antigen
HMGco-A	hydroxy methyl glutaryl coenzyme A
HMSN	hereditary motor and sensory neuropathy
HOCM	hypertrophic obstructive cardiomyopathy
HPOA	hypertrophic pulmonary osteoarthropathy
HRT	hormone replacement therapy
5-HT	serotonin
HTLV	human T-cell lymphotrophic virus
Ig	immunoglobulin
IGF	insulin-like growth factor
IL	interleukin
IRMA	intraretinal microvascular abnormalities
ITU	intensive treatment unit

JCA	juvenile chronic arthritis	**PFR**	peak flow rate
JIA	juvenile idiopathic arthritis	**Ph**	Philadelphia (chromosome)
JVP	jugular venous pressure	**PKD**	polycystic kidney disease
LDH	lactic dehydrogenase	**PUVA**	psoralen and UVA
LDL	low density lipoprotein	**REAL**	Revised European-American
LH	luteinizing hormone		Lymphoma (classification)
LP	lumbar puncture	**SACD**	subacute combined degeneration of the
LPL	lipoprotein lipase		cord
MCP	metacarpophalangeal	**SBE**	subacute bacterial endocarditis
MEA	multiple endocrine adenopathy	**SLE**	systemic lupus erythematosus
MEN	multiple endocrine neoplasia	**TB**	tuberculosis
MRI	magnetic resonance imaging	**TNF**	tumour necrosis factor
MS	multiple sclerosis	**TOE**	transoesophageal echocardiography
MVP	mitral valve prolapse	**TSH**	thyroid-stimulating hormone
NIDDM	non-insulin-dependent diabetes	**UIP**	usual interstitial pneumonia
	mellitus	**USS**	ultrasound scan
NSAIDs	non-steroidal anti-inflammatory drugs	**UVA**	ultraviolet A
pANCA	perinuclear ANCA	**UVB**	ultraviolet B
PAPS	primary antiphospholipid antibody	**VER**	visual evoked response
	syndrome	**VLDL**	very low density lipoprotein
PBG	porphobilinogen	**VSD**	ventricular septal defect
PEG	percutaneous endoscopic gastrostomy	**WBC**	white blood cell(s)
		WHO	World Health Organisation

Index

Note: Page numbers in **bold** refer to main entries for cases, those followed by n refer to footnotes. Alphabetical order is letter-by-letter.

MRCP — it teaches more than it tests